Non-Invasive Sperm Selection for In Vitro Fertilization

Ashok Agarwal • Edson Borges Jr.
Amanda S. Setti
Editors

Non-Invasive Sperm Selection for In Vitro Fertilization

Novel Concepts and Methods

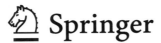

Editors
Ashok Agarwal, PhD, HCLD (ABB), ELD (ACE)
Andrology Center and Center for Reproductive Medicine
Cleveland Clinic
Cleveland, OH, USA

Amanda S. Setti, BSc
Instituto Sapientiae - Centro de Estudos e Pesquisa em Reprodução Assistida
São Paulo, SP, Brazil

Edson Borges Jr., MD, PhD
Fertility - Centro de Fertilização Assistida
São Paulo, SP, Brazil

ISBN 978-1-4939-1410-4   ISBN 978-1-4939-1411-1 (eBook)
DOI 10.1007/978-1-4939-1411-1
Springer New York Heidelberg Dordrecht London

Library of Congress Control Number: 2014942640

© Springer Science+Business Media New York 2015
This work is subject to copyright. All rights are reserved by the Publisher, whether the whole or part of the material is concerned, specifically the rights of translation, reprinting, reuse of illustrations, recitation, broadcasting, reproduction on microfilms or in any other physical way, and transmission or information storage and retrieval, electronic adaptation, computer software, or by similar or dissimilar methodology now known or hereafter developed. Exempted from this legal reservation are brief excerpts in connection with reviews or scholarly analysis or material supplied specifically for the purpose of being entered and executed on a computer system, for exclusive use by the purchaser of the work. Duplication of this publication or parts thereof is permitted only under the provisions of the Copyright Law of the Publisher's location, in its current version, and permission for use must always be obtained from Springer. Permissions for use may be obtained through RightsLink at the Copyright Clearance Center. Violations are liable to prosecution under the respective Copyright Law.
The use of general descriptive names, registered names, trademarks, service marks, etc. in this publication does not imply, even in the absence of a specific statement, that such names are exempt from the relevant protective laws and regulations and therefore free for general use.
While the advice and information in this book are believed to be true and accurate at the date of publication, neither the authors nor the editors nor the publisher can accept any legal responsibility for any errors or omissions that may be made. The publisher makes no warranty, express or implied, with respect to the material contained herein.

Printed on acid-free paper

Springer is part of Springer Science+Business Media (www.springer.com)

Foreword

The fast pace of scientific discovery and technological innovation has greatly affected the care of the infertile couple. As a result, diagnostic and therapeutic options for infertile couples have undergone dramatic evolution in the past three decades, touching the lives of couples for whom few options existed previously. Thirty-five years after the birth of the first child conceived by IVF, we are now able to stimulate ovaries to obtain multiple oocytes, extract sperm from testes of men with severe infertility, inject sperm into oocytes to achieve fertilization, and perform biopsy of embryos for diagnostic purposes. With increasingly complex modalities available for laboratory and clinical aspects of infertility care comes the need for a clear, concise, readable, and practical text to serve as a resource for providers. This book entitled "Non-Invasive Sperm Selection for In-Vitro Fertilization: Novel Concepts and Methods," edited by Drs. Edson Borges Jr. and Ashok Agarwal is an excellent example of this effort directed at the andrology laboratory aspect of infertility care.

The editors are well suited to the purposes of this text. Both are gifted fertility practitioners and physician scientists. Dr. Edson Borges Jr. is the Director of the Fertility—Assisted Fertilization Center, in Sao Paulo, Brazil. He also serves as the Director of the Post-Graduation Course in Human Assisted Reproduction at the Sapientiae Institute. Dr. Ashok Agarwal is the Director of the Center for Reproductive Medicine and the Director of the Andrology Center and Reproductive Tissue Bank at the Cleveland Clinic. They have authored over 600 peer-reviewed publications, garnered multiple research grants, and are internationally recognized for their outstanding contributions in scientific and clinical aspects of reproductive medicine.

Drs. Edson Borges Jr. and Ashok Agarwal have assembled an exciting cast of authors, each an expert in the topics about which they write. The goal of the text is to present strategies for noninvasive sperm selection in IVF. Authors review the existing and emerging technologies in the field including non-apoptotic sperm selection, electrophoretic separation, high-magnification sperm morphology selection, microfluidics, and hyaluronic acid binding. They then discuss the methodology, effectiveness, and safety of the various sperm selection methods. The result is a concise, readable, and highly practical reference guide for scientists, embryologists, infertility specialists, and urologists. For all these reasons I can enthusiastically recommend this textbook to you.

Division of Reproductive Endocrinology and Infertility,
Yale School of Medicine, New Haven, CT, USA   Emre Seli, MD
Yale-New Haven Hospital, New Haven, CT, USA

Preface

In the past three decades or so, there has been tremendous scientific progress in the field of assisted reproduction techniques (ART). These advancements have presented wider options for infertile individuals and strengthened their hope and resolve at having a child of their own. And in tandem with the evolving progress in assisted reproduction techniques, the demand for ART is now greater than ever.

In recent times, significant emphasis is being placed on investigating the characteristics of the human spermatozoon used in assisted reproduction. Identification of the morphological abnormalities of the spermatozoa provides better understanding of the human sperm function and highlights the importance of an adequate sperm selection technique that would greatly contribute to the overall success of the particular assisted reproduction techniques, thereby increasing fertility rates and pregnancy outcome.

Previously, a healthy spermatozoon was considered essential to merely contribute the paternal genome and ensure successful oocyte fertilization. However, the human spermatozoon has now been recognized to play a significant role in key events that occur once fertilization has actually taken place. These events influence not only the fertilization process itself but go on beyond that to contribute to the development of the embryo, and ultimately affect the pregnancy outcome.

This book contains contributions by several key experts who are at the forefront of the field of assisted reproduction. Here, they provide detailed information on the techniques that have been developed to assist in sperm selection for the various ART techniques available—from basic sperm preparation to intracytoplasmic sperm injection (ICSI), to hyaluronic binding assay and physiological intracytoplasmic sperm injection (PICSI), to motile sperm organelle morphology examination (MSOME) and intracytoplasmic morphologically selected sperm injection (IMSI). The implication of the detection of total, partial, irregular, or absent sperm head birefringence, the presence of sperm head vacuoles, and the assessment of sperm chromatin, chromosomal constitution, and DNA integrity through MSOME, in fresh and cryopreserved sperm, is thoroughly explored in this book. Updates on novel sperm tests, sperm selection based on surface charge, and non-apoptotic sperm selection are also delved into.

All in all, this book brings to light the main noninvasive sperm selection techniques that are currently available and those that are being developed to aid in the selection of the best possible sperm for fertilizing the embryo during assisted reproduction. It also contains unique material that will review and assess recent important developments in the selection of sperm for ART, including the advances in the genomics and proteomics eras. Further, this book identifies unresolved issues in assisted reproduction; discuss their feasibility, safety, and effects on sperm quality and ART outcome. Additionally, this book provides recommendations on the clinical application of noninvasive sperm selection techniques and on its future research directions.

We truly believe that this volume will help to clarify the reader on various noninvasive sperm selection techniques available, encourage productive dialogues between reproductive professionals, and serve as a reference guide for all academics, researchers, and professionals in the field of reproductive medicine.

Cleveland, OH, USA	Ashok Agarwal
São Paulo, SP, Brazil	Edson Borges Jr.
São Paulo, SP, Brazil	Amanda S. Setti

Contents

1. **Male Infertility Laboratory Investigation: A Critical Analysis of the 2010 World Health Organization Semen Analysis Guidelines** ... 1
   Khalid Alrabeeah and Armand Zini

2. **Intracytoplasmic Injection with Suboptimal Spermatozoa** ... 7
   Gianpiero D. Palermo and Queenie V. Neri

3. **Novel Sperm Tests and Their Importance** ... 23
   Ralf Henkel

4. **Sperm Selection Based on Surface Electrical Charge** ... 41
   Mohammad Hossein Nasr-Esfahani and Tavalaee Marziyeh

5. **Microfluidics for Sperm Selection** ... 51
   Gary D. Smith, André Monteiro da Rocha, and Laura Keller

6. **Sperm Binding to the Zona Pellucida, Hyaluronic Acid Binding Assay, and PICSI** ... 59
   Sergio C. Oehninger and Dirk Kotze

7. **Non-apoptotic Sperm Selection** ... 69
   Tamer Said, Reda Z. Mahfouz, Iryna Kuznyetsova, and Alfonso P. Del Valle

8. **Motile Sperm Organelle Morphology Examination (MSOME)** ... 81
   José Gonçalves Franco Jr.

9. **Setup of Micromanipulator for Sperm Selection and Injection for IMSI: Configuring the Microscope for Intracytoplasmic Morphology-Selected Sperm Injection (IMSI)** ... 91
   Lynne Chang and Joseph G. LoBiondo

10. **The Technical Background of Advanced IMSI Systems** ... 105
    Mikhail Levtonov, Klaus Rink, and Paul Gassner

11	**Sperm Vacuoles: Origin and Implications**......................................	111
	Pierre Vanderzwalmen, Nicolas Zech, Bernard Lejeune, Anton Neyer, S. Perrier d'Hauterive, Francoise Puissant, Astrid Stecher, Sabine Vanderzwalmen, Barbara Wirleitner, and Olivier Gaspard	
12	**MSOME: Conventional Semen Analysis, Sperm Manipulation, and Cryopreservation**..	123
	Amanda S. Setti and Edson Borges Jr.	
13	**MSOME and Sperm Chromatin Status**......................................	127
	Florence Boitrelle and Martine Albert	
14	**MSOME and Sperm DNA Integrity: Biological and Clinical Considerations**..	137
	Jan Tesarik	
15	**MSOME and Sperm Chromosomal Constitution**......................	149
	Amanda S. Setti and Edson Borges Jr.	
16	**Intracytoplasmic Morphologically Selected Sperm Injection (IMSI): Indications and Clinical Results**....................	157
	Nino Guy Cassuto and André Hazout	
17	**Genomic and Proteomic Approaches in the Diagnosis of Male Infertility**..	167
	Jason R. Kovac, Ryan P. Smith, and Dolores J. Lamb	
Index..		181

Contributors

Ashok Agarwal, PhD, HCLD (ABB), ELD (ACE) Andrology Center and Center for Reproductive Medicine, Cleveland Clinic, Cleveland, OH, USA

Martine Albert, MD Department of Reproductive Biology and Cytogenetics, Poissy General Hospital, Poissy, France

EA 2493, Versailles University of Medicine and Science, Versailles, France

Khalid Alrabeeah, MD, FRCSC Division of Urology, Department of Surgery, McGill University Health Centre, McGill University, Montreal, QC, Canada

Florence Boitrelle, MD Department of Reproductive Biology and Cytogenetics, Poissy General Hospital, Poissy, France

EA 2493, Versailles University of Medicine and Science, Versailles, France

Edson Borges Jr, MD, PhD Fertility - Centro de Fertilização Assistida, São Paulo, SP, Brazil

Nino Guy Cassuto, MD Art Unit, Drouot Laboratory, Paris, France

Lynne Chang, PhD Microscopy Product & Marketing, Nikon Instruments, Inc., Melville, NY, USA

André Monteiro da Rocha, DVM, PhD Department of Obstetrics and Gynecology, University of Michigan Medical School, Ann Arbor, MI, USA

S. Perrier d'Hauterive, MD, PhD Centre de Procréation Médicalement Assistée de l'Université de Liège, CHR de la Citadelle, Boulevard du Douzième de Ligne, Liège, Belgium

Alfonso P. Del Valle, MD, FRCS(C) The Toronto Institute for Reproductive Medicine – ReproMed, Toronto, ON, Canada

José Gonçalves Franco Jr., MD, PhD Center for Human Reproduction 'Professor Franco Jr', Ribeirão Preto, Sao Paulo, Brazil

Olivier Gaspard, BSc Centre de Procréation Médicalement Assistée de l'Université de Liège, CHR de la Citadelle, Liège, Belgium

Paul Gassner, PhD MTG Medical Technology Vertriebs-GmbH, Bruckberg, Germany

André Hazout, MD Art Unit, Drouot Laboratory, Paris, France

Ralf Henkel, PhD, BEd Department of Medical Biosciences, University of the Western Cape, Bellville, South Africa

Laura Keller, AASc Department of Obstetrics and Gynecology, University of Michigan Medical School, Ann Arbor, MI, USA

Dirk Kotze, PhD Department of Obstetrics and Gynecology, The Jones Institute for Reproductive Medicine, Eastern Virginia Medical School, Norfolk, VA, USA

Jason R. Kovac, MD, PhD, FRCSC Scott Department of Urology, Department of Molecular and Cellular Biology, The Center for Reproductive Medicine, Baylor College of Medicine, Houston, TX, USA

Iryna Kuznyetsova, PhD, HCLD Embryology Laboratory, The Toronto Institute for Reproductive Medicine – ReproMed, Toronto, ON, Canada

Dolores J. Lamb, PhD Scott Department of Urology, Department of Molecular and Cellular Biology, The Center for Reproductive Medicine, Baylor College of Medicine, Houston, TX, USA

Bernard Lejeune, MD, PhD Centre de Procréation Médicalement Assistée, Centre Hospitalier Inter Régional Cavell (CHIREC), Braine-l'Alleud, Belgium

Mikhail Levtonov, PhD Octax Microscience GmbH, Bruckberg, Germany

Joseph G. LoBiondo Microscopy Product & Marketing, Nikon Instruments, Inc., Melville, NY, USA

Reda Z. Mahfouz, MD, PhD Translational Haematology/Oncology, Taussig Cancer Institute, Cleveland Clinic, Cleveland, OH, USA

Tavalaee Marziyeh Department of Reproductive Biotechnology at Reproductive Biomedicine Research Center, Royan Institute for Biotechnology, ACECR, Isfahan, Iran

Mohammad Hossein Nasr-Esfahani, PhD Department of Reproductive Biotechnology at Reproductive Biomedicine Research Center, Royan Institute for Biotechnology, ACECR, Isfahan, Iran

Isfahan Fertility and Infertility Center, Isfahan, Iran

Queenie V. Neri, BSc, MSc The Ronald O. Perelman and Claudia Cohen Center for Reproductive Medicine, Weill Cornell Medical College, New York, NY, USA

Anton Neyer, BSc IVF Unit, IVF Centers Prof. Zech, Bregenz, Austria

Sergio C. Oehninger, MD, PhD Department of Obstetrics and Gynecology, The Jones Institute for Reproductive Medicine, Eastern Virginia Medical School, Norfolk, VA, USA

Gianpiero D. Palermo, MD, PhD The Ronald O. Perelman and Claudia Cohen Center for Reproductive Medicine, Weill Cornell Medical College, New York, NY, USA

Francoise Puissant, MD, PhD Centre de Procréation Médicalement Assistée, Centre Hospitalier Inter Régional Cavell (CHIREC), Uccle, Belgium

Klaus Rink, PhD Octax Microscience GmbH, Bruckberg, Germany

Tamer Said, MD, PhD, HCLD/CC Andrology Laboratory & Reproductive Tissue Bank, The Toronto Institute for Reproductive Medicine–ReproMed, Toronto, ON, Canada

Amanda S. Setti, BSc Instituto Sapientiae - Centro de Estudos e Pesquisa em Reprodução Assistida, São Paulo, SP, Brazil

Associação Instituto Sapientiae – Centro de Estudos e Pesquisa em Reprodução Assistida, São Paulo, SP, Brazil

Gary D. Smith, PhD Department of Obstetrics and Gynecology, University of Michigan Medical School, Ann Arbor, MI, USA

Department of Urology, University of Michigan Medical School, Ann Arbor, MI, USA

Department of Molecular and Integrative Physiology, University of Michigan Medical School, Ann Arbor, MI, USA

Reproductive Sciences Program, University of Michigan Medical School, Ann Arbor, MI, USA

Ryan P. Smith, MD The Department of Urology, University of Virginia, Charlottesville, VA, USA

Astrid Stecher, BSc IVF Unit, IVF Centers Prof. Zech, Bregenz, Austria

Jan Tesarik, MD, PhD Molecular Assisted Reproduction and Genetics, MAR&Gen Clinic, Granada, Spain

Pierre Vanderzwalmen, Bio-Eng. IVF Unit, IVF Centers Prof. Zech, Bregenz, Austria

Centre de Procréation Médicalement Assistée, Centre Hospitalier Inter Régional Cavell (CHIREC), Braine l'Alleud, Belgium

Av. Du bois de chapelle, Lasne, Belgium

Sabine Vanderzwalmen, BSc Centre de Procréation Médicalement Assistée, Centre Hospitalier Inter Régional Cavell (CHIREC), Braine l'Alleud, Belgium

Barbara Wirleitner, PhD IVF Unit, IVF Centers Prof. Zech, Bregenz, Austria

Nicolas Zech, MD, PhD IVF Unit, IVF Centers Prof. Zech, Bregenz, Austria

Armand Zini, MD Division of Urology, Department of Surgery, McGill University Health Center, McGill University, Montreal, QC, Canada

Division of Urology, Department of Surgery, St. Mary's Hospital Center, Montreal, QC, Canada

About the Editors

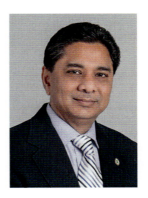

Ashok Agarwal, PhD, HCLD (ABB), ELD (ACE), is a Professor at Lerner College of Medicine, Case Western Reserve University and the head of the Andrology Center. He is the Director of Research at the Center for Reproductive Medicine, Cleveland Clinic, USA. He has researched extensively on oxidative stress and its implications on human fertility and his group has published over 500 research articles. Dr. Agarwal serves on the editorial boards of several key journals in human reproduction. His current research interests are the study of molecular markers of oxidative stress, DNA fragmentation, and apoptosis using proteomics and bioinformatics tools, as well as fertility preservation in patients with cancer, and the efficacy of certain antioxidants in improving male fertility.

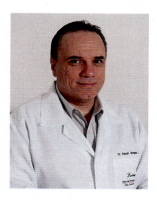

Edson Borges Jr., MD, PhD, is the founding partner of a private assisted reproduction center, the Fertility—Centro de Fertilização Assistida, located in São Paulo, Brazil. He serves this center as the Managing Director and Director of the clinical and scientific departments. He is also the founding partner of a center for research and education in assisted reproduction, the Sapientiae Institute—Centro de Estudos e Pesquisa em Reprodução Assistida, in São Paulo Brazil, where he serves as the Scientific Director and postgraduation course coordinator.

Dr. Edson obtained his M.D. degree in 1984 at the University of Campinas. After that, he received his first Ph.D. in urology in 2005 at the Federal University of São Paulo and the second Ph.D. in gynaecology in 2007 at the Botucatu Medical School in São Paulo State University.

Dr. Edson has published over 130 scientific papers and review articles in peer-reviewed scientific journals, authored over 5 books and 10 book chapters, and presented over 850 papers at both national and international scientific meetings. He is a member of professional societies such as American Society for Reproductive Medicine (ASRM) and European Society of Human Reproduction and Embryology (ESHRE), Sociedade Brasileira de Reprodução Assistida (SBRA), and Sociedade Brasileira de Reprodução Humana (SBRH). He was also a recipient of the 2013 Star Award from the American Society for Reproductive Medicine.

Dr. Edson has trained more than 400 embryologists and doctors from Brazil in his educational center. Dr. Edson is the recipient of many research grants. His research interests include studies on male infertility, oocyte evaluation, endometrial receptivity, and embryo implantation.

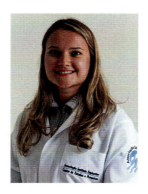

Amanda S. Setti, BSc, is a scientific researcher at a private assisted reproduction center, the Fertility—Centro de Fertilização Assistida, located in São Paulo, Brazil. Also, she serves a researcher of a center for research and education in assisted reproduction, the Sapientiae Institute—Centro de Estudos e Pesquisa em Reprodução Assistida, in São Paulo Brazil.

Amanda Setti obtained her B.Sc. degree in 2005 at the University of Santo Amaro and specialist degree in human assisted reproduction in 2007 at the Sapientiae Institute. In 2007 she was a fellow in the Center for Reproductive Medicine at the Cleveland Clinic. She is currently a master's degree student at Faculdade de Ciências Médicas da Santa Casa de São Paulo.

Amanda has published over 40 scientific papers and review articles in peer reviewed scientific journals, authored 3 book chapters, and presented over 50 papers at both national and international scientific meetings. In 2013, she was a recipient of two awards from the American Society for Reproductive Medicine.

Male Infertility Laboratory Investigation: A Critical Analysis of the 2010 World Health Organization Semen Analysis Guidelines

Khalid Alrabeeah and Armand Zini

Introduction

Infertility is defined as the inability to achieve a natural pregnancy after 1 year of unprotected intercourse and a male component is a contributing factor in roughly 50 % of couple infertility [1]. A cross-sectional study in the United States estimated that approximately 3.3–4.3 million men sought medical advice for infertility evaluation [2]. The evaluation of male factor infertility includes a detailed history, physical examination, and two or three semen analyses performed at 3 months interval.

The semen analysis is one of the most important investigations in the assessment of male fertility potential. The semen analysis provides a global measure of testicular and epididymal function (for sperm production and maturation, respectively), vasal patency (for sperm transport), and accessory sexual gland function (for production and delivery of seminal plasma). The semen parameters that are measured on a basic semen analysis include (1) semen volume, (2) sperm concentration and total count, (3) sperm motility, (4) sperm morphology, (5) sperm viability, (6) semen leukocyte concentration, and (7) semen pH. However, the measurement of all of these parameters on the semen analysis does not allow us to clearly differentiate fertile from infertile men because there is significant overlap in semen parameters between these two groups of men.

The history of the modern semen analysis dates back to the 1920s, when Macomber and Sanders assessed human semen and reported a median sperm concentration of 100 million spermatozoa per milliliter, using blood pipettes and a counting chamber [3]. In the 1950s, Macleod et al. compared the semen analyses of 1,000 fertile and 1,000 infertile couples to assess the differences in semen parameters between the two groups [4–7]. Given the increased demand to standardize the semen analysis worldwide, the World Health Organization (WHO) sets forth to standardize the evaluation and interpretation of the semen analysis and published a first manual on the examination of human semen in 1980. The semen analysis guidelines (and reference values) reported in the first WHO manual (1980) and in the subsequent versions (1987, 1992, and 1999) were largely based on the consensus of a panel of experts. The 1980–1999 WHO manuals were

K. Alrabeeah, MD, FRCSC
Division of Urology, Department of Surgery,
McGill University Health Center, McGill University,
687 Pine Avenue West, Montreal, QC,
Canada H3A1A1
e-mail: alrabeeah@gmail.com

A. Zini, MD (✉)
Division of Urology, Department of Surgery,
McGill University Health Center, McGill University,
687 Pine Avenue West, Montreal, QC,
Canada H3A1A1

Division of Urology, Department of Surgery, St. Mary's Hospital Center, 3830 Lacombe Avenue, Montreal, QC, Canada H3T 1M5
e-mail: ziniarmand@yahoo.com

Table 1.1 Reference studies used to establish the new WHO semen parameters

Study	Countries	Sample size with TTP[a]	Number of semen analysis provided per participant	Sperm morphology evaluation criteria
Bonde et al. (1998) [11]	Denmark	265	1	David
Auger et al. (2001) [19] Jorgensen et al. (2001) [20] Jensen et al. (2001) [23] Slama et al. (2002) [12]	France, Denmark, United Kingdom, Finland	900	1	David, Tygerberg (strict)
Swan et al. (2003) [21]	United States	493	2	Tygerberg (strict)
Haugen et al. (2006) [22]	Norway	89	1	Tygerberg (strict)
Stewart et al. (2009) [18]	Australia	206	2	Tygerberg (strict)

[a]The numbers were adapted from cooper et al. [17]

based on very little data on semen parameters of fertile men (recent fathers) and this has led some centers to view the reference values as either too high or too low [8–12]. Moreover, the authors (expert panel) of the first four editions of the WHO manuals acknowledged that the semen analysis reference values lacked validity because they were not evidence-based [13–16].

WHO 5th Edition Manual for Examining Semen Analysis

The most recent WHO semen analysis manual was published in 2010. Unlike prior WHO semen analysis manuals, the authors of the recent WHO manual (2010) reported evidence-based reference values for semen parameters [17]. The data used to generate the new semen parameter reference values were obtained from multinational studies of recent fathers with a known time to pregnancy (all had a time to pregnancy of 12 months or less). The total dataset was derived from five studies (conducted in seven countries) and included a total of 1,953 semen analyses (Table 1.1) [11, 12, 17–23]. Using the entire dataset of 1,953 semen analyses, the authors of the new WHO semen analysis guidelines set the semen parameter reference values at the lower 5th percentile. As such, according to the new WHO semen analysis guidelines, men who have one or more semen parameters below the lower 5th percentile are deemed to have an abnormal semen analysis. Nonetheless, it is important to remember that all of the 1,953 men from whom the semen parameter reference values were derived had fathered a child, including those men with an abnormal semen analysis.

Table 1.2 Cutoff reference values of the previous and current WHO manuals

Semen characteristics	WHO 1999	WHO 2010
Volume (ml)	2	1.5
Sperm concentration (million per ml)	20	15
Sperm count (million)	40	39
Total motility (%)	50	40
Progressive motility[a] (%)	25 (grade a only)	32 (grade a + b)
Vitality (%)	75	58
Morphology[b] (% of normal sperms)	14	4
Leukocyte count (million per ml)	Less than 1	Less than 1

[a]Grade a is considered rapid progressive motility; grade b is considered sluggish progressive motility
[b]Morphology values using strict criteria

There are several important changes in the current WHO semen analysis guidelines when compared to previous guidelines [17]. One of the notable aspects of the current WHO semen parameter cutoffs is that they are lower than reported in the previous WHO manuals (Table 1.2). These lower reference values in no way indicate a decline in semen quality but, rather, are simply a reflection of the new methods of establishing the cutoff values. Also, the assessment of motility has been simplified to include two motility categories (progressive and nonprogressive) rather than the three categories previously reported: rapid progressive (grade a), slow progressive (grade b), and nonprogressive (grade c) motility. This modification in motility evaluation was meant to allow the technician to assess sperm motility in a more objective manner. However, combining rapid (grade a) and slow progressive motility (grade b) into a single reading is a less accurate means of reporting sperm motility and it is unclear how this will affect management of the infertile male. In the current manual, sperm morphology is reported using strict methods (Tygerberg and David) [24].

ditions or prior exposure that might have affected their reproductive health (e.g., prior chemotherapy, radiotherapy, and cryptorchidism) [12, 20] with an indirect effect on their semen analysis. Lastly, the studies included in the new WHO manual used two different sperm morphology evaluation criteria. Auger et al. [19], Bonde et al. [11], Jorgensen et al. [20], Jensen et al. [23], and Slama et al. [12] all used David sperm morphology criteria method which differs from the strict or Tygerberg sperm morphology used by the other studies. Thus, the latest WHO reference value for sperm morphology do not accurately represent either the strict (Tygerberg) or David methods.

WHO 2010: Limitations

Although the new WHO manual semen parameter reference values are evidence-based (derived from controlled studies of recent fathers), these reference values have several limitations. One of the notable limitations is that the sample size ($n = 1953$) from which these reference values were derived is relatively small. Also, the mean age of the fathers was 31 years with only ten men above the age of 45 years, thereby limiting the relevance of these reference values to older men [17]. Another limitation is that the men who were tested came from seven countries and three continents, with 55 % of the population originating from western European cities. This means that in the development of the new reference values, there was clear overrepresentation from some continents (Europe) and no representation from others (e.g., Africa, Asia). This is an important limitation because regional differences in semen parameters between different European cities have been reported [20]. Moreover, Swan et al. [21] have also observed differences in semen parameters between different cities in the United States.

The reference values are based on studies that included men who had submitted only one semen analysis [12]. It is well known that the results of the semen analysis can vary markedly both between different men as well as between different ejaculates from the same man [25, 26]. Also, a fair number of men included in these studies had con-

Impact of the New WHO Reference Values on Clinical Practice

Establishing a Correct Diagnosis of Male Factor Infertility

The male partner evaluation of an infertile couple includes a detailed history, physical examination, and two or more semen analyses. Although the semen analysis represents a key component of the male evaluation, it is important to recognize that this test does not discriminate infertile from fertile men [27]. The semen parameter reference values reported in the new WHO semen analysis manual provide a more objective framework with which a clinician can gauge a man's fertility potential because these reference values are evidence-based. However, as with the reference values reported in the previous editions of the WHO manuals, the new WHO reference values also fail to discriminate infertile from fertile men. Therefore, using the lower 5th percentile (of semen parameters) as a threshold to assign or not to assign a diagnosis of male infertility is too simplistic and probably incorrect. Using the 50th percentile, which represents the median value of the reference population, together with the 5th percentile may be a better way to gauge the relative fertility potential of the infertile man as suggested by Esteves et al. [28]. As such, it is important that clinicians integrate clinical parameters (e.g., history, physical examination, other laboratory

Table 1.3 Distribution of semen parameters of fertile men whose partner had achieved pregnancy within 12 months or less

Percentile	5th centile	25th centile	50th centile	75th centile	95th centile
Semen volume (ml)	1.5	2.7	3.7	4.8	6.8
Sperm concentration (million/ml)	15	41	73	116	213
Sperm count (million/ejaculate)	39	142	255	422	802
Total motility (PR + NP%)[a]	40	53	61	69	78
Progressive motility (PR%)[a]	32	47	55	62	72
Normal forms (%)[b]	4	9	15	24.5	44
Vitality (%)	58	72	79	84	91

The table was adapted from cooper et al. [17]
[a] *PR* progressive motility, *NP* nonprogressive motility
[b] According to Tygerberg strict criteria

evaluation) as well as a general sense of the distribution of semen parameter values (e.g., 5th and 50th percentiles) before establishing a diagnosis of male factor infertility (Table 1.3).

If clinicians (e.g., urologists, gynecologists, reproductive endocrinologists) misinterpret the new semen parameter reference values and solely rely on the lower 5th percentile as a threshold to assign a diagnosis of male infertility, it is likely that a large number of couples with male factor infertility will be incorrectly classified as having unexplained infertility because the new (5th edition) WHO semen parameter reference values are lower than the previous WHO reference values. As a result of misinterpreting the new semen parameter reference values, many of these infertile couples will not proceed to a male partner evaluation. For some of these couples, the male evaluation may be postponed until subsequent semen analyses demonstrate abnormal sperm parameters or until other therapies have failed (e.g., assisted reproduction). It is unclear whether this re-classification will be more or less cost-effective but it is likely that assisted reproductive technologies utilization will increase as a result of an increased number of couples now being classified as having unexplained infertility [29].

Impact of the New WHO Reference Values on Treatment of Clinical Varicocele

A clinical varicocele is detected in approximately 35 % of men presenting for infertility evaluation [30] and many of these men have normal or low-normal semen parameters [31]. It has been shown that varicocele repair will result in improved semen parameters and sperm DNA integrity, and in lower seminal oxidative stress [32–36]. Moreover, repair of clinical varicocele may increase pregnancy rates although the number of high-quality studies supporting this premise is low [37, 38].

The current AUA guidelines suggest treating a varicocele if it is clinically palpable and associated with couple infertility and abnormal semen parameters (based on the 4th edition WHO guidelines) [39]. If clinicians adopt and misinterpret the new semen parameter reference values, and, solely rely on the lower 5th percentile as a threshold to assign a diagnosis of male infertility, there will be fewer candidates for varicocele repair because the new (5th edition) WHO semen parameter reference values are lower than the previous WHO reference values. This suggests that many infertile couples with clinical varicocele and normal or low-normal semen parameters (based on the previous, 4th edition, WHO guidelines) will potentially be denied a varicocele repair. Yet, several studies have demonstrated that adults can present with palpable varicocele and normal semen parameters but have abnormal sperm function tests, such as high levels of sperm DNA damage or seminal oxidative stress [33, 40]. Moreover, couples in whom men have clinical varicocele and mild oligozoospermia or normozoospermia will achieve greater spontaneous pregnancy rates after varicocele repair than similar couples with moderate or severe oligozoospermia. Therefore, denying these couples (with clinical varicocele and mild oligozoospermia or normozoospermia) a varicocele repair would be deemed poor clinical practice [41, 42]. Nonetheless, the exact semen parameter thresholds below which an infertile couple with a clinical varicocele is deemed to benefit from varicocele repair remain unknown. Additional prospective studies on the effect of varicocelectomy in infertile couples with clinical varicocele and low-normal semen parameters are needed to address this question, and in particular the relevance of the new WHO reference values in the management of clinical varicocele.

Impact of the New WHO Reference Values on Assisted Reproductive Technologies (ART)

The effect of applying the new reference values into clinical practice on ARTs has not been studied extensively. However, if clinicians use the lower 5th percentile as a threshold to assign a diagnosis of male infertility, it is likely that ART utilization will increase because the new (5th edition) WHO semen parameter reference values are lower than the previous WHO reference values and a greater number of couples will now be classified as having unexplained infertility. Using the 4th edition WHO guidelines, couples with borderline or subnormal semen parameters (e.g., sperm concentration between 15 and 20 million per ml) would have been classified as having male factor infertility, and in many cases would have been offered male-specific therapy. Using the new, 5th edition WHO guidelines, these same couples with borderline or subnormal semen parameters would now be offered ARTs rather than male-specific therapy, if the lower 5th percentile is used as a threshold to assign a diagnosis of male infertility. As such, it is likely that utilization of intrauterine insemination (IUI) and intracytoplasmic sperm injection (ICSI) will increase because there will be larger pool of couples with unexplained infertility. Although many of the couples with borderline or subnormal semen parameters will be offered IUI first, those couples who fail IUI will then likely proceed to ICSI [43–45].

Conclusion

The latest WHO manual is a valuable resource for laboratories analyzing semen samples and clinicians alike. However, it is important to recognize that the new reference values cannot differentiate between fertile and infertile men and the evaluation of the infertile man also needs to include a detailed history and physical examination. There is concern that many infertile men will be exempt from having timely and necessary male evaluation because the new WHO reference limits are lower (compared to prior WHO guidelines) and may be used incorrectly to establish or exclude a diagnosis of male factor infertility. As a result, clinicians will delay male-specific treatments or altogether fail to treat a potentially correctable cause of male factor infertility. The development of new markers of male factor infertility (e.g., sperm function tests or new biomarkers) may help clarify the clinical importance of the semen analysis in the evaluation of the infertile couple.

References

1. Practice Committee of American Society for Reproductive Medicine. Definitions of infertility and recurrent pregnancy loss: a committee opinion. Fertil Steril. 2013;99(1):63.
2. Anderson JE, et al. Infertility services reported by men in the United States: national survey data. Fertil Steril. 2009;91(6):2466–70.
3. Macomber D, Sanders MB. The spermatozoa count. N Engl J Med. 1929;200(19):981–4.
4. Macleod JF, Gold RZ. The male factor in fertility and infertility. III. An analysis of motile activity in the spermatozoa of 1000 fertile men and 1000 men in infertile marriage. Fertil Steril. 1951;2:187–204.
5. Macleod JF, Gold RZ. The male factor in fertility and infertility. II. Spermatozoon counts in 1000 men of known fertility and in 1000 cases of infertile marriage. J Urol. 1951;66:436–9.
6. Mac LJ. The male factor in fertility and infertility; an analysis of ejaculate volume in 800 fertile men and in 600 men in infertile marriage. Fertil Steril. 1950;1(4):347–61.
7. MacLeod JF, Gold RZ. The male factor in fertility and infertility. IV. Sperm morphology in fertile and infertile marriage. Fertil Steril. 1951;2(5):394–414.
8. Barratt CL, Dunphy BC, et al. Semen characteristics of 49 fertile males. Andrologia. 1988;20(3):264–9.

9. Chia SE, Tay SK, Lim ST. What constitutes a normal seminal analysis? Semen parameters of 243 fertile men. Hum Reprod. 1998;13(12):3394–8.
10. Nallella KP, Sharma RK, et al. Significance of sperm characteristics in the evaluation of male infertility. Fertil Steril. 2006;85(3):629–34.
11. Bonde JP, Ernst E, et al. Relation between semen quality and fertility: a population-based study of 430 first-pregnancy planners. Lancet. 1988;352(9135):1172–7.
12. Slama R, Eustache F, et al. Time to pregnancy and semen parameters: a cross-sectional study among fertile couples from four European cities. Hum Prod. 2002;17(2):503–15.
13. W.H. Organization. WHO laboratory manual for the examination of human semen and sperm-cervical mucus interaction. 2nd ed. Cambridge: Cambridge University Press; 1987.
14. W.H. Organization. WHO laboratory manual for the examination of human semen and sperm-cervical mucus interaction. 3rd ed. Cambridge: Cambridge University Press; 1992.
15. W.H. Organization. WHO laboratory manual for the examination of human semen and sperm-cervical mucus interaction. 4th ed. Cambridge: Cambridge University Press; 1999.
16. W.H. Organization. WHO laboratory manual for the examination of human semen and semen-cervical mucus interaction. 1st ed. Singapore: Press Concern; 1980.
17. Cooper TG, Noonan E, et al. World Health Organization reference values for human semen characteristics. Hum Reprod Update. 2010;16(3):231–45.
18. Stewart TM, Liu DY, et al. Associations between andrological measures, hormones and semen quality in fertile Australian men: inverse relationship between obesity and sperm output. Hum Reprod. 2009;24(7):1561–8.
19. Auger J, Eustache F, et al. Sperm morphological defects related to environment, lifestyle and medical history of 1001 male partners of pregnant women from four European cities. Hum Reprod. 2001;16(12):2710–7.
20. Jorgensen N, Andersen AG, et al. Regional differences in semen quality in Europe. Hum Reprod. 2001;16(5):1012–9.
21. Swan SH, Brazil C, et al. Geographic differences in semen quality of fertile U.S. males. Environ Health Perspect. 2003;114(4):414–20.
22. Haugen TB, Egeland T, Magnus T. Semen parameters in Norwegian fertile men. J Androl. 2006;27(1):66–71.
23. Jensen TK, Slama R, et al. Regional differences in waiting time to pregnancy among fertile couples from four European cities. Hum Reprod. 2002;16:2697–704.
24. W.H.Organization. WHO Laboratory Manual for the Examination and Processing of Human Semen. 5th ed. Geneva: WHO Press; 2010. p. 287.
25. Keel BA. Within- and between-subject variation in semen parameters in infertile men and normal semen donors. Fertil Steril. 2006;85(1):128–34.
26. Amann RP. Considerations in evaluating human spermatogenesis on the basis of total sperm per ejaculate. J Androl. 2009;30(6):626–41.
27. Guzick DS, Overstreet JW, et al. Sperm morphology, motility, and concentration in fertile and infertile men. N Engl J Med. 2001;345(19):1388–93.
28. Esteves SC, Zini A, et al. Critical appraisal of World Health Organization's new reference values for human semen characteristics and effect on diagnosis and treatment of subfertile men. Urology. 2012;79(1):16–22.
29. Meacham RB, Joyce GF, et al. Male infertility. J Urol. 2007;177:2058–66.
30. Greenberg SH, Lipshultz LI, Wein AJ. Experience with 425 subfertile male patients. J Urol. 1978;119(4):507–10.
31. Bm A-A, Marszalek M, et al. Clinical parameters and semen analysis in 716 Austrian patients with varicocele. Urology. 2010;75(5):1069–73.
32. Zini A, Blumenfeld A, et al. Beneficial effect of microsurgical varicocelectomy on human sperm DNA integrity. Hum Reprod. 2005;20(4):1018–21.
33. Agarwal A, Deepinder F, et al. Efficacy of varicocelectomy in improving semen parameters: new meta-analytical approach. Urology. 2007;70(3):532–8.
34. Smit M, Romijn JC, et al. Decreased sperm DNA fragmentation after surgical varicocelectomy is associated with increased pregnancy rate. J Urol. 2010;183(1):270–4.
35. Esteves SC, Oliveira FV, Bertolla RP. Clinical outcome of intracytoplasmic sperm injection in infertile men with treated and untreated clinical varicocele. J Urol. 2010;184(4):1442–6.
36. Schlesinger MH, Wilets IF, Nagler HM. Treatment outcome after varicocelectomy. A critical analysis. Urol Clin North Am. 1994;21(3):517–29.
37. Baazeem A, Belzile E, et al. Varicocele and male factor infertility treatment: a new meta-analysis and review of the role of varicocele repair. Eur Urol. 2011;60(47):796–808.
38. Kroese AC, de Lange NM, et al. Varicocele surgery, new evidence. Hum Reprod Update. 2013;19(4):317.
39. Report on varicocele and infertility. Fertil Steril. 2008;90(5):247–9.
40. Bertolla RP, Cedenho AP, et al. Sperm nuclear DNA fragmentation in adolescents with varicocele. Fertil Steril. 2006;85(3):625–8.
41. Kamal KM, Jarvi K, Zini A. Microsurgical varicocelectomy in the era of assisted reproductive technology: influence of initial semen quality on pregnancy rates. Fertil Steril. 2001;75(5):1013–6.
42. Richardson I, Grotas M, Nagler HM. Outcomes of varicocelectomy treatment: an updated critical analysis. Urol Clin North Am. 2008;35(2):191–209.
43. Smith S, Pfeifer SM, Collins JA. Diagnosis and management of female infertility. JAMA. 2003;290(13):1767–70.
44. Nuojua-Huttunen S, Gissler M, et al. Obstetric and perinatal outcome of pregnancies after intrauterine insemination. Hum Reprod. 1999;14(8):2110–5.
45. Murray KS, James A, et al. The effect of the new 2010 World Health Organization criteria for semen analyses on male infertility. Fertil Steril. 2012;98(6):1428–31.

Intracytoplasmic Injection with Suboptimal Spermatozoa

Gianpiero D. Palermo and Queenie V. Neri

Background

Since the report of the first birth with in vitro fertilization (IVF) in 1978, this procedure has been used extensively for the alleviation of human infertility [1]. However, because spermatozoa cannot fertilize in many cases of male factor indication, a number of supplementary techniques emerged to overcome this inability, and these are generally referred to as assisted fertilization, microsurgical fertilization, or simply gamete micromanipulation. The application of microscopic surgery to human gametes has allowed the achievement of fertilization in cases of severe oligo-astheno-terato-zoospermia and with dysfunctional spermatozoa. In addition, it has served as a powerful tool for a comprehensive understanding of the basic elements of oocyte maturation, fertilization, and early conceptus development. Gamete micromanipulation techniques now permit the diagnosis and at times even the correction of genetic anomalies, as well as optimization of embryo implantation chances in selected cases.

When sperm density, motility, and morphology are inadequate, various techniques have been proposed to bypass the zona pellucida. Zona drilling (ZD) [2] involved the creation of a circumscribed opening in the zona by acid Tyrode's solution delivered through a fine glass micropipette. It inevitably became clear that the use of an acidic medium had a deleterious effect on the one-celled egg—an effect not reported in cleavage-stage embryos using the "hatching" procedure. Alternative procedures were zona cracking in which the zona was breached mechanically with two fine glass hooks [3] and zona softening performed by a brief exposure to trypsin [4] or pronase. Partial zona dissection (PZD) [5] involved slicing of the zona with glass needles prior to exposure of the treated oocytes to spermatozoa. The above listed approaches carried a distinct risk of injury to the oocytes and aimed at producing an opening in the zona of proper size to facilitate penetration of spermatozoa in the perivitelline space and then fusion with the oolemma. Localized laser photoablation of the zona was even tested in this regard to produce a gap of precise dimensions within the zona, and this has resulted in a few offspring [6, 7]. However, not only did all these early procedures brought a modest and inconsistent fertilization, with PZD being the most used in that regard, but they were plagued by an unacceptably higher incidence of polyspermy. The mechanical insertion of spermatozoa directly into the perivitelline space—subzonal sperm injection (SUZI) [8]—was introduced as another option of overcoming inadequacies of sperm concentration and motility, and

G.D. Palermo, MD, PhD (✉)
Q.V. Neri, BSc, MSc
The Ronald O. Perelman and Claudia Cohen Center for Reproductive Medicine, Weill Cornell Medical College, 1305 York Avenue, Suite 720, New York, NY 10021, USA
e-mail: gdpalerm@med.cornell.edu

this proved to be more effective than ZD or PZD, particularly following prior induction of the acrosome reaction [9, 10]. However, SUZI also remained limited by the inability to overcome acrosomal abnormalities or dysfunction of the sperm–oolemma fusion process, and, ultimately, by disappointingly low fertilization rates.

Because ICSI involves insertion of a single selected spermatozoon directly into the oocyte, this bypasses all the preliminary steps of fertilization. The technique was initially attempted in lower organisms, such as the sea urchin [11] and then in mammalian oocytes [12] with the observation of a sperm nucleus decondensing after its microinjection into hamster eggs [13] with subsequent male pronucleus formation [14, 15]. This approach obviously caused oocyte injury and lysis [16], and in early studies only about 30 % of injected mouse eggs survived the procedure, even when supposedly fine micropipettes were used [17].

Because the gamete fusion step in ICSI fertilization is bypassed, male pronucleus development generally requires oocyte activation in most species tested and this can be granted by energetic suction of some cytoplasm immediately before or during sperm nucleus insertion [18]. The first live offspring using sperm injection were obtained in the rabbit following the transfer of the so inseminated oocytes into the oviduct of a pseudopregnant female [19], and soon after a single live birth was reported in the bovine [20]. Although applied to human gametes some years earlier [21], the first human pregnancies with ICSI occurred only in 1992 [22].

When Is ICSI Used?

The intracytoplasmic sperm injection (ICSI) procedure entails the deposition of a single spermatozoon directly into the cytoplasm of the oocyte, thus bypassing the ZP and the oolemma. The ability of ICSI to achieve higher fertilization and pregnancy rates regardless of sperm characteristics makes it the most powerful micromanipulation procedure yet with which to treat male factor infertility. However, no universal standards for patient selection have been defined for ICSI. The general consensus is that ICSI may be adopted when an extremely poor sperm sample is noted or following fertilization failure using in vitro insemination techniques.

Although oocytes that failed to fertilize with standard IVF techniques can be reinseminated by ICSI, this introduces a risk of fertilizing aged eggs [23]. In our own limited experience, six of eight pregnancies established by micromanipulation of such oocytes miscarried, and cytogenetic studies performed on conceptuses provided evidence of chromosomal abnormalities. Thus, notwithstanding reports of normal pregnancies [24, 25] the reinsemination of unfertilized oocytes is currently not advisable for routine clinical application.

When initial sperm concentration in the ejaculate is $<5 \times 10^6$/ml, the likelihood of fertilization with standard IVF is significantly reduced [26], and therefore such couples should be considered unsuitable for this technique, particularly where <1 % normal forms are observed. However, fertilization of mature oocytes may still fail to occur in the presence of normal sperm [27] because of the hardening of the zona pellucida [28], or when oocytes reveal ooplasmic inclusions [29, 30]. Abnormalities of the zona pellucida prevent sperm fusion with the oolemma [31] thus justifying sperm injection. In most instances, however, failure of fertilization is due to coexisting sperm abnormalities presenting ICSI as the only treatment option [32].

Early experience showed that isolated nuclei of testicular and epididymal hamster spermatozoa decondensed soon after injection into mature hamster oocytes, and formed pronuclei in activated eggs [33]. Although in vitro fertilization of human oocytes was accomplished with epididymal spermatozoa in men with obstructive azoospermia [34, 35], only with the advent of ICSI it was possible to obtain consistent fertilization with each gamete source [36–38]. Testicular biopsy was employed to retrieve sperm cells from men who had a scarred epididymis and therefore, no chance of retrieval through that route [39, 40]. However, the therapeutic possibilities of ICSI go even further since immotile testicular spermatozoa and supposedly even spermatids have been successfully used [41].

Some men produce only round-headed spermatozoa which have no acrosome and can neither bind to nor penetrate zona-free hamster oocytes [42, 43]. However, ICSI has enabled even such acrosomeless spermatozoa to establish pregnancies [44–48]. Moreover, ICSI's dependability has broadened its initial use from a technique capable of overriding the dysfunctionality of spermatozoa to one that may partly compensate for problems with the egg. Indeed, ICSI has allowed successful fertilization when only a few and/or abnormal oocytes were available [49]. Stripping cumulus cells from the oocytes allows a direct assessment of maturation, thus offering a woman with a limited number of oocytes a much greater chance of successful fertilization. In fact, the availability of ICSI has been instrumental in some European countries that include Italy and Germany in circumventing restrictive legislation that limits the number of oocytes inseminated or embryos to be replaced [50–52].

ICSI made it possible to have more consistent fertilization when injecting cryopreserved oocytes [53]—overcoming the problem that freezing can lead to premature exocytosis of cortical granules, resulting in zona hardening and inhibition of natural sperm penetration [54–57]. ICSI is also the preferred conception method during the application of preimplantation genetic diagnosis (PGD) because it avoids DNA contamination from additional sperm adhering to the zona and it enhances the number of fertilizable oocytes and ultimately embryos available for screening [58].

ICSI also has an impact in the arena of HIV infection in serodiscordant couples. Three-quarters of individuals infected by HIV or HCV are in their reproductive years. Male-to-female transmission of HIV is estimated to be only 1 per 1,000 acts of unprotected intercourse [59] and even higher in HCV infected patients [60]. Moreover, because of antiretroviral therapies, the course of HIV-1 infection has shifted from a lethal acquired immunodeficiency syndrome to a chronic manageable disease. In such cases, intrauterine insemination (IUI) with spermatozoa processed by double gradient centrifugation followed by swim up has been the suggested method of treating couples with an HIV-1-infected male partner [61]. However, the use of ICSI has been proposed by several groups because of its negligible oocyte exposure to semen, thereby reducing the risk of viral transmission [62, 63]. Advantages of ICSI over IUI also include the considerably higher success rate [62], requiring fewer attempts to achieve pregnancy while reducing viral exposure [64]. Fortunately, so far, no seroconversions have been reported following ART treatments including IUIs [65, 66].

Finally, because only a single spermatozoon is needed for each egg, ICSI has allowed treatment of men who are virtually azoospermic (also defined as cryptozoospermic) [67]. Such cases of spermatogenic arrest have necessarily involved the injection of immature spermatozoa or even spermatogonia [40, 41, 68, 69]. Nonetheless, where fertilization occurs in ICSI cases, conception is accomplished with an embryo implantation that follows a success pattern, at least in our experience, comparable to that seen with standard in vitro insemination.

Clinical Outcome

In the last 19 years at Cornell, we have performed a total of 34,425 ART cycles. Of those, 31.7 % (10,898) included the standard in vitro insemination cycles; the average maternal age was 37.6 ± 4 years and paternal age of 39.6 ± 6 years that resulted in a fertilization rate of 60.5 % and a clinical pregnancy rate of 37.6. In vitro insemination was generally performed in patients with ideal semen parameters, while ICSI has been used to treat couples with suboptimal spermatozoa, a history of poor fertilization, and/or limited numbers of oocytes.

ICSI was performed in 21,302 cycles with ejaculated spermatozoa with a mean maternal age of 36.9 ± 5 years and paternal age of 40.8 ± 8 years. In our patient population 18,757 of our men had at least one abnormal semen parameter according to the WHO 2010 criteria. In these suboptimal sperm cohort, of the 175,833 MII oocyte injected, 5.1 % lysed and those that survived yielded 79.2 % (132,183/166,796)

Table 2.1 Fertilization and pregnancy rates according to semen origin

No. of	Spermatozoa Ejaculated	Surgically retrieved
Maternal age (M±SD years)	36.9±5[a]	35.1±5[a]
Cycles	21,302	2,225
Fertilization (%)	132,183/166,796 (79.2)[a]	12,922/20,779 (62.2)[a]
Clinical pregnancies (%)	8,404 (39.5)[b]	993 (44.6)[b]

[a]χ^2, 2×2, 1 df, effect of spermatozoal source on fertilization rate, $P=0.0001$
[b]χ^2, 2×2, 1 df, effect of spermatozoal source on clinical pregnancy rate, $P=0.0001$

Table 2.2 Spermatozoal parameters and intracytoplasmic sperm injection (ICSI) outcome according to retrieval sites and specimen condition

No. of	Spermatozoa Epididymal Fresh	Frozen/thawed	Testicular Fresh	Frozen/thawed
Cycles	342	624	917	342
Density (10^6/ml±SD)	45.8±47	26.6±32	0.4±2	0.2±0.7
Motility (%±SD)	19.0±17[a]	4.1±8[a]	3.1±7	1.2±4
Morphology (%±SD)	1.7±2.3	1.2±2	0	0
Fertilization (%)	2,515/3,473 (72.4)	4,104/5,779 (71.0)	4,894/8,568 (57.1)[b]	1,406/2,959 (47.6)[b]

[a]Student's t-test, two independent samples, effect of epididymal cryopreservation on sperm motility, $P<0.0001$
[b]χ^2, 2×2, 1 df, effect of testicular cryopreservation on fertilization rates, $P=0.0001$

zygotes. Of the oocytes that abnormally fertilized, 4,170 (2.5 %) displayed 1PN and 5,838 (3.5 %) were 3PN. The clinical pregnancy rate, as detected by the presence of at least one fetal heartbeat, was 39.5 % (Table 2.1).

When more immature forms of spermatozoa were utilized, for example those surgically retrieved, the fertilization rate of 62.5 % and although satisfactory was lower than that achieved with ejaculated spermatozoa ($P=0.0001$) (Table 2.1). In contrast, the clinical pregnancy rate appeared lower in the ejaculated group in comparison to the surgically retrieved spermatozoa; this difference may be attributed to the younger maternal age in the latter cohort.

In situations where no spermatozoa were found in the ejaculate after two semen analyses, patients opted to undergo epididymal or testicular sperm retrieval. In 2,225 cycles with surgically retrieved spermatozoa, the mean maternal age was 35.1±5 years. A total of 966 cycles were performed with epididymal specimens and 1,259 cycles with testicular samples. When looking at men with obstructive azoospermia that used spermatozoa retrieved from the epididymis, those diagnosed with congenital absence of the vas ($n=524$) had superior fertilization (72.1 % vs. 70.9 %; $P=0.0001$) as well as higher clinical pregnancies (54.0 % vs. 46.8 %; $P=0.03$) in comparison to those that had an acquired vas obstruction ($n=442$). In cycles that used testicular sampling, we divided them according to their etiology as being obstructive ($n=228$) or nonobstructive ($n=1,031$). In these cases, the fertilization rate was superior in the obstructive cohort when compared to the nonobstructive group (64.5 % vs. 52.7 %; $P=0.0001$) but resulting in comparable clinical pregnancies (45.2 % vs. 38.8 %).

When the fertilization and pregnancy characteristics were analyzed according to whether the sample was cryopreserved, we observed that after cryopreservation epididymal samples had lower motility parameters ($P<0.0001$; Table 2.2) as well as pregnancy outcome ($P=0.0001$; Fig. 2.1), though without affecting fertilization rate (Table 2.2). When testicular samples were used for ICSI, the situation was reversed with zygote

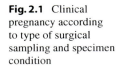

Fig. 2.1 Clinical pregnancy according to type of surgical sampling and specimen condition

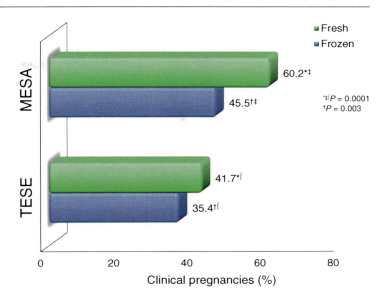

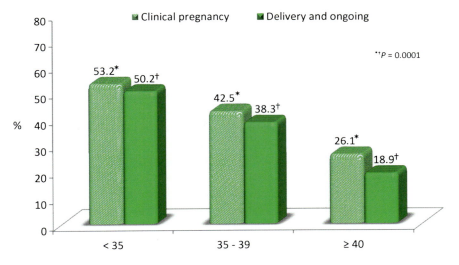

Fig. 2.2 Clinical outcome per oocyte retrieval grouped according to maternal age. Clinical pregnancy is considered as the presence of at least one fetal heartbeat

formation being higher in the fresh specimens ($P=0.03$) as well as the ability of the embryo to implant ($P=0.0001$; Table 2.2; Fig. 2.1).

When 21,028 ICSI cycles (after exclusion of the donor egg cycles) were plotted as a function of increasing maternal age, there was a progressive decrease in pregnancy ($P=0.0001$; Fig. 2.2) and consequently in delivery rates ($P=0.0001$). As predicted, there was a higher incidence of miscarriages, therapeutic abortions, and overall pregnancy losses as a function of the age of the female partner ($P=0.0001$), pregnancy wastage being 2.6 times greater in women ≥40 years compared to those of <35 years.

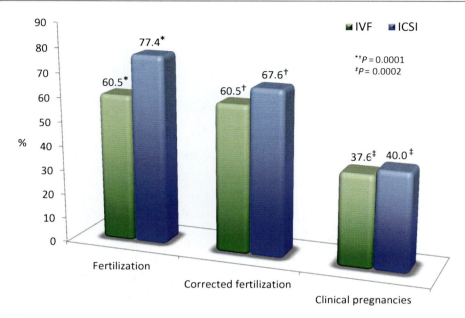

Fig. 2.3 Fertilization and clinical pregnancy reported at Cornell following standard in vitro insemination and ICSI. To better compare fertilization success between the two insemination methods, we have corrected fertilization with ICSI using the total number of oocytes retrieved as the denominator

A total of 7,422 ICSI patients delivered 9,150 babies comprising 4,606 males and 4,521 females (with 23 unknown genders). A total of 3.6 % (330) exhibited congenital abnormalities at birth, of which 174 (1.9 %) were major and 156 (1.7 %) were minor. IVF children ($n = 5,183$) had a comparable overall malformation rate (104 major and 83 minor).

To evaluate differences in performance between insemination methods, we compared embryological outcomes and clinical pregnancy rates between standard in vitro insemination and ICSI. While it appeared that fertilization was lower in IVF than with ICSI ($P = 0.0001$; Fig. 2.3), after correcting for all retrieved oocytes and not for metaphase II injected, ICSI still yielded more oocytes fertilized (60.5 % vs. 67.6 %; $P = 0.0001$). Furthermore, the ability to generate term pregnancies was also higher with the ICSI cohort ($P = 0.0002$). However, as in all fields of reproductive medicine, the limiting factor remains to be maternal age (Fig. 2.2), as evidenced by an inverse relationship between delivery rate and female age [70].

The Quest for the Ideal Spermatozoon

While ICSI has been the gold standard for most IVF centers for more than 20 years with no proven significant or attributable side effects, some researchers still question the possible deleterious effects of a technique that bypasses the natural gamete selection processes typical of in vivo reproduction. Towards that goal, several methods have been introduced that expound upon the procedures of ICSI with additional protocols aimed at finding the optimal spermatozoon to inseminate an oocyte.

It is difficult to select spermatozoa in terms of morphology while they are in motion and without the use of stains. However, selection of normally shaped spermatozoa can be accomplished to a certain extent by observing their shape, light refraction, and motion patterns while screening them in a viscous medium.

Initial preparation methods were based on a simple separation of spermatozoa from the seminal fluid referred to as "washing technique" [71].

Subsequently, the spermatozoa were selected according to sperm motility by the migration or swim up method [72]. Later methods were mainly based on sperm density (mass/volume) in order to select viable and motile spermatozoa with normal morphology. These methods have been mainly referred to as density gradient centrifugation (DGC) techniques that are commonly used for sperm processing in different centers [73]. Alternative methods infrequently used are mostly based on forcing spermatozoa to swim through a variety of artificially created hurdle paths such as glass wool filtration [74], Tea-Jondet Tube [75], and Wang's Tube [76] and Sephadex [77], just to name a few.

The majority of these techniques not only recover viable spermatozoa with normal morphology, but it is believed that they can also, to different degrees, recover mature spermatozoa with intact chromatin and DNA [78]. Because spermatozoa contribute to approximately half of the genome of the next generation, selection of spermatozoa with intact chromatin for the ICSI procedure should become mandatory. Sperm DNA integrity is currently assessed by destructive methods such as TUNEL, COMET, sperm chromatin dispersion (SCD) test, or by a sperm chromatin structural assay (SCSA). However, all of these require fixation and so loss of the sperm cell being evaluated [79]. As assessment of chromatin integrity while observing sperm viability is not plausible, researchers have tried to select spermatozoa mainly based on their surface characteristics and attempted to establish a relationship with sperm genetics and epigenetic traits such as DNA integrity or ploidy.

Recently, our attention has been directed towards the unicellular approach for studying the male gamete aiming at reading its chromosomal constitution [80–82] or its chromatinic integrity [83–85]. Suspending spermatozoa in viscous medium allows the observation of their 3D kinetic patterns [86, 87] and to evaluate their morphological characteristics at high magnification [88, 89]. While new insights are being established on surface markers of the spermatozoon [90–92], a clearer understanding of the conformational chromatin structure characterized by the two forms of DNA present (protamine and histone bound) and the recent recognition of small noncoding RNA [93–95] will guide the treatment of infertility through the next generation.

It has been postulated that fertile men with normal semen parameters almost uniformly have low levels of DNA breakage, whereas infertile men with compromised semen parameters presumably present with nicks and breaks in their sperm chromatin. However, in these men spermatozoa with compromised DNA integrity, measured by the most popular methods, do not seem to correlate with sperm concentration and morphology [96, 97]. In a systematic observation carried out in our laboratory, instead we have reported a strong inverse correlation between DNA fragmentation (measured by SCSA and TUNEL) and kinetic characteristics [98]—as motility decreases, there was an increase in DNA fragmentation. Perhaps this may explain why there is a lack of predictability between DNA integrity and pregnancy outcome with ICSI inseminations [99] because of the fact that only motile spermatozoa are utilized for injection regardless of their number.

The pledge for the ideal spermatozoon has been perceived as a surface scrutiny under high magnification of the individual sperm cell dubbed "motile sperm organellar morphology examination" (MSOME) [88]. This hinted to "intracytoplasmic morphologically selected sperm injection" (IMSI) that claimed to yield superior clinical outcomes than conventional ICSI [88, 89]. IMSI promised higher fertilization, implantation, clinical pregnancy rates along with lower pregnancy losses and healthy offspring in a series of studies [100–103]. Higher magnification screening of sperm surface irregularities, however, did not prove the asserted amelioration of clinical outcome in independent investigations. This has been true for male factor couples, at first or repeated ART attempts [87]. Moreover, light microscopic observations of surface sperm head irregularities or vacuoles are almost ubiquitous once higher level examination, i.e., by transmission electron microscopy (TEM), scanning electron microscopy (SEM), and confocal microscopy suggesting a paraphysiologic nature of these entities [87, 104–106]. In fact, these vacuole-like structures, or as more appropriately described craters, appear in over 90 % of spermatozoa from fertile donors with normal semen parameters [107, 108]. The whole concept of IMSI may possibly be suited for cases where millions of morphologically normal spermatozoa are available for selection, but in fact cannot practically be employed in severe oligozoospermic cases where cryptozoospermia and nonobstructive azoospermia only yield scarce viable cells.

A connection between a specific phenotype and the intrinsic chromosomal/chromatinic integrity of the spermatozoa has also been attempted through the hyaluronic acid binding characteristics appearing on the surface of the mature sperm cells [90–92]. This biochemical marker was verisimilarly used to identify the most viable mature spermatozoa with intact DNA, euploid, and restricted amount of histones, and achieve embryo developmental competence [90–92] to be used for ICSI. However, this concept is somewhat contradicted by the observation that immature spermatozoa, such as those retrieved from epididymis and testes, are capable of generating high fertilization and pregnancy rates in a comparable manner to their ejaculated counterparts (see Table 2.2; Fig. 2.1). PICSI, or "Physiologic ICSI," makes use of hyaluronic acid (HA), a substance naturally present in the human body [109]. HA can be found in the cumulus oophorus around the oocyte and represents a barrier to the immature gametes by only relenting to "mature" spermatozoa. These putatively ready spermatozoa that have undergone the complete process of plasma membrane remodeling, cytoplasmic extrusion, and nuclear maturity will have a significantly higher number of HA receptors and binding sites. Two methods have been proposed on how to perform PICSI. The first is an ICSI dish coated with microdots of hyaluronic acid hydrogel that allow HA-bound spermatozoa to be recovered using a standard ICSI injection pipette [92]. The other method is represented by a viscous medium composed partially of HA [109] that also fully replaces PVP. Some studies have shown that spermatozoa capable of HA binding have lower DNA fragmentation than simple post-swim-up spermatozoa. In addition, nucleus normalcy rate (according to MSOME criteria) has been shown to be higher in spermatozoa bound to HA as compared to spermatozoa in PVP [109]. However, PICSI correlations to pregnancy or delivery rates or malformation incidence have been inconsistent. In a systematic observation performed in our laboratory we carried out the selection of spermatozoa that exhibit HA binding sites on which we assessed chromosomal status and chromatinic competence. HA-bound and HA-unbound sperm cells were individually picked up by an ICSI pipette and assessed by Diff-Quik™, Aniline Blue, SCD, TUNEL, and FISH (Fig. 2.4). Male gamete genetic and epigenetic characteristics according to the expression of HA-binding sites are illustrated in Fig. 2.5. Surprisingly, the arrays of assays were within the expected limits for each individual test thresholds and across the HA expression characteristics. Although there were some improvements in the outcome of the tested parameters of the spermatozoa selected upon their motility characteristics, HA selection technique did not seem to add any further advantage [110]. Ultimately, PICSI is still impacted by the same major drawbacks as IMSI, represented by cases where extremely few sperm cells are present and therefore, rendering unworkable the putative selection.

ICSI with Unselected Spermatozoa

ICSI was exclusively developed to assist those with severe male factor infertility and this can include a wide variety of spermatogenic defects as often seen in cryptozoospermic and azoospermic men. In the latter case, the solution is to extract spermatozoa directly from the seminiferous tubules. In the micro-testicular sperm extraction (micro-TESE) procedure performed at our facility, the larger opaque seminiferous tubule is selected for excision [111]. This novel approach has greatly enhanced the chances of identifying spermatozoa in comparison to a random testicular sperm extraction while limiting scarring. Even with this targeted sampling approach, testicular surgery carries surgical and anesthesiological risks and those factors need to be carefully evaluated and discussed with patients particularly when seldom ejaculated spermatozoa are present. Independently of the technique used for the

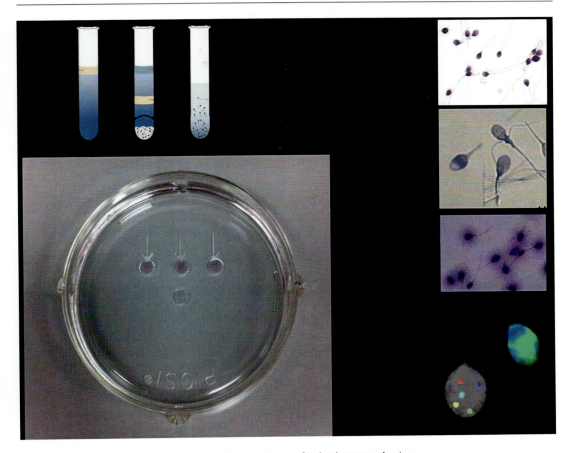

Fig. 2.4 Genetic and epigenetic assessment of spermatozoa after hyaluronan selection

retrieval of spermatozoa in men with compromised spermatogenesis, the minute amount of sperm cells available requires an exhaustive search for the much needed gamete to inseminate all oocytes. At times these extreme searches do not yield enough spermatozoa and often cryopreservation of the surplus oocytes need to be contemplated.

To provide an idea of the results obtained following the gargantuous effort during an extended sperm quest carried out on an inverted microscope while searching in droplets under oil by several embryologists, we grouped these cases according to time, 30 min–1 h, 1–2 h, 2–3 h, and >3 h, and compared to a control requiring less than 30 min [112]. Embryo development and implantation were recorded for the different sperm quest times. Independently of the source whether ejaculated or surgically retrieved, an exhaustive search for spermatozoa is needed to retrieve all spermatozoa for injection. In spite of the increasing search time and the extremely limited number of sperm cells identified, when oocytes were finally injected, fertilization did not dramatically differ in function of time and/or sperm source (control 58.9 % TESE vs. 75.6 % Ejac, $P<0.0001$; 30 min–1 h was 55.6 % TESE vs. 56.2 % Ejac; 1–2 h was 50.5 % TESE vs. 52.5 % Ejac; 2–3 h was 32.7 % TESE vs. 33.9 % Ejac; and >3 h was 27.8 % TESE vs. 33.3 % Ejac). Similarly, for both gamete provenance clinical pregnancies maintained a satisfactory clinical profile in spite of the increasing time spent to identify the spermatozoa (30 min–1 h was 51.6 % TESE vs. 35.4 % Ejac; 1–2 h was 44.6 % TESE vs. 57.1 % Ejac; 2–3 h was 34.4 % TESE vs. 0 % Ejac; and >3 h was 26.7 TESE vs. 100 % Ejac) [113].

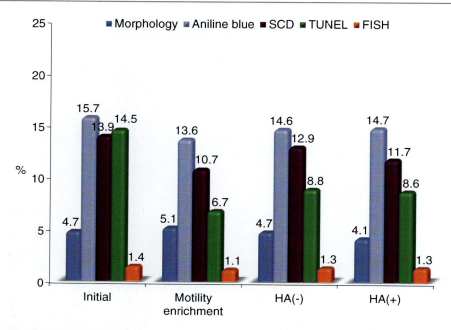

Fig. 2.5 Assessment of spermatozoa in raw semen, after sperm selection by density gradient, and after microtool pick-up of spermatozoa that were either bound to hyaluronan (HA+) or unbound (HA−)

Safety and Conclusions

Since the early establishment of in vitro insemination it became clear that a large portion of couples would not be capable of achieving fertilization. We have been involved since the early efforts in devising methods for assisted fertilization to allow men with subfertile spermatozoa to generate conceptuses once in vitro insemination of their partner oocytes failed in previous attempts. It quickly became evident that among the different approaches the direct injection of a spermatozoon would be the most effective way to solve male gamete dysfunction. Now ICSI is generously applied worldwide for a variety of indications and not exclusively for male factor infertility. ICSI has been shown to be the procedure of choice when spermatozoa, such as in azoospermic men, are directly retrieved from the epididymis and the testis. In fact in these men, as long as a viable spermatozoon is isolated, there is a chance of generating a conceptus. The fertilization achieved with surgically retrieved specimens matches those seen with optimal ejaculated gametes and similarly, embryo development is uncompromised.

Concerns raised by this invasive procedure where a gamete is arbitrarily selected have proved to be mainly unfounded as the health and developmental potential of offspring born from ICSI are comparable to those born after standard in vitro insemination. The real concerns erupt from the fact that infertile men carry a higher incidence of chromosomal defects and, particularly in azoospermic men, even meaningful microdeletion(s) on a gonosome may be present. Likewise, azoospermia itself is associated with a higher incidence of aneuploidy in the germ cells due to meiotic errors and with possible increase in autosomal/gonosomal disomies.

Notwithstanding the large number of babies born following ICSI worldwide, concerns still exist as to whether the use of suboptimal spermatozoa can result in genomic or phenotypic abnormalities in the progeny [114]. In one of the earlier studies on the evolution of pregnancies after ICSI, it was observed that the rate of malformation was

2.6 % after ICSI [115]. An extension of the Cornell series which included a total of 14,333 ART children examined found that the incidence of overall malformation was comparable between the IVF and ICSI [70]. Evidence regarding the outcome of singletons born at term following ART is generally reassuring [116]. The increased risk of perinatal morbidity and mortality associated with singleton births has been linked to the infertility of the couple rather than the ART techniques used [117].

The specific concerns in regard to ICSI, whether real or theoretical [118–121], involve the insemination method, the use of spermatozoa with genetic or structural defects, and the possible introduction of foreign genes.

In summary, the most palpable factor that can lead to adverse outcomes in offspring conceived by IVF or ICSI is the high and higher gestational order. The occurrence of this phenomenon has induced the consideration of single embryo transfer policies to address this considerably. Small for gestational age and prematurity confirmed in the ART population also appears to find an explanation in the higher order of embryos transferred and therefore implanted. Once ART reigns in the incidence of multiple gestations, the health of ART offspring seems comparable to those spontaneously conceived even considering the older age of the female partners. Although perinatal outcomes such as prematurity, low birth weight, perinatal mortality, and increased incidence of malformations that have been observed with ART techniques, it is clear that the main culprit is related to infertility itself [70]. Overall, studies of children ranging from newborn to 14 years of age [122–129] have been reassuring in terms of perinatal outcome, IQ, and physical development [116]. Further follow-up on ICSI teenagers into adulthood should be continued to better understand the reproductive capacity of these youngsters.

Acknowledgements We are most grateful to the Andrology and Embryology Laboratories and particularly to the clinicians, scientists, and nursing staff of The Ronald O. Perelman & Claudia Cohen Center for Reproductive Medicine.

References

1. Steptoe PC, Edwards RG. Birth after the reimplantation of a human embryo. Lancet. 1978;2:366.
2. Gordon JW, Talansky BE. Assisted fertilization by zona drilling: a mouse model for correction of oligospermia. J Exp Zool. 1986;239:347–54.
3. Odawara Y, Lopata A. A zona opening procedure for improving in vitro fertilization at low sperm concentrations: a mouse model. Fertil Steril. 1989;51:699–704.
4. Gordon JW, Grunfeld L, Garrisi GJ, Talansky BE, Richards C, et al. Fertilization of human oocytes by sperm from infertile males after Zona Pellucida drilling. Fertil Steril. 1988;50:68–73.
5. Cohen J, Malter H, Fehilly C, Wright G, Elsner C, et al. Implantation of embryos after partial opening of oocyte Zona Pellucida to facilitate sperm penetration. Lancet. 1988;2:162.
6. Antinori S, Versaci C, Fuhrberg P, Panci C, Caffa B, et al. Seventeen live births after the use of an erbium-yytrium aluminum garnet laser in the treatment of male factor infertility. Hum Reprod. 1994;9:1891–6.
7. Feichtinger W, Strohmer H, Fuhrberg P, Radivojevic K, Antinori S, et al. Photoablation of oocyte zona pellucida by erbium-YAG laser for in-vitro fertilisation in severe male infertility. Lancet. 1992;339:811.
8. Laws-King A, Trounson A, Sathananthan H, Kola I. Fertilization of human oocytes by microinjection of a single spermatozoon under the zona pellucida. Fertil Steril. 1987;48:637–42.
9. Palermo G, Joris H, Devroey P, Van Steirteghem AC. Induction of acrosome reaction in human spermatozoa used for subzonal insemination. Hum Reprod. 1992;7:248–54.
10. Palermo G, Van Steirteghem A. Enhancement of acrosome reaction and subzonal insemination of a single spermatozoon in mouse eggs. Mol Reprod Dev. 1991;30:339–45.
11. Hiramoto Y. Microinjection of the live spermatozoa into sea urchin eggs. Exp Cell Res. 1962;27:416–26.
12. Lin TP. Microinjection of mouse eggs. Science. 1966;151:333–7.
13. Uehara T, Yanagimachi R. Microsurgical injection of spermatozoa into hamster eggs with subsequent transformation of sperm nuclei into male pronuclei. Biol Reprod. 1976;15:467–70.
14. Naish SJ, Perreault SD, Foehner AL, Zirkin BR. DNA synthesis in the fertilizing hamster sperm nucleus: sperm template availability and egg cytoplasmic control. Biol Reprod. 1987;36:245–53.
15. Perreault SD, Wolff RA, Zirkin BR. The role of disulfide bond reduction during mammalian sperm nuclear decondensation in vivo. Dev Biol. 1984;101:160–7.
16. Laufer N, Pratt BM, DeCherney AH, Naftolin F, Merino M, et al. The in vivo and in vitro effects of clomiphene citrate on ovulation, fertilization, and

16. development of cultured mouse oocytes. Am J Obstet Gynecol. 1983;147:633–9.
17. Thadani VM. Injection of sperm heads into immature rat oocytes. J Exp Zool. 1979;210:161–8.
18. Perreault SD, Zirkin BR. Sperm nuclear decondensation in mammals: role of sperm-associated proteinase in vivo. J Exp Zool. 1982;224:253–7.
19. Iritani A, Utsumi K, Miyake M, Hosoi Y, Saeki K. In vitro fertilization by a routine method and by micromanipulation. Ann N Y Acad Sci. 1988;541:583–90.
20. Goto K, Kinoshita A, Takuma Y, Ogawa K. Fertilization of bovine oocytes by the injection of immobilized, killed spermatozoa. Vet Rec. 1990;127:517–20.
21. Lanzendorf SE, Maloney MK, Veeck LL, Slusser J, Hodgen GD, et al. A preclinical evaluation of pronuclear formation by microinjection of human spermatozoa into human oocytes. Fertil Steril. 1988;49:835–42.
22. Palermo G, Joris H, Devroey P, Van Steirteghem AC. Pregnancies after intracytoplasmic injection of single spermatozoon into an oocyte. Lancet. 1992;340:17–8.
23. Nagy ZP, Staessen C, Liu J, Joris H, Devroey P, et al. Prospective, auto-controlled study on reinsemination of failed-fertilized oocytes by intracytoplasmic sperm injection. Fertil Steril. 1995;64:1130–5.
24. Morton PC, Yoder CS, Tucker MJ, Wright G, Brockman WD, et al. Reinsemination by intracytoplasmic sperm injection of 1-day-old oocytes after complete conventional fertilization failure. Fertil Steril. 1997;68:488–91.
25. Zhu L, Xi Q, Nie R, Chen W, Zhang H, et al. Rescue intracytoplasmic sperm injection: a prospective randomized study. J Reprod Med. 2011;56:410–4.
26. Yovich JL, Stanger JD. The limitations of in vitro fertilization from males with severe oligospermia and abnormal sperm morphology. J In Vitro Fert Embryo Transf. 1984;1:172–9.
27. Chia CM, Sathananthan H, Ng SC, Law HY, Edirisinghe WR. Ultrastructural investigation of failed in vitro fertilisation in idiopathic subfertility. Proceedings 18th Singapore-Malaysia Congress of Medicine. Singapore: Academy of Medicine; 1984.
28. Defelici M, Siracusa G. Spontaneous hardening of the zona pellucida of mouse oocytes during invitro culture. Gamete Res. 1982;6:107–13.
29. Bedford JM, Kim HH. Sperm/egg binding patterns and oocyte cytology in retrospective analysis of fertilization failure in vitro. Hum Reprod. 1993;8:453–63.
30. Vanblerkom J, Henry G. Oocyte dysmorphism and aneuploidy in meiotically mature human oocytes after ovarian stimulation. Hum Reprod. 1992;7:379–90.
31. Lalonde L, Langlais J, Antaki P, Chapdelaine A, Roberts KD, et al. Male infertility associated with round-headed acrosomeless spermatozoa. Fertil Steril. 1988;49:316–21.
32. Palermo GD, Cohen J, Rosenwaks Z. Intracytoplasmic sperm injection: a powerful tool to overcome fertilization failure. Fertil Steril. 1996;65:899–908.
33. Uehara T, Yanagimachi R. Behavior of nuclei of testicular, caput and cauda epididymal spermatozoa injected into hamster eggs. Biol Reprod. 1977;16:315–21.
34. Silber S, Ord T, Borrero C, Balmaceda J, Asch R. New treatment for infertility due to congenital absence of vas deferens. Lancet. 1987;2:850–1.
35. Temple-Smith PD, Southwick GJ, Yates CA, Trounson AO, de Kretser DM. Human pregnancy by in vitro fertilization (IVF) using sperm aspirated from the epididymis. J In Vitro Fert Embryo Transf. 1985;2:119–22.
36. Palermo GD, Cohen J, Alikani M, Adler A, Rosenwaks Z. Development and implementation of intracytoplasmic sperm injection (ICSI). Reprod Fertil Dev. 1995;7:211–7. discussion 217–8.
37. Silber SJ, Nagy ZP, Liu J, Godoy H, Devroey P, et al. Conventional in-vitro fertilization versus intracytoplasmic sperm injection for patients requiring microsurgical sperm aspiration. Hum Reprod. 1994;9:1705–9.
38. Tournaye H, Devroey P, Liu JE, Nagy Z, Lissens W, et al. Microsurgical epididymal sperm aspiration and intracytoplasmic sperm injection—a new effective approach to infertility as a result of congenital bilateral absence of the vas-deferens. Fertil Steril. 1994;61:1045–51.
39. Craft I, Bennett V, Nicholson N. Fertilising ability of testicular spermatozoa. Lancet. 1993;342:864.
40. Fishel S, Green S, Bishop M, Thornton S, Hunter A, et al. Pregnancy after intracytoplasmic injection of spermatid. Lancet. 1995;345:1641–2.
41. Tesarik J, Mendoza C, Testart J. Viable embryos from injection of round spermatids into oocytes. N Engl J Med. 1995;333:525.
42. Lanzendorf S, Maloney M, Ackerman S, Acosta A, Hodgen G. Fertilizing potential of acrosome-defective sperm following microsurgical injection into eggs. Gamete Res. 1988;19:329–37.
43. Lundin K, Sjogren A, Nilsson L, Hamberger L. Fertilization and pregnancy after intracytoplasmic microinjection of acrosomeless spermatozoa. Fertil Steril. 1994;62:1266–7.
44. Egashira A, Murakami M, Haigo K, Horiuchi T, Kuramoto T. A successful pregnancy and live birth after intracytoplasmic sperm injection with globozoospermic sperm and electrical oocyte activation. Fertil Steril. 2009;2037(92):e5–9.
45. Heindryckx B, Van der Elst J, De Sutter P, Dhont M. Treatment option for sperm- or oocyte-related fertilization failure: assisted oocyte activation following diagnostic heterologous ICSI. Hum Reprod. 2005;20:2237–41.
46. Liu J, Nagy Z, Joris H, Tournaye H, Devroey P, et al. Successful fertilization and establishment of pregnancies after intracytoplasmic sperm injection in patients with globozoospermia. Hum Reprod. 1995;10:626–9.

47. Taylor SL, Yoon SY, Morshedi MS, Lacey DR, Jellerette T, et al. Complete globozoospermia associated with PLCzeta deficiency treated with calcium ionophore and ICSI results in pregnancy. Reprod Biomed Online. 2010;20:559–64.
48. Tejera A, Molla M, Muriel L, Remohi J, Pellicer A, et al. Successful pregnancy and childbirth after intracytoplasmic sperm injection with calcium ionophore oocyte activation in a globozoospermic patient. Fertil Steril. 2008;90:1202 e1–5.
49. Ludwig M, al-Hasani S, Kupker W, Bauer O, Diedrich K. A new indication for an intracytoplasmic sperm injection procedure outside the cases of severe male factor infertility. Eur J Obstet Gynecol Reprod Biol. 1997;75:207–10.
50. Ludwig M, Schopper B, Al-Hasani S, Diedrich K. Clinical use of a pronuclear stage score following intracytoplasmic sperm injection: impact on pregnancy rates under the conditions of the German embryo protection law. Hum Reprod. 2000;15:325–9.
51. Ludwig M, Strik D, Al-Hasani S, Diedrich K. No transfer in a planned ICSI cycle: we cannot overcome some basic rules of human reproduction. Eur J Obstet Gynecol Reprod Biol. 1999;87:3–11.
52. Benagiano G, Gianaroli L. The new Italian IVF legislation. Reprod Biomed Online. 2004;9:117–25.
53. Porcu E, Fabbri R, Seracchioli R, Ciotti PM, Magrini O, et al. Birth of a healthy female after intracytoplasmic sperm injection of cryopreserved human oocytes. Fertil Steril. 1997;68:724–6.
54. Johnson MH. The effect on fertilization of exposure of mouse oocytes to dimethyl sulfoxide: an optimal protocol. J In Vitro Fert Embryo Transf. 1989;6:168–75.
55. Schalkoff ME, Oskowitz SP, Powers RD. Ultrastructural observations of human and mouse oocytes treated with cryopreservatives. Biol Reprod. 1989;40:379–93.
56. Vincent C, Pickering SJ, Johnson MH. The hardening effect of dimethylsulphoxide on the mouse zona pellucida requires the presence of an oocyte and is associated with a reduction in the number of cortical granules present. J Reprod Fertil. 1990;89:253–9.
57. Van Blerkom J, Davis PW. Cytogenetic, cellular, and developmental consequences of cryopreservation of immature and mature mouse and human oocytes. Microsc Res Tech. 1994;27:165–93.
58. Harton GL, De Rycke M, Fiorentino F, Moutou C, SenGupta S, et al. ESHRE PGD consortium best practice guidelines for amplification-based PGD. Hum Reprod. 2011;26:33–40.
59. de Vincenzi I. A longitudinal study of human immunodeficiency virus transmission by heterosexual partners. European Study Group on Heterosexual Transmission of HIV. N Engl J Med. 1994;331:341–6.
60. Garrido N, Meseguer M, Simon C, Pellicer A, Remohi J. Assisted reproduction in HIV and HCV infected men of serodiscordant couples. Arch Androl. 2004;50:105–11.
61. Bujan L, Daudin M, Pasquier C. Choice of ART programme for serodiscordant couples with an HIV infected male partner. Hum Reprod. 2006;21:1332–3. author reply 1333-4.
62. Mencaglia L, Falcone P, Lentini GM, Consigli S, Pisoni M, et al. ICSI for treatment of human immunodeficiency virus and hepatitis C virus-serodiscordant couples with infected male partner. Hum Reprod. 2005;20:2242–6.
63. Sauer MV, Chang PL. Establishing a clinical program for human immunodeficiency virus 1-seropositive men to father seronegative children by means of in vitro fertilization with intracytoplasmic sperm injection. Am J Obstet Gynecol. 2002;186:627–33.
64. Pena JE, Klein J, Thornton 2nd M, Chang PL, Sauer MV. Successive pregnancies with delivery of two healthy infants in a couple who was discordant for human immunodeficiency virus infection. Fertil Steril. 2002;78:421–3.
65. van Leeuwen E, Repping S, Prins JM, Reiss P, van der Veen F. Assisted reproductive technologies to establish pregnancies in couples with an HIV-1-infected man. Neth J Med. 2009;67:322–7.
66. Vitorino RL, Grinsztejn BG, de Andrade CA, Hokerberg YH, de Souza CT, et al. Systematic review of the effectiveness and safety of assisted reproduction techniques in couples serodiscordant for human immunodeficiency virus where the man is positive. Fertil Steril. 2011;95:1684–90.
67. Bendikson KA, Neri QV, Takeuchi T, Toschi M, Schlegel PN, et al. The outcome of intracytoplasmic sperm injection using occasional spermatozoa in the ejaculate of men with spermatogenic failure. J Urol. 2008;180:1060–4.
68. Edwards RG, Tarin JJ, Dean N, Hirsch A, Tan SL. Are spermatid injections into human oocytes now mandatory? Hum Reprod. 1994;9:2217–9.
69. Tsai MC, Takeuchi T, Bedford JM, Reis MM, Rosenwaks Z, et al. Alternative sources of gametes: reality or science fiction? Hum Reprod. 2000;15:988–98.
70. Palermo GD, Neri QV, Takeuchi T, Squires J, Moy F, et al. Genetic and epigenetic characteristics of ICSI children. Reprod Biomed Online. 2008;17:820–33.
71. Edwards RG, Bavister BD, Steptoe PC. Early stages of fertilization in vitro of human oocytes matured in vitro. Nature. 1969;221:632–5.
72. Mahadevan M, Baker G. Assessment and preparation of semen for in vitro fertilization. In: Wood C, Trounson A, editors. Clinical in vitro fertilization. Berlin: Springer; 1984. p. 83–97.
73. Pousette A, Akerlof E, Rosenborg L, Fredricsson B. Increase in progressive motility and improved morphology of human spermatozoa following their migration through Percoll gradients. Int J Androl. 1986;9:1–13.
74. van der Ven HH, Jeyendran RS, Al-Hasani S, Tunnerhoff A, Hoebbel K, et al. Glass wool column

filtration of human semen: relation to swim-up procedure and outcome of IVF. Hum Reprod. 1988;3:85–8.
75. Tea NT, Jondet M, Scholler R. A migration-gravity sedimentation method for collecting motile spermatozoa from human semen. In: Harrison RF, Bonnar J, Thompson W, editors. In vitro fertilization, embryo transfer and early pregnancy. Lancaster: MTP Press; 1984. p. 117–20.
76. Wang FN, Lin CT, Hong CY, Hsiung CH, Su TP, et al. Modification of the Wang tube to improve in vitro semen manipulation. Arch Androl. 1992; 29:267–9.
77. Drobnis EZ, Zhong CQ, Overstreet JW. Separation of cryopreserved human semen using Sephadex columns, washing, or Percoll gradients. J Androl. 1991;12:201–8.
78. Henkel RR, Schill WB. Sperm preparation for ART. Reprod Biol Endocrinol. 2003;1:108.
79. Zini A, Sigman M. Are tests of sperm DNA damage clinically useful? Pros and cons. J Androl. 2009; 30:219–29.
80. Colombero LT, Hariprashad JJ, Tsai MC, Rosenwaks Z, Palermo GD. Incidence of sperm aneuploidy in relation to semen characteristics and assisted reproductive outcome. Fertil Steril. 1999;72:90–6.
81. Hu JCY, Monahan D, Neri QV, Rosenwaks Z, Palermo GD. The role of sperm aneuploidy assay. Fertil Steril. 2011;96:S24–5.
82. Palermo GD, Colombero LT, Hariprashad JJ, Schlegel PN, Rosenwaks Z. Chromosome analysis of epididymal and testicular sperm in azoospermic patients undergoing ICSI. Hum Reprod. 2002;17:570–5.
83. Bungum M, Humaidan P, Spano M, Jepson K, Bungum L, et al. The predictive value of sperm chromatin structure assay (SCSA) parameters for the outcome of intrauterine insemination, IVF and ICSI. Hum Reprod. 2004;19:1401–8.
84. Evenson D, Jost L. Sperm chromatin structure assay is useful for fertility assessment. Methods Cell Sci. 2000;22:169–89.
85. Fernandez-Gonzalez R, Moreira PN, Perez-Crespo M, Sanchez-Martin M, Ramirez MA, et al. Long-term effects of mouse intracytoplasmic sperm injection with DNA-fragmented sperm on health and behavior of adult offspring. Biol Reprod. 2008;78:761–72.
86. Palermo GD, Cohen J, Alikani M, Adler A, Rosenwaks Z. Intracytoplasmic sperm injection: a novel treatment for all forms of male factor infertility. Fertil Steril. 1995;63:1231–40.
87. Palermo GD, Hu JCY, Rienzi L, Maggiulli R, Takeuchi T, et al. Thoughts on IMSI. In: Racowsky C, Schlegel PN, Fauser BC, Carrell DT, editors. Biennial review of infertility, vol. 2. New York: Springer; 2011. p. 296.
88. Bartoov B, Berkovitz A, Eltes F. Selection of spermatozoa with normal nuclei to improve the pregnancy rate with intracytoplasmic sperm injection. N Engl J Med. 2001;345:1067–8.
89. Bartoov B, Berkovitz A, Eltes F, Kogosowski A, Menezo Y, et al. Real-time fine morphology of motile human sperm cells is associated with IVF-ICSI outcome. J Androl. 2002;23:1–8.
90. Huszar G, Ozenci CC, Cayli S, Zavaczki Z, Hansch E, et al. Hyaluronic acid binding by human sperm indicates cellular maturity, viability, and unreacted acrosomal status. Fertil Steril. 2003;79 Suppl 3:1616–24.
91. Jakab A, Sakkas D, Delpiano E, Cayli S, Kovanci E, et al. Intracytoplasmic sperm injection: a novel selection method for sperm with normal frequency of chromosomal aneuploidies. Fertil Steril. 2005; 84:1665–73.
92. Yagci A, Murk W, Stronk J, Huszar G. Spermatozoa bound to solid state hyaluronic acid show chromatin structure with high DNA chain integrity: an acridine orange fluorescence study. J Androl. 2011;31:566–72.
93. Hamatani T. Spermatozoal RNA, profiling towards a clinical evaluation of sperm quality. Reprod Biomed Online. 2011;22:103–5.
94. Krawetz SA, Kruger A, Lalancette C, Tagett R, Anton E, et al. A survey of small RNAs in human sperm. Hum Reprod. 2011;26:3401–12.
95. Miller D, Ostermeier GC, Krawetz SA. The controversy, potential and roles of spermatozoal RNA. Trends Mol Med. 2005;11:156–63.
96. Spano M, Bonde JP, Hjollund HI, Kolstad HA, Cordelli E, et al. Sperm chromatin damage impairs human fertility. The Danish First Pregnancy Planner Study Team. Fertil Steril. 2000;73:43–50.
97. Zini A, Bielecki R, Phang D, Zenzes MT. Correlations between two markers of sperm DNA integrity, DNA denaturation and DNA fragmentation, in fertile and infertile men. Fertil Steril. 2001;75:674–7.
98. Chen C, Hu JCY, Neri QV, Rosenwaks Z, Palermo GD. Kinetic characteristics and DNA integrity of human spermatozoa. Hum Reprod. 2011;19:i30.
99. Evenson DP, Wixon R. Clinical aspects of sperm DNA fragmentation detection and male infertility. Theriogenology. 2006;65:979–91.
100. Antinori M, Licata E, Dani G, Cerusico F, Versaci C, et al. Intracytoplasmic morphologically selected sperm injection: a prospective randomized trial. Reprod Biomed Online. 2008;16:835–41.
101. Bartoov B, Berkovitz A, Eltes F, Kogosovsky A, Yagoda A, et al. Pregnancy rates are higher with intracytoplasmic morphologically selected sperm injection than with conventional intracytoplasmic injection. Fertil Steril. 2003;80:1413–9.
102. Berkovitz A, Eltes F, Yaari S, Katz N, Barr I, et al. The morphological normalcy of the sperm nucleus and pregnancy rate of intracytoplasmic injection with morphologically selected sperm. Hum Reprod. 2005;20:185–90.
103. Hazout A, Dumont-Hassan M, Junca AM, Cohen Bacrie P, Tesarik J. High-magnification ICSI overcomes paternal effect resistant to conventional ICSI. Reprod Biomed Online. 2006;12:19–25.
104. Fawcett DW, Ito S. Observations on the cytoplasmic membranes of testicular cells, examined by phase contrast and electron microscopy. J Biophys Biochem Cytol. 1958;4:135–42.

105. Baccetti B, Burrini AG, Collodel G, Magnano AR, Piomboni P, et al. Crater defect in human spermatozoa. Gamete Res. 1989;22:249–55.
106. Kacem O, Sifer C, Barraud-Lange V, Ducot B, De Ziegler D, et al. Sperm nuclear vacuoles, as assessed by motile sperm organellar morphological examination, are mostly of acrosomal origin. Reprod Biomed Online. 2010;20:132–7.
107. Tanaka A, Nagayoshi M, Awata S, Tanaka I, Kusunoki H, et al. Are crater defects in human sperm heads physiological changes during spermiogenesis? Fertil Steril. 2009;92:S165.
108. Watanabe S, Tanaka A, Fujii S, Misunuma H. No relationship between chromosome aberrations and vacuole-like structures on human sperm head. Hum Reprod. 2009;24:i94–6.
109. Parmegiani L, Cognigni GE, Bernardi S, Troilo E, Ciampaglia W, et al. "Physiologic ICSI": hyaluronic acid (HA) favors selection of spermatozoa without DNA fragmentation and with normal nucleus, resulting in improvement of embryo quality. Fertil Steril. 2010;93:598–604.
110. Hu JCY, Seo BK, Neri QV, Rosenwaks Z, Palermo GD. The role of HA selection on spermatozoon competence. Hum Reprod. 2012;27:i121.
111. Schlegel PN. Nonobstructive azoospermia: a revolutionary surgical approach and results. Semin Reprod Med. 2009;27:165–70.
112. Fields T, Neri QV, Rosenwaks Z, Palermo GD. Extreme ICSI. Hum Reprod. 2013;28:i258.
113. Palermo GD, Neri QV, Schlegel PN, Rosenwaks Z. Extreme ICSI. Fertil Steril. 2013 submitted.
114. Ludwig M, Katalinic A. Malformation rate in fetuses and children conceived after ICSI: results of a prospective cohort study. Reprod Biomed Online. 2002;5:171–8.
115. Palermo GD, Colombero LT, Schattman GL, Davis OK, Rosenwaks Z. Evolution of pregnancies and initial follow-up of newborns delivered after intracytoplasmic sperm injection. JAMA. 1996;276:1893–7.
116. Basatemur E, Sutcliffe A. Follow-up of children born after ART. Placenta. 2008;29(Suppl B):135–40.
117. Steel AJ, Sutcliffe A. Long-term health implications for children conceived by IVF/ICSI. Hum Fertil (Camb). 2009;12:21–7.
118. Cummins JM, Jequier AM. Treating male infertility needs more clinical andrology, not less. Hum Reprod. 1994;9:1214–9.
119. de Kretser DM. The potential of intracytoplasmic sperm injection (ICSI) to transmit genetic defects causing male infertility. Reprod Fertil Dev. 1995;7:137–41. discussion 141–2.
120. De Rycke M, Liebaers I, Van Steirteghem A. Epigenetic risks related to assisted reproductive technologies: risk analysis and epigenetic inheritance. Hum Reprod. 2002;17:2487–94.
121. Edwards RG, Ludwig M. Are major defects in children conceived in vitro due to innate problems in patients or to induced genetic damage? Reprod Biomed Online. 2003;7:131–8.
122. Basatemur E, Shevlin M, Sutcliffe A. Growth of children conceived by IVF and ICSI up to 12years of age. Reprod Biomed Online. 2010;20:144–9.
123. Belva F, Bonduelle M, Schiettecatte J, Tournaye H, Painter RC, et al. Salivary testosterone concentrations in pubertal ICSI boys compared with spontaneously conceived boys. Hum Reprod. 2011;26:438–41.
124. Belva F, Henriet S, Liebaers I, Van Steirteghem A, Celestin-Westreich S, et al. Medical outcome of 8-year-old singleton ICSI children (born >or=32 weeks' gestation) and a spontaneously conceived comparison group. Hum Reprod. 2007;22:506–15.
125. Belva F, Roelants M, Painter R, Bonduelle M, Devroey P, et al. Pubertal development in ICSI children. Hum Reprod. 2012;27:1156–61.
126. Carson C, Sacker A, Kelly Y, Redshaw M, Kurinczuk JJ, et al. Asthma in children born after infertility treatment: findings from the UK Millennium Cohort Study. Hum Reprod. 2013;28:471–9.
127. Goldbeck L, Gagsteiger F, Mindermann I, Strobele S, Izat Y. Cognitive development of singletons conceived by intracytoplasmic sperm injection or in vitro fertilization at age 5 and 10 years. J Pediatr Psychol. 2009;34:774–81.
128. Knoester M, Helmerhorst FM, Vandenbroucke JP, van der Westerlaken LA, Walther FJ, et al. Perinatal outcome, health, growth, and medical care utilization of 5- to 8-year-old intracytoplasmic sperm injection singletons. Fertil Steril. 2008;89:1133–46.
129. Leunens L, Celestin-Westreich S, Bonduelle M, Liebaers I, Ponjaert-Kristoffersen I. Follow-up of cognitive and motor development of 10-year-old singleton children born after ICSI compared with spontaneously conceived children. Hum Reprod. 2008;23:105–11.

Novel Sperm Tests and Their Importance

Ralf Henkel

Introduction

Within living memory, human fertility has always been associated with special fertility symbols such as the prehistoric Venus of Willendorf symbolizing female fertility, which dates back to between 24,000 and 22,000 years BC, or phalli as a male fertility symbol. Such symbols and rituals were thought to have magic effects and thus used by all cultures around the world to assure fecundity in groups or individuals. In this context, infertility is being perceived as a stigma and leads, although mostly not painful, to psychological disorders [1]. Even though women carry the reproductive burden in most societies, men also experience psychological trauma, which leads to damaged self-esteem, inadequacy in the relation, and ridicule [2–4].

Worldwide, an estimated 80 million people are affected by infertility, thus resulting in a prevalence of infertility of 9 % [5]. Initially, the male contribution to infertility was largely ignored because the focus was rather on female infertility. In addition, the male ego and self-image, which, particularly in African and Asian societies, attribute women a low status and regard reproduction related issues as a female duty, whereas the male contribution to human reproduction is either totally underestimated or barely acknowledged. Yet about 50 % of the causes for couple infertility is attributed or partly attributed to male infertility [6]. However, since the advent of assisted reproduction and the improvement of its techniques, scientists increasingly realized that a basic semen analysis, which is still regarded a cornerstone of andrological diagnosis, is sufficient to predict neither the fertilizing potential of a single ejaculate nor the fertility of an individual man. However, although parameters like sperm count or motility or normal sperm morphology are related to fertilization success, results of a standard semen analysis have to be used with caution as they do not necessarily predict the outcome of the assisted reproduction treatment [7, 8].

The reasons for this are manifold and include the fact that the fertilization process in itself is multifactorial and can therefore be limited by numerous sperm parameters [9, 10]. In addition, the quality of ejaculates and the functional parameters of the male germ cell vary on a daily basis and do not necessarily reflect the situation on the day of insemination in an assisted reproduction program [10]. Furthermore, although the number of treatment procedures in assisted reproduction has increased over the past 30 years, pregnancy rates for both in vitro fertilization (IVF) and intracytoplasmic sperm injection (ICSI) remain within a range of 29–33 %, relatively low, [11] and has not significantly increased during that time [12].

R. Henkel, PhD, BEd (✉)
Department of Medical Biosciences, University of the Western Cape, Private Bag X17, Robert Sobukwe Road, Bellville, 7535, Western Cape Province, South Africa
e-mail: rhenkel@uwc.ac.za

Since standard semen analysis is incomplete and does neither provide information about the functional capacity of the male germ cell, nor shows low variability of the individual parameters such as sperm count or motility, scientists were urged to find other solutions to the problem of accurately predicting male fertility. Yet even parameters with a low biological variability like normal sperm morphology [10] or sperm DNA fragmentation [13] do not detect sperm abnormalities in about 20 % of infertile men, high prevalence of idiopathic infertility is observed [14]. Therefore, some laboratories incorporated advanced sperm tests to determine the functionality of the acrosome, chromatin condensation, or DNA fragmentation into andrological diagnostics. Particularly, the latter one together with high resolution morphological analysis (motile sperm organelle morphology examination; MSOME) has been identified as a valuable parameter [15–17]. In addition, except for MSOME all other methods used to diagnose the male fertility capacity are consumptive, i.e., spermatozoa are used and by the very nature of the procedures involved are devitalized and therefore not suitable for fertilization anymore. Nevertheless, the progress made in improving, standardizing, and validating the methodologies for various male fertility parameters including sperm DNA damage [18, 19], the prediction of male fertility remains controversial [20, 21], and the emphasis for new techniques to predict the male fertility potential is not only on the identification of parameters with low biological variation and the standardization, reliability, repeatability, and validation of the relevant techniques, but also on cost-effectiveness, time consumption as well as the application of non-consumptive tests where the sperm cells can then still be used for insemination purposes.

Techniques that have been shown to have significant importance in the diagnosis of sperm fertilizing potential include sperm DNA fragmentation, mitochondrial membrane potential, sperm binding to hyaluronic acid, MSOME, the determination of reactive oxygen species (ROS), and the total antioxidant capacity (TAC) in the seminal plasma. Furthermore, newly developed techniques that might become important to test male fertility potential are sperm birefringence, proteomics, and DNA microarrays.

Current Techniques

DNA Fragmentation

Sperm nuclear DNA damage has repeatedly been shown to be associated with male infertility and recurrent pregnancy failure [22, 23] and poor seminal parameters such as motility, abnormal sperm morphology or sperm-head morphology [24–26]. On the other hand, sperm nuclear DNA damage is not only limited to infertile or subfertile patients, but incidences of up to 43 % of the ejaculates showing spermatozoa with DNA damage where the seminal parameters were normal [27]. Nevertheless, concerns were raised about the impact and validity of this parameter on fertilization and pregnancy as conflicting studies from different groups have been reported for IVF and ICSI. While researchers like Sun et al. [28], Benchaib et al. [29], or Huang et al. [30] found a relationship between sperm DNA fragmentation and fertilization rates after IVF, others [31–33] could not find an association with fertilization but with embryo formation and pregnancy rates. This finding was confirmed in a meta-analysis by Li et al. [34] is most probably due to the fact that the male genome with its subsequent gene expression is only switched on as from the four- to eight-cell stage [31, 35] and highlights early and late paternal effects on the embryo.

For ICSI, some studies [32, 36, 37] indicate a predictive value of sperm nuclear DNA fragmentation for pregnancy rates. However, in a subsequent meta-analysis based on 14 studies [38], this could not be confirmed. Instead, sperm DNA fragmentation was rather associated with increased pregnancy loss. This discrepancy might be related to the fact that for ICSI a careful selection of morphologically normal spermatozoa is performed, which might reduce the probability of injecting DNA-damaged sperm into the oocyte [39], seeing normal sperm morphology, particularly in p-pattern sperm morphology patients and as evaluated under high magnification using MSOME, is negatively related to DNA damage [[26, 40–42], Henkel and Menkveld, unpublished]. It further underlines the possibility that male germ cells with abnormal genetic material are able to fertilize oocytes, thereby posing the risk that such damaged genomes can be manifested in the germ line and contribute to aneuploidy, malformations, miscarriages, and development of early childhood cancer [43–49], particularly after ICSI. Whereas cytoplasmic sperm defects can be repaired by the oocyte immediately after gamete fusion, this appears not to be possible for sperm nuclear damages as they will only be detected once the paternal genome is switched on [50].

Despite the criticism of sperm DNA damage as a prognostic parameter to predict fertilization outcome in assisted reproduction in terms of standardization, reliability, repeatability, and validation of the methods that can be used as "gold-standard" for clinical practice [20, 21], the currently most commonly used techniques, TUNEL (terminal deoxynucleotidyl transferase-mediated dUTP nick-end labeling) assay, sperm chromatin structure assay (SCSA), COMET assay, and the sperm chromatin dispersion (SCD) test, have been shown to be sensitive and produced clinical thresholds for diagnosis and prediction of success [31, 51–55]. With regard to the mentioned methods, however, one must also keep in mind that they determine different aspects of sperm DNA fragmentation [56], namely "real" DNA damage for the TUNEL assay and "potential" DNA damage in terms of susceptibility to DNA denaturation for the SCSA. Thus, one should clearly distinguish between the different assays, not only practically and methodologically but also linguistically. Therefore, further refinement is necessary. The first steps in this regard have been done for the TUNEL and COMET assay [55, 57].

On the other hand, 8-hydroxy-2-deoxyguanosine (8-OHdG) as one of the major ROS-induced DNA damage products [58], which is mutagenic and cancerogenic [59, 60], has also been shown to be closely linked with oxidative stress (OS) [61], poor sperm quality [62, 63] and function [64]. Several methodologies to detect 8-OHdG including high-performance liquid chromatography (HPLC) and immunofluorescence using microscopic or flow-cytometric analysis are available. While the measurement with HPLC is a rather large-scaled procedure, the determination of the percentage of 8-OHdG-positive cells employing fluorescence methods is easier and has been shown to be effective in predicting clinical pregnancy after intrauterine insemination, but not after ICSI [65]. The reason for this discrepancy might lie in the selection process of spermatozoa for ICSI as indicated above. Nevertheless, the possibility for flow-cytometric analysis is also available and has been shown to be rapid, reproducible, and highly accurate [66]. Yet the latter still needs to be evaluated in an assisted reproduction program for IVF and ICSI.

Mitochondrial Membrane Potential

Spermatozoa and essentially their functions depend on the functionality of the mitochondria, which can be measured by determining the inner mitochondrial membrane potential ($\Delta\psi_m$). The $\Delta\psi_m$ has been described as a sensitive indicator of mitochondrial function in terms of the functionality of the mitochondrial electron transfer chain [67]. Therefore, $\Delta\psi_m$ has been widely used in cell biology to investigate metabolism, viability and cell functionality including apoptosis. Several cationic lipophilic dyes have been used to determine the $\Delta\psi_m$. One of those dyes that were originally used is rhodamine 123 (Rh123). However, mitochondria have been found to have several energy-dependent Rh123-binding sites [68], which render this probe not very useful for the determination of $\Delta\psi_m$. In contrast, 5,5′,6,6′-tetrachloro-1,1′,3,3′-tetraethylbenzimiddazolyl-carbocyanine iodide (JC-1) was found to evaluate changes in $\Delta\psi_m$ accurately [69] and specifically [70].

In spermatozoa, $\Delta\psi_m$ has repeatedly been associated with poor sperm motility, elevated levels of sperm ROS production, and parameters of apoptosis such as annexin V-binding, DNA fragmentation or caspase activity [71–75]. In two separate studies including 28 and 91 patients, respectively, Marchetti and coworkers [70] revealed a positive and significant relationship between sperm $\Delta\psi_m$ and the fertilization rate in vitro after IVF. Although the correlation coefficients in both studies were relatively low ($r=0.36$ and $r=0.24$, respectively), the test was suggested to as one of the most sensitive parameters of functional quality of spermatozoa and therefore useful in diagnosis of male factor infertility and the prediction of fertilization in IVF [74, 76–78]. On the other hand, a recent study by Zorn et al. [79] comparing various clinical and sperm parameters including sperm DNA damage and $\Delta\psi_m$ revealed that the DNA damage predicted the occurrence of natural pregnancy better than all other parameters investigated. Thus, more work has to be carried out in order to evaluate and most importantly standardize and validate this certainly important functional parameter of spermatozoa.

Hyaluronic Acid (Hyaluronan) Binding

Hyaluronan is the main glycosaminoglycan secreted by the cumulus mass [80] which spermatozoa have to penetrate before reaching the oocyte. During this process, interaction between the male germ cell and the female organism takes place and spermatozoa are thought to bind to hyaluronan via a receptor on their membranes [81]. Considering that this appears as an essential step in the fertilization process, sperm able to bind to hyaluronan are regarded as mature [82] and have been shown to have normal general and nuclear morphology and functions. Moreover, they exhibit lower rates of aneuploidies and DNA damage [83–85]. Interestingly, the physiologic response of human spermatozoa in terms of tyrosine phosphorylation patterns does not differ after sperm binding to zona pellucida or hyaluronan. In turn, immature sperm fail to execute this important physiologic process [86].

ICSI performed with hyaluronan-selected sperm resulted in high quality embryos and improved life birth rates [87, 88] and Worrilow et al. [89] showed in a multicenter, double-blinded, randomized controlled study that ICSI with spermatozoa from men who were prescreened with less than 65 % hyaluronan-bound spermatozoa had a significantly higher chance of an ongoing pregnancy after ICSI if spermatozoa were selected by means of hyaluronan-binding. Nevertheless, the test is not without any criticism by well-known scientists. Van den Bergh et al. [90] found no significant differences in fertilization rates and zygote scores by hyaluronan-bound and non-hyaluronan-bound spermatozoa in their controversially received study [91]. On the other hand, other recent studies revealed that hyaluronan-binding was not able to predict the results of the sperm penetration assay [92], pregnancy rates in intrauterine insemination cycles [93], and IVF [94].

The failure of the hyaluronan binding test to predict fertility indicates only a limited role of isolated hyaluronan in sperm selection [95] because both components of the cumulus, the extracellular matrix with its hyaluronan content, and the cumulus cells with their conversion of glycodelin-A and -F into glycodelin-C contribute to the male germ cells' ability to penetrate the cumulus and modulate sperm functions [96, 97]. The reason for this failure of hyaluronan-separated spermatozoa to achieve higher implantation rates might reside in the nature of the method because other factors such as glycodelin-C are missing.

Motile Sperm Organelle Morphological Examination (MSOME)

Normal sperm morphology has been regarded as a good predictor of male fertility potential, particularly if a strict evaluation approach is followed [98–100]. Nevertheless, this classic methodology of assessing normal sperm morphology is a relatively large-scaled procedure and consumptive, i.e., the spermatozoa that are assessed are no longer available for fertilization. In addition, the evaluation must be carried out in a semen sample different from that used for insemination. These obvious disadvantages can be overcome by a method developed by Bartoov et al. [101], which evaluates sperm morphology at higher, digital magnification (6,300×) using Nomarski interference contrast. Using this technique, a finer morphological status of acrosome, post-acrosomal lamina, neck, mitochondria, flagellum, and the nucleus can be examined. For the latter, the shape, as well as the presence and size of vacuoles, is observed. Since MSOME identifies objects undetectable by light microscopy, such as nuclear vacuoles, which are indicative of abnormal chromatin packaging [102], this method is regarded more stringent than the evaluation of sperm morphology according to strict criteria [103].

High resolution of specific morphologic features like nuclear vacuolization and sperm head morphometry as evaluated by MSOME has been shown to correlate very well with various other sperm parameters including sperm concentration and motility [26], capacitation and acrosomal status [104], and DNA integrity [42, 105, 106]. Since MSOME is thought to identify good quality spermatozoa, the technique has been included in ICSI protocols in an increasing number of groups (intracytoplasmic morphologically selected sperm injection; IMSI). In turn, using IMSI, not only fertilization rates but also implantation and pregnancy rates could be improved [107, 108]. These results were confirmed in a recent meta-analysis [109]. On the other hand, Balaban et al. [110] restrict the beneficial effects of IMSI to selected male factor patients and only with lower rates of aneuploidy and miscarriage [109, 111].

In contrast to these positive results, other studies indicate that the association of the occurrence of large nuclear vacuoles with sperm DNA damage is only valid if the nuclear vacuoles are taking up more than 50 % of the nuclear volume [112]. This assumption is supported by Watanabe et al. [113] showing that only 7 (=3.1 %) of spermatozoa with large vacuoles out 227 were TUNEL-positive suggesting that ICSI using spermatozoa selected for injection by MSOME from patients with high quality semen is not necessary. This assumption can be supported by the study of Tanaka et al. [114] who showed that sperm head vacuoles do not affect the outcome of ICSI. Although this methodology is appealing because it is non-consumptive, the procedure, for diagnostic (MSOME) and treatment (IMSI), is time consuming and little practical for routine semen testing. In addition, MSOME has not been properly validated yet.

Reactive Oxygen Species (ROS)/Total Antioxidant Capacity (TAC)

Reactive oxygen species (ROS) are highly reactive radical derivatives of oxygen that are produced by any living cell, including spermatozoa, in the mitochondria. These molecules are chemical intermediates that have one or more unpaired electrons, which causes them to be highly labile and results in extreme reactivity. Examples of biologically relevant ROS are hydroxyl radicals ($\cdot$OH), superoxide anion ($\cdot O_2^-$), or hydrogen peroxide (H_2O_2). ROS have a high oxidative potential and therefore very short half life-times in the nanosecond (10^{-9} s) ($\cdot$OH; hydroxyl radicals) to millisecond range (10^{-3} s) ($\cdot O_2^-$; superoxide anion) [115]. Consequently, these molecules essentially react at the site of generation.

Considering that male germ cells exhibit a specially composed plasma membrane with an extraordinary high amount of polyunsaturated fatty acids, which is essential for normal sperm functions, spermatozoa are very sensitive to oxidative damage by ROS [for review see: [116]]. Despite the detrimental effect that ROS have on spermatozoa causing lipid peroxidation or DNA fragmentation by means of oxidative stress (OS), ROS also exert important physiologic roles by triggering cellular events such as sperm capacitation, hyperactivation, and the penetration of the zona pellucida [117–119], and thereby modulating acrosome reaction as key event in the fertilization process [120, 121].

Considering the two important features of ROS, namely, causing OS if present in excessive amounts [116, 122–125], thus having detrimental effects, and on the other hand, having beneficial effects by triggering essential cellular functions, the male and female organisms must counteract excessive OS for spermatozoa. For this purpose, seminal plasma contains more antioxidant compounds than any other physiological fluid, including vitamins C and E

[126, 127], superoxide dismutase [128], glutathione [129], glutathione peroxidase [130], or uric acid [131]. Except for the semen-specific polyamines spermine and spermidine [132], the female organism also provides these radical scavengers [133, 134], and a lack thereof will result in disturbed reproductive functions [135, 136]. Thus, finding the correct balance between oxidation and reduction is crucial for normal sperm function and fertilization [137, 138] as reductive stress is as dangerous as OS [116, 139].

This has serious consequences for andrological diagnostics as both parameters, sperm ROS levels [137, 140] as well as the so-called total antioxidant capacity (TAC) [141, 142], have to be tested in order to obtain a picture of the seminal redox status reflecting the seminal OS. This concept also explains the inconsistency reported in the literature about the impact and importance of ROS as well as that of leukocytes. Therefore, it is not sufficient to measure only one of these parameters, the ROS levels or seminal TAC, because both parameters may vary between different patients. For example, a patient might have high numbers of leukocytes present in the ejaculate, but if the patient also shows high levels of TAC, the seminal redox status and therefore the fertility might not be compromised. On the other hand, a patient might have low numbers of activated seminal leukocytes, but a very low TAC which do not scavenge ROS production sufficiently. In the latter case, the patient might be infertile as the system between oxidation and reduction is not in balance. Thus, for spermatozoa this system is like a "balancing act", they will only have functional competence if the system of seminal oxidants and antioxidants as a whole does not deviate to either side [116, 137, 138].

For ROS, the most commonly used test system is based on chemiluminescence with luminol [140] or lucigenin [143] as probes. The difference between these two chemiluminescent probes is that chemiluminescence of luminol appears to be dependent on the myeloperoxidase-H_2O_2-Cl^- system [144], hydroxyl radicals in vivo [145], or neutrophils in vitro [146], while lucigenin is rather specific for extracellularly released superoxide [147–149]. Furthermore, lucigenin rather measures extracellular ROS production, which is clinically more important as they are capable of damaging surrounding spermatozoa and might therefore be more suitable as a diagnostic tool [147]. Nevertheless, numerous groups are using luminol as chemiluminescent probe as it is cheaper and easy to use. Thus, the determination of ROS in seminal fluid is recommended by a number of groups to improve the management of male infertility [150–152], particularly if measured in neat semen [153]. Higher seminal ROS levels were not only significantly negatively correlated with sperm motility and concentration [154], but also with fertilization and pregnancy rates as well as embryo quality after IVF and ICSI [155].

On the other hand, Yeung et al. [156] concluded that the determination of ROS in a sperm suspension after swim-up has no diagnostic impact. In contrast, it might even play a positive role for fertilization, which then refers to the beneficial aspects of ROS. This is in line with data of Henkel and coworkers (unpublished) who showed that ROS in the medium after sperm separation is weakly, but significantly correlated with fertilization after IVF ($r=0.148$; $P=0.0454$; $n=183$). Furthermore, a positive trend was observed between sperm ROS production after sperm separation and the 4-cell stage formation ($r=0.135$, $P=0.0695$; $n=183$), possibly retrospectively reflecting the sperm cells' ability to undergo capacitation and acrosome reaction. The latter events are triggered by ROS physiologically produced by spermatozoa [121].

For the analysis of the antioxidative protection system for spermatozoa provided by seminal plasma several techniques are available including the oxygen radical absorbance capacity (ORAC) [157], ferric reducing ability (FRAP) [158], phycoerythrin fluorescence-based assay (PEFA) [159], and Trolox-equivalent antioxidant capacity (TEAC) [160]. While the latter test is most frequently used [141, 161, 162], the ORAC is high specificity and responds to numerous antioxidants [157]. On the other hand, the chemiluminescent detection of the antioxidant capacity and subsequent comparison to the water-soluble tocopherol equivalent Trolox is also time-consuming and requires fresh preparation of chemicals each time the assay is run. Milner and coworkers [163] developed an inexpensive colorimetric alternative using 2,2′-azinobis-(3-ethyl-benzothiazoline-6-sulfonic acid) (ABTS) and was commercialized. Said et al. [164] compared both assays, the chemiluminescent and colorimetric, and concluded that the colorimetric measurement is reliable and accurate and might therefore be an easy-to-perform, rapid, and cheap alternative. Yet none of these techniques has been evaluated with regard to its predictivity of male fertility.

TAC as measured by means of the FRAP method has been shown to correlate significantly with seminal parameters such as sperm concentration ($r=0.533$), motility ($r=0.530$), and normal sperm morphology ($r=0.533$) [165]. In addition, this group confirmed earlier data by Mahfouz et al. [142] using the colorimetric TEAC that TAC levels in abnormal ejaculates or from infertile patients were significantly lower. These authors also calculated a cut-off of 1,420 μM Trolox equivalent with a sensitivity of the assay of 76 % and as specificity of 64 %. Considering that there are significant correlations between TAC and serum prolactin and tetraiodothyronine levels, but not with gonadotropins, testosterone, or estradiol, Manchini et al. [166] suggest that systemic hormones might play a role in the regulation of seminal TAC.

Birefringence

A technique that can evaluate life sperm cells is polarization microscopy. In this approach, which was pioneered by Baccetti [167] to identify functional spermatozoa for ICSI, the birefringence (double refraction) of light caused by the anisotropic properties of the compact textures of the sperm nucleus, acrosome, and flagella permits the evaluation of the organelle structure of the male germ cell. Gianaroli et al. [168, 169] used the technique to distinguish acrosome-reacted from non-reacted spermatozoa. In a more recent report from the same group, Magli et al. [170] showed a strong relationship between partial birefringence and acrosome reaction. Yet the patterns of birefringence, total or partial, depends to some extend on motility and normal sperm morphology.

Collodel et al. [171] tried to evaluate the diagnostic value of the technique and used sperm birefringence to estimate viability and normal morphology. The morphology was compared with the standard technique after Papanicolaou (PAP) staining. Although there was no significant difference ($P=0.308$) between PAP and the evaluation with polarization microscopy, receiver operating characteristics (ROC) curves always showed a greater area under the curve for polarization microscopy than for PAP staining, indicating a better a higher diagnostic value. The authors suggest a cutoff value of 20 % of spermatozoa showing birefringence as indicator for fertility.

Later, Collodel and coworkers [172] confirmed positive relationships between sperm cell birefringence and motility as well as the fertility index calculated by a mathematical formula after transmission electron microscopy [173]. The authors concluded that polarization microscopy offers several advantages and that it should be considered in sperm analysis [172].

Contrary, Petersen et al. [174] challenged the positive reports with regard to sperm DNA fragmentation. These authors showed a significantly higher percentage of sperm with DNA damage in sperm presenting with total head birefringence than in those with partial head birefringence. This was in support of findings by Vagnini et al. [175] that the patterns of birefringence (total or partial) could not discriminate between sperm with normal and abnormal chromatin packaging. Gianaroli et al. [169] report significantly higher implantation, clinical pregnancy and ongoing pregnancy rates in ICSI cycles where spermatozoa selected by means of polarization microscopy were injected. The authors conclude that injection of acrosome-reacted spermatozoa seems to result in more viable embryos. Nevertheless, as reported for other tests systems, a proper clinical evaluation of the technique in terms of the establishment of reliable cutoff values has not been carried out yet.

"Omics" as Molecular Techniques

In the light of the limited predictive value of the currently used parameters, scientists started to look at biomarkers as a novel approach to identify infertile men, in recent years. Biomarkers are "distinctive biological or biologically derived indicators (as a biochemical metabolite in the body) of a process, event, or condition (as aging, disease, or exposure to a toxic substance)" that can be utilized as an objective and quantitative measure to identify infertile patients [176]. In addition, for clinical application, these biomarkers should be able to indentify infertile me easily, accurately, and cost-effectively [177]. Principally, this identification can make use of genomic, proteomic, or metabolomic techniques.

Proteomics

Considering that RNA is translated into proteins and sperm proteins not only come from the testis but are also derived from the epididymis or other accessory sex glands, and are modified and incorporated into sperm surface [178, 179], the actual protein expression in spermatozoa differs from their gene expression [177, 180, 181], this approach is of particular importance. However, scientists are facing grave problems as two compartments of the semen can be analyzed, namely, the seminal fluid and the male germ cell itself. With regard to the seminal plasma, the protein composition has multiple origin as the seminal fluid is composed of secretions from testis (about 5 %), seminal vesicles (about 60 %), prostate (about 30 %), and the bulbo-urethral glands (about 5 %) [182]. Therefore, seminal plasma markers might rather reflect pathologies of the respective glands, which, of course, can also contribute or be a cause of male infertility. In addition, the composition of seminal fluid also depends on other factors such as the general health of a particular man; for example diabetes, flu, alcohol consumption, or smoking can cause variability of the seminal fluid [8, 183]. All this makes the analysis and identification of specific male "infertility markers" in seminal plasma rather difficult [184]. Nevertheless, a number of recent studies report on the proteomic analysis of seminal plasma and found relevant differences between fertile and infertile men.

Proteomic Analysis of Seminal Plasma

Seminal plasma is abundantly available in both donors and patients and its protein concentration is with about 58 mg/mL approximately as high as in serum. The concentration of albumin, however, is markedly lower [185] and one of the major components are seminogelin I (MM 49.9 kDa) and II (MM 63.5 kDa), which are involved in the gel formation [186]. Seminal plasma is a rich source of thousands of proteins mainly belonging to three major groups; proteins carrying fibronectin type II modules, spermadhesins, cysteine-rich secretory proteins (CRISPs) [187], and approximately 25 % of the proteins are secretory [188, 189].

In an in-depth analysis of human seminal plasma, Rolland and coworkers [190] initially identified 699 proteins. However, in a subsequent comparison with previous descriptions, 2,545 unique proteins were identified, of which 83 were of testicular origin, 42 derived from the epididymis, 7 from the seminal vesicles, and 17 from the prostate. For the testis-specific proteins, three (TKTLI, LDHC, and PGK2) germ cell expression was confirmed and a difference in their expression between fertile and infertile men was established, thus highlighting these proteins as possible diagnostic biomarkers. Similarly, Milardi et al. [181] identified 83 seminal plasma proteins, including seminogelin I and II, olfactory receptor 5R1, lactoferrin, hCAP18, spindlin, and clusterin as possible target proteins to identify infertile patients. Other proteins were specifically identified in subgroups of patients showing a high percentage of DNA damage [15], an important aspect of sperm function. These proteins were associated with increased immune response, sperm motility, or inhibition of mitochondrial apoptosis.

Although the proteomic analysis of seminal plasma is a good approach for andrological diagnostics as it is non-consumptive of spermatozoa, the methodology is still in its infancy and specific marker proteins still have to be validated for their use. Eventually, normal values have to be established.

Proteomic Analysis of Spermatozoa

On the other hand, the analysis of the sperm cells themselves might give a better idea of the actual fertilizing potential of spermatozoa from a specific man. Considering that the male germ cell is highly specialized and differentiated, and has also to interact not only with the female reproductive tract [for review see [191]], but also with the cumulus oophorus, the zona pellucida, and the oolemma, this approach would make spermatozoa a primary target for a proteomic analysis. In this context, sperm surface proteins are of particular interest as the interaction between spermatozoa and the female genital tract as well as the oocyte must take place at this level for the female to select the most capable spermatozoon to fertilize the oocyte. This natural selection process is most stringent as it selects only one spermatozoon out of about 10^7 spermatozoa that are ejaculated into the upper part of the vagina.

In contrast to the analysis of seminal plasma, proteomic analysis of spermatozoa is more difficult and might therefore be limited for various reasons. In spermatozoa, not only the protein concentration is much less than for seminal plasma, but the number of spermatozoa available for the analysis varies individually and might even reach the detection limit if the seminal sperm count is very low, particularly in patient samples. Moreover, the risk of contamination of the samples by leukocytes or other non-sperm cells is high, and therefore the probability of a detection of non-sperm proteins, if the spermatozoa are not properly separated from the seminal plasma and debris prior to the analysis [192].

For human spermatozoa, the number of identified proteins varies considerably from 1,760 [193] to 4,675 of which 227 were shown to be testis-specific [194]. In a very recent literature review analyzing 30 studies, Amaral et al. [195] even report a total number of identified sperm proteins of 6,198 of which about 30 % are of testicular origin. This high number of proteins indicates the complex composition and function of the male germ cell and the proteins showed to be associated with various essential cellular functions such as sperm motility, capacitation, sperm–oocyte binding, metabolism, apoptosis, cell cycle, or membrane trafficking [195, 196]. It also makes the task of identifying highly specific diagnostic markers difficult. Nevertheless, using MALDI-TOF/TOF analysis of protein spots after 2D-gel electrophoresis, Xu et al. [197] identified 24 differentially expressed proteins in infertile patients, of which 9 (including TGF-β1, MYC, MYCN, TP53) are involved in main physiological pathways. With respect to seminal oxidative stress, Hamada et al. [198] revealed a significantly different expression of proteins related to the protection against oxidants, with 6 proteins decreased and 25 proteins increased in patients exhibiting seminal oxidative stress. Yet the methodology for a diagnostic approach has still to be standardized as the use of different detergents for the solubilization of membrane proteins results in different proteins that can be detected after electrophoresis (Fortuin and Henkel, unpublished). Moreover, none of the currently employed proteomics methodologies is properly evaluated for clinical use.

Genomics

DNA Microarrays

The progress in genomic biotechnology revealed genetic testing to be a viable alternative in andrological diagnostics, particularly as the prevalence of genetic abnormalities causing male infertility was found to between 15 and 30 % [199]. Due to the rapid improvement of technologies, which make it possible that very small genomic regions can now be analyzed and have already been found to be responsible for infertility [200–202], it is likely that this number would increase in near future since even single nucleotide modifications can be detected [201].

Currently, two main genetic tests are carried out, karyotyping and fluorescence in situ hybridization (FISH). While these techniques are limited in their ability to diagnose and specifically identify larger numbers of infertile men, and need a specific sequence of interest before determining this region in specific patients, respectively, microarrays not only allow the examination of a higher number of men but also the detection of copy number variations, gene expression levels, and single nucleotide polymorphisms [177]. Using the microarray technology, Park et al. [203] and Lee et al. [204] were able to identify copy number variations and Y-chromosomal microdeletions outside the AZF regions.

Spermatozoa do not only store and transport the male genetic material in form of DNA, but RNA obtained from ejaculated spermatozoa also reflects gene expression during spermatogenesis [205, 206]. Although spermatozoa are transcriptionally silent [207], spermatozoa RNAs play a vital role not only in the development of the male germ cells but also in early embryo development [208, 209], which lead to the development of novel approaches in the diagnostics of male infertility using microarrays [210]. In fact, Ostermeier and coworkers [211] were able to distinguish between sperm populations exhibiting rapidly degrading and stable spermatozoa RNAs. Following this initial discovery, Krawetz et al. [212] revealed a complex population of small noncoding RNA (sncRNA) that is available at fertilization. MicroRNA (miRNA), which is a subclass of sncRNA, appears to play a modifying role in early post-fertilization [213–215]. In infertile patients, Montjean and coworkers [216] found a 33-fold lower gene expression of genes involved in spermatogenesis and sperm motility. These authors conclude that the spermatozoal transcription profile in idiopathic infertility differs significantly from that in fertile men. Although these technologies seem to be appealing for diagnostic purposes, they are still in infancy stages as relevant biomarkers have yet to be identified and validated.

Conclusion

Considering that standard semen analysis fails to predict male fertility in up to about 40 % of the cases, scientists searched for novel parameters and methodologies to close this obvious gap in andrological diagnostics. Requirements for such new tests are that they should not only be reproducible, effective, properly validated and cost-effective and time-effective, but also be non-consumptive and stable. Particularly, the latter represents an essential condition and might even be one of the biggest challenges for novel sperm tests, as the diagnostics are carried out way before assisted reproduction treatment, and standard semen parameters vary considerably, even on a daily basis. Techniques such as determination of sperm DNA fragmentation, mitochondrial membrane potential, and hyaluronan binding refer to essential sperm functions and have been investigated for a number of years already. Attempts have been made to establish clinically significant cutoff values. However, except for the hyaluronan binding test, the consumptive nature of these test parameters still remains unexposed. Novel nonconsumptive parameters such as the high resolution evaluation of sperm morphology by MSOME, the determination of seminal ROS and/or TAC, as well as the evaluation of the birefringence of spermatozoa seem to point to alternative ways. Yet proper determination of clinical significance in terms of the fertilizing capacity of spermatozoa and valuation thereof are also still outstanding. In recent years, new promising molecular approaches to identify biomarkers of male fertility in terms of proteomic or genomic analyses of the male germ cells and seminal plasma, respectively, have been made available. On the other hand, some researchers were able to distinguish between fertile and infertile men using DNA/RNA microarrays. However, although "omics" approaches in the male infertility diagnostics are very appealing, both proteomic and genomic methodologies are still lacking the indubitable identification of markers that meet all the criteria for a good clinical marker as well as the necessary validation. Therefore, the implementation of these novel techniques in clinical routine will still take some time.

References

1. Cousineau TM, Domar AD. Psychological impact of infertility. Best Pract Res Clin Obstet Gynaecol. 2007;21:293–308.
2. Wright J, Duchesne C, Sabourin S, Bissonnette F, Benoit J, Girard Y. Psychosocial distress and infertility: men and women respond differently. Fertil Steril. 1991;55:100–8.

3. Carmeli YS, Birenbaum-Carmeli D. The predicament of masculinity: towards understanding the male experience of infertility treatments. Sex Roles. 1994;30:663–77.
4. Dyer S, Lombard C, Van der Spuy Z. Psychological distress among men suffering from couple infertility in South Africa: a quantitative assessment. Hum Reprod. 2009;24:2821–6.
5. Boivin J, Bunting L, Collins JA, Nygren KG. International estimates of infertility prevalence and treatment-seeking: potential need and demand for infertility medical care. Hum Reprod. 2007;22:1506–12.
6. World Health Organization. Towards more objectivity in diagnosis and management of male infertility. Int J Androl. 1987;7(Suppl):1–53.
7. Bonde JP, Ernst E, Jensen TK, Hjollund NH, Kolstad H, Henriksen TB, Scheike T, Giwercman A, Olsen J, Skakkebaek NE. Relation between semen quality and fertility: a population-based study of 430 first-pregnancy planners. Lancet. 1998;352:1172–7.
8. Guzick DS, Overstreet JW, Factor-Litvak P, Brazil CK, Nakajima ST, Coutifaris C, Carson SA, Cisneros P, Steinkampf MP, Hill JA, Xu D, Vogel DL, National Cooperative Reproductive Medicine Network. Sperm morphology, motility, and concentration in fertile and infertile men. N Engl J Med. 2001;345:1388–93.
9. Amann RP, Hammerstedt RH. *In vitro* evaluation of sperm quality: an opinion. J Androl. 1993;14:397–406.
10. Henkel R, Maaß G, Bödeker R-H, Scheibelhut C, Stalf T, Mehnert C, Schuppe HC, Jung A, Schill W-B. Sperm function and assisted reproduction technology. Reprod Med Biol. 2005;4:7–30.
11. de Mouzon J, Goossens V, Bhattacharya S, Castilla JA, Ferraretti AP, Korsak V, Kupka M, Nygren KG, Nyboe Andersen A, European IVF-monitoring (EIM) Consortium, for the European Society of Human Reproduction and Embryology (ESHRE). Assisted reproductive technology in Europe, 2006: results generated from European registers by ESHRE. Hum Reprod. 2010;25:1851–62.
12. Land JA, Evers JL. Risks and complications in assisted reproduction techniques: report of an ESHRE consensus meeting. Hum Reprod. 2003;18:455–7.
13. Zini A, Kamal K, Phang D, Willis J, Jarvi K. Biologic variability of sperm DNA denaturation in infertile men. Urology. 2001;58:258–61.
14. Brugh 3rd VM, Lipshultz LI. Male factor infertility: evaluation and management. Med Clin North Am. 2004;88:367–85.
15. Intasqui P, Camargo M, Del Giudice PT, Spaine DM, Carvalho VM, Cardozo KHM, Zylbersztejn DS, Bertolla RP. Sperm nuclear DNA fragmentation rate is associated with differential protein expression and enriched functions in human seminal plasma. BJU Int. 2013;112:835–43. doi:10.1111/bju.12233.
16. Lewis SE, John Aitken R, Conner SJ, Iuliis GD, Evenson DP, Henkel R, Giwercman A, Gharagozloo P. The impact of sperm DNA damage in assisted conception and beyond: recent advances in diagnosis and treatment. Reprod Biomed Online. 2013;27:325–37. doi:10.1016/j.rbmo.2013.06.014. pii: S1472-6483(13)00363-5.
17. Setti AS, Paes de Almeida Ferreira Braga D, Iaconelli Jr A, Aoki T, Borges Jr E. Twelve years of MSOME and IMSI: a review. Reprod Biomed Online. 2013;27:338–52.
18. World Health Organization. WHO laboratory manual for the examination and processing of human semen. 5th ed. Geneva, Switzerland: WHO; 2010.
19. De Jonge C. Semen analysis: looking for an upgrade in class. Fertil Steril. 2012;97:260–6.
20. Practice Committee of American Society for Reproductive Medicine. The clinical utility of sperm DNA integrity testing. Fertil Steril. 2008;90(5 Suppl):S178–80.
21. Practice Committee of the American Society for Reproductive Medicine. The clinical utility of sperm DNA integrity testing: a guideline. Fertil Steril. 2013;99:673–7.
22. Lewis SE, Agbaje I, Alvarez J. Sperm DNA tests as useful adjuncts to semen analysis. Syst Biol Reprod Med. 2008;54:111–25.
23. Ribas-Maynou J, Garcia-Peiro A, Fernandez-Encinas A, Amengual MJ, Prada E, Cortes P, Navarro J, Benet J. Double stranded sperm DNA breaks, measured by Comet assay, are associated with unexplained recurrent miscarriage in couples without a female factor. PLoS One. 2012;7:e44679.
24. Lopes S, Sun JG, Jurisicova A, Meriano J, Casper RF. Sperm deoxyribonucleic acid fragmentation is increased in poor-quality semen samples and correlates with failed fertilization in intracytoplasmic sperm injection. Fertil Steril. 1998;69:528–32.
25. Muratori M, Piomboni P, Baldi E, Filimberti E, Pecchioli P, Moretti E, Gambera L, Baccetti B, Biagiotti R, Forti G, Maggi M. Functional and ultrastructural features of DNA-fragmented human sperm. J Androl. 2000;21:903–12.
26. Cassuto NG, Hazout A, Hammoud I, Balet R, Bouret D, Barak Y, Jellad S, Plouchart JM, Selva J, Yazbeck C. Correlation between DNA defect and sperm-head morphology. Reprod Biomed Online. 2012;24:211–8.
27. Saleh A, Agarwal A, Nelson DR, Nada EA, El-Tonsy MH, Alvarez JG, Thomas AJ, Sharma RK. Increased sperm nuclear DNA damage in normozoospermic infertile men: a prospective study. Fertil Steril. 2002;78:313–8.
28. Sun JG, Jurisicova A, Casper RF. Detection of deoxyribonucleic acid fragmentation in human sperm: correlation with fertilization *in vitro*. Biol Reprod. 1997;56:602–7.
29. Benchaib M, Braun V, Lornage J, Hadj S, Salle B, Lejeune H, Guerin JF. Sperm DNA fragmentation

decreases the pregnancy rate in an assisted reproductive technique. Hum Reprod. 2003;18:1023–8.
30. Huang CC, Lin DP, Tsao HM, Cheng TC, Liu CH, Lee MS. Sperm DNA fragmentation negatively correlates with velocity and fertilization rates but might not affect pregnancy rates. Fertil Steril. 2005;84:130–40.
31. Henkel R, Hajimohammad M, Stalf T, Hoogendijk C, Mehnert C, Menkveld R, Gips H, Schill W-B, Kruger TF. Influence of deoxyribonucleic acid damage on fertilization and pregnancy. Fertil Steril. 2004;81:965–72.
32. Borini A, Tarozzi N, Bizzaro D, Bonu MA, Fava L, Flamigni C, Coticchio G. Sperm DNA fragmentation: paternal effect on early post-implantation embryo development in ART. Hum Reprod. 2006;21: 2876–81.
33. Benchaib M, Lornage J, Mazoyer C, Lejeune H, Salle B, Guerin JF. Sperm deoxyribonucleic acid fragmentation as a prognostic indicator of assisted reproductive technology outcome. Fertil Steril. 2007; 87:93–100.
34. Li Z, Wang L, Cai J, Huang H. Correlation of sperm DNA damage with IVF and ICSI outcomes: a systematic review and meta-analysis. J Assist Reprod Genet. 2006;23:367–76.
35. Braude P, Bolton V, Moore S. Human gene expression first occurs between the four- and eight-cell stages of preimplantation development. Nature. 1988;332:459–61.
36. Henkel R, Kierspel E, Hajimohammad M, Stalf T, Hoogendijk C, Mehnert C, Menkveld R, Schill WB, Kruger TF. DNA fragmentation of spermatozoa and assisted reproduction technology. RBM Online. 2003;7(Comp 1):44–51.
37. Tarozzi N, Nadalini M, Stronati A, Bizzaro D, Dal Prato L, Coticchio G, Borini A. Anomalies in sperm chromatin packaging: implications for assisted reproduction techniques. Reprod Biomed Online. 2009;18:486–95.
38. Zini A. Are sperm chromatin and DNA defects relevant in the clinic? Syst Biol Reprod Med. 2011;57: 78–85.
39. Gandini L, Lombardo F, Paoli D, Caruso F, Eleuteri P, Leter G, Ciriminna R, Culasso F, Dondero F, Lenzi A, Spano M. Full-term pregnancies achieved with ICSI despite high levels of sperm chromatin damage. Hum Reprod. 2004;19:1409–17.
40. Henkel R, Bastiaan HS, Schuller S, Hoppe I, Starker W, Menkveld R. Leukocytes and intrinsic ROS production may be factors compromising sperm chromatin condensation status. Andrologia. 2010;42:69–75.
41. Wilding M, Coppola G, di Matteo L, Palagiano A, Fusco E, Dale B. Intracytoplasmic injection of morphologically selected spermatozoa (IMSI) improves outcome after assisted reproduction by deselecting physiologically poor quality spermatozoa. J Assist Reprod Genet. 2011;28:253–62.
42. Utsuno H, Oka K, Yamamoto A, Shiozawa T. Evaluation of sperm head shape at high magnification revealed correlation of sperm DNA fragmentation with aberrant head ellipticity and angularity. Fertil Steril. 2013;99:1573–80.
43. Ahmadi A, Ng SC. Developmental capacity of damaged spermatozoa. Hum Reprod. 1999;14:2279–85.
44. Aitken RJ, Krausz C. Oxidative stress, DNA damage and the Y chromosome. Reproduction. 2001;122: 497–506.
45. Lathi RB, Milki AA. Rate of aneuploidy in miscarriages following *in vitro* fertilization and intracytoplasmic sperm injection. Fertil Steril. 2004;81: 1270–2.
46. Barroso G, Valdespin C, Vega E, Kershenovich R, Avila R, Avendano C, Oehninger S. Developmental sperm contributions: fertilization and beyond. Fertil Steril. 2009;92:835–48.
47. Funke S, Flach E, Kiss I, Sandor J, Vida G, Bodis J, Ertl T. Male reproductive tract abnormalities: more common after assisted reproduction? Early Hum Dev. 2010;86:547–50.
48. Robinson L, Gallos ID, Conner SJ, Rajkhowa M, Miller D, Lewis S, Kirkman-Brown J, Coomarasamy A. The effect of sperm DNA fragmentation on miscarriage rates: a systematic review and meta-analysis. Hum Reprod. 2012;27:2908–17.
49. Zwink N, Jenetzky E, Schmiedeke E, Schmidt D, Märzheuser S, Grasshoff-Derr S, Holland-Cunz S, Weih S, Hosie S, Reifferscheid P, Ameis H, Kujath C, Rissmann A, Obermayr F, Schwarzer N, Bartels E, Reutter H, Brenner H, CURE-Net Consortium. Assisted reproductive techniques and the risk of anorectal malformations: a German case-control study. Orphanet J Rare Dis. 2012;7:65.
50. Tesarik J. Paternal effects on cell division in the human preimplantation embryo. Reprod Biomed Online. 2005;10:370–5.
51. Aitken RJ, De Iuliis GN. Origins and consequences of DNA damage in male germ cells. Reprod Biomed Online. 2007;14:727–33.
52. Bungum M, Humaidan P, Axmon A, Spano M, Bungum L, Erenpreiss J, Giwercman A. Sperm DNA integrity assessment in prediction of assisted reproduction technology outcome. Hum Reprod. 2007;22:174–9.
53. Velez de la Calle JF, Muller A, Walschaerts M, Clavere JL, Jimenez C, Wittemer C, Thonneau P. Sperm deoxyribonucleic acid fragmentation as assessed by the sperm chromatin dispersion test in assisted reproductive technology programs: results of a large prospective multicenter study. Fertil Steril. 2008;90:1792–9.
54. Sharma RK, Sabanegh E, Mahfouz R, Gupta S, Thiyagarajan A, Agarwal A. TUNEL as a test for sperm DNA damage in the evaluation of male infertility. Urology. 2010;76:1380–6.
55. Ribas-Maynou J, Garcia-Peiro A, Fernandez-Encinas A, Abad C, Amengual MJ, Prada E, Navarro J, Benet J. Comprehensive analysis of sperm DNA fragmentation by five different assays: TUNEL assay, SCSA, SCD test and alkaline and neutral Comet assay. Andrology. 2013;1:715–22.

56. Henkel R, Hoogendijk CF, Bouic PJ, Kruger TF. TUNEL assay and SCSA determine different aspects of sperm DNA damage. Andrologia. 2010;42:305–13.
57. Mitchell LA, De Iuliis GN, Aitken RJ. The TUNEL assay consistently underestimates DNA damage in human spermatozoa and is influenced by DNA compaction and cell vitality: development of an improved methodology. Int J Androl. 2011;34:2–13.
58. Von Sonntag C. The chemical basis of radiation biology. London, UK: Taylor and Francis; 1987.
59. Floyd RA. The role of 8-hydroxyguanine in carcinogenesis. Carcinogenesis. 1990;11:1447–50.
60. Shibutani S, Takeshita M, Grollman AP. Insertion of specific base during DNA synthesis past the oxidation-damaged base 8-oxodG. Nature. 1991;349:431–4.
61. Aitken RJ, De Iuliis GN, Finnie JM, Hedges A, McLachlan RI. Analysis of the relationships between oxidative stress, DNA damage and sperm vitality in a patient population: development of diagnostic criteria. Hum Reprod. 2010;25:2415–26.
62. Ni ZY, Liu YQ, Shen HM, Chia SE, Ong CN. Does the increase of 8-hydroxydeoxyguanosine lead to poor sperm quality? Mutat Res. 1997;381:77–82.
63. Kao SH, Chao HT, Chen HW, Hwang TI, Liao TL, Wei YH. Increase of oxidative stress in human sperm with lower motility. Fertil Steril. 2008;89:1183–90.
64. Shen H, Ong C. Detection of oxidative DNA damage in human sperm and its association with sperm function and male infertility. Free Radic Biol Med. 2000;28:529–36.
65. Thomson LK, Zieschang JA, Clark AM. Oxidative deoxyribonucleic acid damage in sperm has a negative impact on clinical pregnancy rate in intrauterine insemination but not intracytoplasmic sperm injection cycles. Fertil Steril. 2011;96:843–7.
66. Cambi M, Tamburrino L, Marchiani S, Olivito B, Azzari C, Forti G, Baldi E, Muratori M. Development of a specific method to evaluate 8-hydroxy, 2-deoxyguanosine in sperm nuclei: relationship with semen quality in a cohort of 94 subjects. Reproduction. 2013;45:227–35.
67. Ly JD, Grubb DR, Lawen A. The mitochondrial membrane potential (deltapsi(m)) in apoptosis: an Update. Apoptosis. 2003;8:115–20.
68. Lopez-Mediavilla C, Orfao A, Gonzalez M, Medina JM. Identification by flow cytometry of two distinct rhodamine-123-stained mitochondrial populations in rat liver. FEBS Lett. 1989;254:115–20.
69. Salvioli S, Ardizzoni A, Franceschi C, Cossarizza A. JC-1, but not DiOC6(3) or rhodamine 123, is a reliable fluorescent probe to assess delta psi changes in intact cells: implications for studies on mitochondrial functionality during apoptosis. FEBS Lett. 1997;411:77–82.
70. Marchetti C, Jouy N, Leroy-Martin B, Defossez A, Formstecher P, Marchetti P. Comparison of four fluorochromes for the detection of the inner mitochondrial membrane potential in human spermatozoa and their correlation with sperm motility. Hum Reprod. 2004;19:2267–76.
71. Troiano L, Granata AR, Cossarizza A, Kalashnikova G, Bianchi R, Pini G, Tropea F, Carani C, Franceschi C. Mitochondrial membrane potential and DNA stainability in human sperm cells: a flow cytometry analysis with implications for male infertility. Exp Cell Res. 1998;241:384–93.
72. Donnelly ET, O'Connell M, McClure N, Lewis SE. Differences in nuclear DNA fragmentation and mitochondrial integrity of semen and prepared human spermatozoa. Hum Reprod. 2000;15:1552–61.
73. Wang X, Sharma RK, Gupta A, George V, Thomas AJ, Falcone T, Agarwal A. Alterations in mitochondria membrane potential and oxidative stress in infertile men: a prospective observational study. Fertil Steril. 2003;80 Suppl 2:844–50.
74. Marchetti C, Gallego MA, Defossez A, Formstecher P, Marchetti P. Staining of human sperm with fluorochrome-labeled inhibitor of caspases to detect activated caspases: correlation with apoptosis and sperm parameters. Hum Reprod. 2004;19:1127–34.
75. Lee TH, Liu CH, Shih YT, Tsao HM, Huang CC, Chen HH, Lee MS. Magnetic-activated cell sorting for sperm preparation reduces spermatozoa with apoptotic markers and improves the acrosome reaction in couples with unexplained infertility. Hum Reprod. 2010;25:839–46.
76. Kasai T, Ogawa K, Mizuno K, Nagai S, Uchida Y, Ohta S, Fujie M, Suzuki K, Hirata S, Hoshi K. Relationship between sperm mitochondrial membrane potential, sperm motility, and fertility potential. Asian J Androl. 2002;4:97–103.
77. Marchetti C, Obert G, Deffosez A, Formstecher P, Marchetti P. Study of mitochondrial membrane potential, reactive oxygen species, DNA fragmentation and cell viability by flow cytometry in human sperm. Hum Reprod. 2002;17:1257–65.
78. Marchetti P, Ballot C, Jouy N, Thomas P, Marchetti C. Influence of mitochondrial membrane potential of spermatozoa on in vitro fertilisation outcome. Andrologia. 2012;44:136–41.
79. Zorn B, Golob B, Ihan A, Kopitar A, Kolbezen M. Apoptotic sperm biomarkers and their correlation with conventional sperm parameters and male fertility potential. J Assist Reprod Genet. 2012;29:357–64.
80. Kim E, Yamashita M, Kimura M, Honda A, Kashiwabara S, Baba T. Sperm penetration through cumulus mass and zona pellucida. Int J Dev Biol. 2008;52:677–82.
81. Ranganathan S, Ganguly AK, Datta K. Evidence for presence of hyaluron binding protein on spermatozoa and its possible involvement in sperm function. Mol Reprod Dev. 1994;38:69–76.
82. Huszar G, Ozenci CC, Cayli S, Zavaczki Z, Hansch E, Vigue L. Hyaluronic acid binding by human sperm indicates cellular maturity, viability, and unreacted acrosomal status. Fertil Steril. 2003;79 Suppl 3:1616–24.

83. Jakab A, Sakkas D, Delpiano E, Cayli S, Kovanci E, Ward D, Ravelli A, Huszar G. Intracytoplasmic sperm injection: a novel selection method for sperm with normal frequency of chromosomal aneuploidies. Fertil Steril. 2005;84:1665–73.
84. Parmegiani L, Cognigni GE, Bernardi S, Troilo E, Ciampaglia W, Filicori M. "Physiologic ICSI": hyaluronic acid (HA) favors selection of spermatozoa without DNA fragmentation and with normal nucleus, resulting in improvement of embryo quality. Fertil Steril. 2010;93:598–604.
85. Yagci A, Murk W, Stronk J, Huszar G. Spermatozoa bound to solid state hyaluronic acid show chromatin structure with high DNA chain integrity: an acridine orange fluorescence study. J Androl. 2010;31:566–72.
86. Sati L, Cayli S, Delpiano E, Sakkas D, Huszar G. The pattern of tyrosine phosphorylation in human sperm in response to binding to zona pellucida or hyaluronic acid. Reprod Sci. 2013;21:573–81.
87. Nasr-Esfahani MH, Razavi S, Vahdati AA, Fathi F, Tavalaee M. Evaluation of sperm selection procedure based on hyaluronic acid binding ability on ICSI outcome. J Assist Reprod Genet. 2008;25:197–203.
88. Parmegiani L, Cognigni GE, Ciampaglia W, Pocognoli P, Marchi F, Filicori M. Efficiency of hyaluronic acid (HA) sperm selection. J Assist Reprod Genet. 2010;27:13–6.
89. Worrilow KC, Eid S, Woodhouse D, Perloe M, Smith S, Witmyer J, Ivani K, Khoury C, Ball GD, Elliot T, Lieberman J. Use of hyaluronan in the selection of sperm for intracytoplasmic sperm injection (ICSI): significant improvement in clinical outcomes–multicenter, double-blinded and randomized controlled trial. Hum Reprod. 2013;28:306–14.
90. Van Den Bergh MJ, Fahy-Deshe M, Hohl MK. Pronuclear zygote score following intracytoplasmic injection of hyaluronan-bound spermatozoa: a prospective randomized study. Reprod Biomed Online. 2009;19:796–801.
91. Parmegiani L, Cognigni GE, Filicori M. Risks in injecting hyaluronic acid non-bound spermatozoa. Reprod Biomed Online. 2010;20:437–8.
92. Lazarevic J, Wikarczuk M, Somkuti SG, Barmat LI, Schinfeld JS, Smith SE. Hyaluronan binding assay (HBA) vs. sperm penetration assay (SPA): can HBA replace the SPA test in male partner screening before in vitro fertilization? J Exp Clin Assist Reprod. 2010;7:2.
93. Boynukalin FK, Esinler I, Guven S, Gunalp S. Hyaluronan binding assay does not predict pregnancy rates in IUI cycles in couples with unexplained infertility. Arch Gynecol Obstet. 2012;286:1577–80.
94. Kovacs P, Kovats T, Sajgo A, Szollosi J, Matyas S, Kaali SG. The role of hyaluronic acid binding assay in choosing the fertilization method for patients undergoing IVF for unexplained infertility. J Assist Reprod Genet. 2011;28:49–54.
95. Nijs M, Creemers E, Cox A, Janssen M, Vanheusden E, Van der Elst J, Ombelet W. Relationship between hyaluronic acid binding assay and outcome in ART: a pilot study. Andrologia. 2010;42:291–6.
96. Hong SJ, Chiu PC, Lee KF, Tse JY, Ho PC, Yeung WS. Cumulus cells and their extracellular matrix affect the quality of the spermatozoa penetrating the cumulus mass. Fertil Steril. 2009;92:971–8.
97. Yeung WS, Lee KF, Koistinen R, Koistinen H, Seppälä M, Chiu PC. Effects of glycodelins on functional competence of spermatozoa. J Reprod Immunol. 2009;83:26–30.
98. Menkveld R. Clinical significance of the low normal sperm morphology value as proposed in the fifth edition of the WHO Laboratory Manual for the Examination and Processing of Human Semen. Asian J Androl. 2010;12:47–58.
99. Menkveld R, Holleboom CA, Rhemrev JP. Measurement and significance of sperm morphology. Asian J Androl. 2011;13:59–68.
100. Abu Hassan Abu D, Franken DR, Hoffman B, Henkel R. Accurate sperm morphology assessment predicts sperm function. Andrologia. 2012;44 Suppl 1:571–7.
101. Bartoov B, Berkovitz A, Eltes F, Kogosowski A, Menezo Y, Barak Y. Real-time fine morphology of motile human sperm cells is associated with IVF-ICSI outcome. J Androl. 2002;23:1–8.
102. Franco Jr JG, Mauri AL, Petersen CG, Massaro FC, Silva LF, Felipe V, Cavagna M, Pontes A, Baruffi RL, Oliveira JB, Vagnini LD. Large nuclear vacuoles are indicative of abnormal chromatin packaging in human spermatozoa. Int J Androl. 2012;35:46–51.
103. Oliveira JB, Massaro FC, Mauri AL, Petersen CG, Nicoletti AP, Baruffi RL, Franco Jr JG. Motile sperm organelle morphology examination is stricter than Tygerberg criteria. Reprod Biomed Online. 2009;18:320–6.
104. Montjean D, Belloc S, Benkhalifa M, Dalleac A, Menezo Y. Sperm vacuoles are linked to capacitation and acrosomal status. Hum Reprod. 2012;27:2927–32.
105. Hammoud I, Boitrelle F, Ferfouri F, Vialard F, Bergere M, Wainer B, Bailly M, Albert M, Selva J. Selection of normal spermatozoa with a vacuole-free head (x6300) improves selection of spermatozoa with intact DNA in patients with high sperm DNA fragmentation rates. Andrologia. 2013;45:163–70.
106. Maettner R, Sterzik K, Isachenko V, Strehler E, Rahimi G, Alabart JL, Sánchez R, Mallmann P, Isachenko E. Quality of human spermatozoa: relationship between high-magnification sperm morphology and DNA integrity. Andrologia. 2013;46:547–55. doi:10.1111/and.12114.
107. Bartoov B, Berkovitz A, Eltes F, Kogosovsky A, Yagoda A, Lederman H, Artzi S, Gross M, Barak Y. Pregnancy rates are higher with intracytoplasmic morphologically selected sperm injection than with conventional intracytoplasmic injection. Fertil Steril. 2003;80:1413–9.
108. Hazout A, Dumont-Hassan M, Junca AM, Cohen Bacrie P, Tesarik J. High-magnification ICSI

overcomes paternal effect resistant to conventional ICSI. Reprod Biomed Online. 2006;12:19–25.
109. Souza Setti A, Ferreira RC, de Almeida P, Ferreira Braga D, de Cassia Savio Figueira R, Iaconelli Jr A, Borges Jr E. Intracytoplasmic sperm injection outcome versus intracytoplasmic morphologically selected sperm injection outcome: a meta-analysis. Reprod Biomed Online. 2010;21:450–5.
110. Balaban B, Yakin K, Alatas C, Oktem O, Isiklar A, Urman B. Clinical outcome of intracytoplasmic injection of spermatozoa morphologically selected under high magnification: a prospective randomized study. Reprod Biomed Online. 2011;22:472–6.
111. de Cassia Savio Figueira R, Braga DP, Setti AS, Iaconelli Jr A, Borges Jr E. Morphological nuclear integrity of sperm cells is associated with preimplantation genetic aneuploidy screening cycle outcomes. Fertil Steril. 2011;95:990–3.
112. Oliveira JB, Massaro FC, Baruffi RL, Mauri AL, Petersen CG, Silva LF, Vagnini LD, Franco Jr JG. Correlation between semen analysis by motile sperm organelle morphology examination and sperm DNA damage. Fertil Steril. 2010;94:1937–40.
113. Watanabe S, Tanaka A, Fujii S, Mizunuma H, Fukui A, Fukuhara R, Nakamura R, Yamada K, Tanaka I, Awata S, Nagayoshi M. An investigation of the potential effect of vacuoles in human sperm on DNA damage using a chromosome assay and the TUNEL assay. Hum Reprod. 2011;26:978–86.
114. Tanaka A, Nagayoshi M, Tanaka I, Kusunoki H. Human sperm head vacuoles are physiological structures formed during the sperm development and maturation process. Fertil Steril. 2012;98:315–20.
115. Halliwell B, Gutteridge JMC. Free radicals in biology and medicine. 2nd ed. Oxford: Clarendon; 1989.
116. Henkel R. Leukocytes and oxidative stress: dilemma for sperm function and male fertility. Asian J Androl. 2011;13:43–52.
117. De Lamirande E, Gagnon C. Human sperm hyperactivation and capacitation as parts of an oxidative process. Free Radic Biol Med. 1993;14:157–66.
118. de Lamirande E, Gagnon C. A positive role for the superoxide anion in triggering hyperactivation and capacitation of human spermatozoa. Int J Androl. 1993;16:21–5.
119. Stauss CR, Votta TJ, Suarez SS. Sperm motility hyperactivation facilitates penetration of the hamster zona pellucida. Biol Reprod. 1995;53:1280–5.
120. Dorval V, Dufour M, Leclerc P. Role of protein tyrosine phosphorylation in the thapsigargin-induced intracellular Ca^{2+} store depletion during human sperm acrosome reaction. Mol Hum Reprod. 2003;9:125–31.
121. O'Flaherty C, de Lamirande E, Gagnon C. Reactive oxygen species modulate independent protein phosphorylation pathways during human sperm capacitation. Free Radic Biol Med. 2006;40:1045–55.
122. Sies H. Oxidative stress: oxidants and antioxidants. Exp Physiol. 1997;82:291–5.
123. Aitken RJ, Gordon E, Harkiss D, Twigg JP, Milne P, Jennings Z, Irvine DS. Relative impact of oxidative stress on the functional competence and genomic integrity of human spermatozoa. Biol Reprod. 1998;59:1037–46.
124. Agarwal A, Said TM. Oxidative stress, DNA damage and apoptosis in male infertility: a clinical approach. BJU Int. 2005;95:503–7.
125. Aitken RJ, Baker MA. Oxidative stress, sperm survival and fertility control. Mol Cell Endocrinol. 2006;250:66–9.
126. Chow CK. Vitamin E and oxidative stress. Free Radic Biol Med. 1991;11:215–32.
127. Niki E. Action of ascorbic acid as a scavenger of active and stable oxygen radicals. Am J Clin Nutr. 1991;54:1119S–24.
128. Kobayashi T, Miyazaki T, Natori M, Nozawa S. Protective role of superoxide dismutase in human sperm motility: superoxide dismutase activity and lipid peroxide in human seminal plasma and spermatozoa. Hum Reprod. 1991;6:987–91.
129. Li TK. The glutathione and thiol content of mammalian spermatozoa and seminal plasma. Biol Reprod. 1975;12:641–6.
130. Drevet JR. The antioxidant glutathione peroxidase family and spermatozoa: a complex story. Mol Cell Endocrinol. 2006;250:70–9.
131. Grootveldt M, Halliwell B. Measurement of allantoin and uric acid in human body fluids. Biochem J. 1987;242:803–8.
132. Ha HC, Sirisoma NS, Kuppusamy P, Zweier JL, Woster PM, Casero Jr RA. The natural polyamine spermine functions directly as a free radical scavenger. Proc Natl Acad Sci U S A. 1998;95:11140–5.
133. Paszkowski T, Traub AI, Robinson SY, McMaster D. Selenium dependent glutathione peroxidase activity in human follicular fluid. Clin Chim Acta. 1995;236:173–80.
134. Knapen MF, Zusterzeel PL, Peters WH, Steegers EA. Glutathione and glutathione-related enzymes in reproduction. A review. Eur J Obstet Gynecol Reprod Biol. 1999;82:171–84.
135. Oyawoye O, Abdel Gadir A, Garner A, Constantinovici N, Perrett C, Hardiman P. Antioxidants and reactive oxygen species in follicular fluid of women undergoing IVF: relationship to outcome. Hum Reprod. 2003;18:2270–4.
136. Gupta S, Surti N, Metterle L, Chandra A, Agarwal A. Antioxidants and female reproductive pathologies. Arch Med Sci. 2009;5(1A):S151–73.
137. Aitken J, Fisher H. Reactive oxygen species generation and human spermatozoa: the balance of benefit and risk. Bioessays. 1994;16:259–67.
138. Kothari S, Thompson A, Agarwal A, du Plessis S. Free radicals: their beneficial and detrimental effects on sperm function. Indian J Exp Biol. 2010;48:425–35.
139. Brewer A, Banerjee Mustafi S, Murray TV, Namakkal Soorappan R, Benjamin I. Reductive

stress linked to small HSPs, G6PD and NRF2 pathways in heart disease. Antioxid Redox Signal. 2013;18:1114–27.
140. Iwasaki A, Gagnon C. Formation of reactive oxygen species in spermatozoa of infertile patients. Fertil Steril. 1992;57:409–16.
141. Lewis SEM, Boyle PM, McKinney KA, Young IS, Thompson W. Total antioxidant capacity of seminal plasma is different in fertile and infertile men. Fertil Steril. 1995;64:868–70.
142. Mahfouz R, Sharma R, Sharma D, Sabanegh E, Agarwal A. Diagnostic value of the total antioxidant capacity (TAC) in human seminal plasma. Fertil Steril. 2009;91:805–11.
143. Aitken RJ, Buckingham DW, West KM. Reactive oxygen species and human spermatozoa: analysis of the cellular mechanisms involved in luminol- and lucigenin-dependent chemiluminescence. J Cell Physiol. 1992;151:466–77.
144. McNally JA, Bell AL. Myeloperoxidase-based chemiluminescence of polymorphonuclear leukocytes and monocytes. J Biolumin Chemilumin. 1996;11:99–106.
145. Oldenburg B, van Kats-Renaud H, Koningsberger JC, van Berge Henegouwen GP, van Asbeck BS. Chemiluminescence in inflammatory bowel disease patients: a parameter of inflammatory activity. Clin Chim Acta. 2001;310:151–6.
146. Nemeth K, Furesz J, Csikor K, Schweitzer K, Lakatos S. Luminol-dependent chemiluminescence is related to the extracellularly released reactive oxygen intermediates in the case of rat neutrophils activated by formyl-methionyl-leucyl-phenylalanine. Haematologia. 2002;31:277–85.
147. McKinney KA, Lewis SEM, Thompson W. Reactive oxygen species generation in human sperm: luminol and lucigenin chemiluminescence probes. Arch Androl. 1996;36:119–25.
148. Halliwell B, Gutteridge JMC. Free radicals in biology and medicine. New York, NY: Oxford University Press; 1999.
149. Myhre O, Andersen JM, Aarnes H, Fonnum F. Evaluation of the probes 2′,7′-dichlorofluorescin diacetate, luminol, and lucigenin as indicators of reactive species formation. Biochem Pharmacol. 2003;65:1575–82.
150. Zalata A, Hafez T, Comhaire F. Evaluation of the role of reactive oxygen species in male infertility. Hum Reprod. 1995;10:1444–51.
151. Alkan I, Simsek F, Haklar G, Kervancioglu E, Ozveri H, Yalcin S, Akdas A. Reactive oxygen species production by the spermatozoa of patients with idiopathic infertility: relationship to seminal plasma antioxidants. J Urol. 1997;157:140–3.
152. Said TM, Agarwal A, Sharma RK, Mascha E, Sikka SC, Thomas Jr AJ. Human sperm superoxide anion generation and correlation with semen quality in patients with male infertility. Fertil Steril. 2004; 82:871–7.
153. Venkatesh S, Shamsi MB, Dudeja S, Kumar R, Dada R. Reactive oxygen species measurement in neat and washed semen: comparative analysis and its significance in male infertility assessment. Arch Gynecol Obstet. 2011;283:121–6.
154. Henkel R, Schill WB. Sperm separation in patients with urogenital infections. Andrologia. 1998;30 Suppl 1:91–7.
155. Zorn B, Vidmar G, Meden-Vrtovec H. Seminal reactive oxygen species as predictors of fertilization, embryo quality and pregnancy rates after conventional in vitro fertilization and intracytoplasmic sperm injection. Int J Androl. 2003;26:279–85.
156. Yeung CH, De Geyter C, De Geyter M, Nieschlag E. Production of reactive oxygen species by and hydrogen peroxide scavenging activity of spermatozoa in an IVF program. J Assist Reprod Genet. 1996;13:495–500.
157. Cao G, Prior RL. Comparison of different analytical methods for assessing total antioxidant capacity of human serum. Clin Chem. 1998;44(6 Pt 1):1309–15.
158. Benzie IF, Strain JJ. The ferric reducing ability of plasma (FRAP) as a measure of "antioxidant power": the FRAP assay. Anal Biochem. 1996;239:70–6.
159. Glazer AN. Phycoerythrin fluorescence-based assay for reactive oxygen species. Methods Enzymol. 1990;186:161–8.
160. Whitehead TP, Thorpe GHG, Maxwell SRJ. Enhanced chemiluminescent assay for antioxidant capacity in biological fluids. Anal Chim Acta. 1992;266:265–77.
161. Kolettis PN, Sharma RK, Pasqualotto FF, Nelson D, Thomas Jr AJ, Agarwal A. Effect of seminal oxidative stress on fertility after vasectomy reversal. Fertil Steril. 1999;71:249–55.
162. Sharma RK, Pasqualotto AE, Nelson DR, Thomas Jr AJ, Agarwal A. Relationship between seminal white blood cell counts and oxidative stress in men treated at an infertility clinic. J Androl. 2001;22:575–83.
163. Milner NJ, Rice-Evans C, Davies MJ, Gopinathan V, Milner A. A novel method for measuring antioxidant capacity and its application to monitoring the antioxidant status in premature neonates. Clin Sci. 1993;84:407–12.
164. Said TM, Kattal N, Sharma RK, Sikka SC, Thomas Jr AJ, Mascha E, Agarwal A. Enhanced chemiluminescence assay vs colorimetric assay for measurement of the total antioxidant capacity of human seminal plasma. J Androl. 2003;24:676–80.
165. Pahune PP, Choudhari AR, Muley PA. The total antioxidant power of semen and its correlation with the fertility potential of human male subjects. J Clin Diagn Res. 2013;7:991–5.
166. Mancini A, Festa R, Silvestrini A, Nicolotti N, Di Donna V, La Torre G, Pontecorvi A, Meucci E. Hormonal regulation of total antioxidant capacity in seminal plasma. J Androl. 2009;30:534–40.
167. Baccetti B. Microscopical advances in assisted reproduction. J Submicrosc Cytol Pathol. 2004; 36:333–9.
168. Gianaroli L, Magli MC, Collodel G, Moretti E, Ferraretti AP, Baccetti B. Sperm head's birefringence: a new criterion for sperm selection. Fertil Steril. 2008;90:104–12.

169. Gianaroli L, Magli MC, Ferraretti AP, Crippa A, Lappi M, Capitani S, Baccetti B. Birefringence characteristics in sperm heads allow for the selection of reacted spermatozoa for intracytoplasmic sperm injection. Fertil Steril. 2010;93:807–13.
170. Magli MC, Crippa A, Muzii L, Boudjema E, Capoti A, Scaravelli G, Ferraretti AP, Gianaroli L. Head birefringence properties are associated with acrosome reaction, sperm motility and morphology. Reprod Biomed Online. 2012;24:352–9.
171. Collodel G, Federico MG, Pascarelli NA, Geminiani M, Moretti E. Natural sperm birefringence can be used to estimate sperm viability and morphology. Syst Biol Reprod Med. 2010;56:465–72.
172. Collodel G, Iacoponi F, Mazzi L, Terzuoli G, Pascarelli NA, Moretti E. Light, polarizing, and transmission electron microscopy: three methods for the evaluation of sperm quality. Syst Biol Reprod Med. 2013;59:27–33.
173. Baccetti B, Mirolli M. Notulae seminologicae. 3. Mathematical diagnosis from TEM seminological detection. Andrologia. 1994;26:47–9.
174. Petersen CG, Vagnini LD, Mauri AL, Massaro FC, Cavagna M, Baruffi RL, Oliveira JB, Franco Jr JG. Relationship between DNA damage and sperm head birefringence. Reprod Biomed Online. 2011; 22:583–9.
175. Vagnini LD, Petersen CG, Mauri AL, Massaro FC, Junta CM, Silva LFI, Nicoletti APM, Cavagna M, Pontes A, Baruffi RLR, Oliveira JBA, Franco Jr JG. Can sperm-head birefringence indicate sperm chromatin-packaging abnormalities? Hum Reprod. 2010;25 Suppl 1:i279.
176. Merriam-Webster (2013); Merriam-Webster dictionary. Accessed on 18 November 2013 (http://www.merriam-webster.com/dictionary/biomarker)
177. Kovac JR, Pastuszak AW, Lamb DJ. The use of genomics, proteomics, and metabolomics in identifying biomarkers of male infertility. Fertil Steril. 2013;99:998–1007.
178. James P. Protein identification in the post-genome era: the rapid rise of proteomics. Q Rev Biophys. 1997;30:279–331.
179. Blackstock WP, Weir MP. Proteomics: quantitative and physical mapping of cellular proteins. Trends Biotechnol. 1999;17:121–7.
180. Drabovich AP, Jarvi K, Diamandis EP. Verification of male infertility biomarkers in seminal plasma by multiplex selected reaction monitoring assay. Mol Cell Proteomics. 2011;10:M110.004127.
181. Milardi D, Grande G, Vincenzoni F, Messana I, Pontecorvi A, De Marinis L, Castagnola M, Marana R. Proteomic approach in the identification of fertility pattern in seminal plasma of fertile men. Fertil Steril. 2012;97:67–73.
182. Krause W, Rothauge C-F. Andrologie, Krankheiten der männlichen Geschlechtsorgane. 2nd ed. Stuttgart: Ferdinand Enke Verlag; 1991.
183. Kovac JR, Flood D, Mullen JB, Fischer MA. Diagnosis and treatment of azoospermia resulting from testicular sarcoidosis. J Androl. 2012;33:162–6.
184. Duncan MW, Thompson HS. Proteomics of semen and its constituents. Proteomics Clin Appl. 2007;1: 861–75.
185. Henkel R. Ejakulat. In: Krause W, Weidner W, Diemer T, Sperling H, editors. Andrologie - Krankheiten der männlichen Geschlechtsorgane. 4th ed. Stuttgart, Germany: Georg Thieme Verlag; 2011. p. 27–40.
186. Aumüller G, Riva A. Morphology and functions of the human seminal vesicle. Andrologia. 1992;24: 183–96.
187. Kelly VC, Kuy S, Palmer DJ, Xu Z, Davis SR, Cooper GJ. Characterization of bovine seminal plasma by proteomics. Proteomics. 2006;6:5826–33.
188. Pilch B, Mann M. Large-scale and high-confidence proteomic analysis of human seminal plasma. Genome Biol. 2006;7:R40–9.
189. Batruch I, Lecker I, Kagedan D, Smith CR, Mullen BJ, Grober E, Lo KC, Diamandis EP, Jarvi KA. Proteomic analysis of seminal plasma from normal volunteers and post-vasectomy patients identifies over 2000 proteins and candidate biomarkers of the urogenital system. J Proteome Res. 2011;10:941–53.
190. Rolland AD, Lavigne R, Dauly C, Calvel P, Kervarrec C, Freour T, Evrard B, Rioux-Leclercq N, Auger J, Pineau C. Identification of genital tract markers in the human seminal plasma using an integrative genomics approach. Hum Reprod. 2013;28:199–209.
191. Henkel R. Sperm preparation: state-of-the-art—physiological aspects and application of advanced sperm preparation methods. Asian J Androl. 2012; 14:260–9.
192. Rodriguez-Martinez H, Larsson B, Pertoft H. Evaluation of sperm damage and techniques for sperm clean-up. Reprod Fertil Dev. 1997;9:297–308.
193. Johnston DS, Wooters J, Kopf GS, Qiu Y, Roberts KP. Analysis of the human sperm proteome. Ann N Y Acad Sci. 2005;1061:190–202.
194. Wang G, Guo Y, Zhou T, Shi X, Yu J, Yang Y, Wu Y, Wang J, Liu M, Chen X, Tu W, Zeng Y, Jiang M, Li S, Zhang P, Zhou Q, Zheng B, Yu C, Zhou Z, Guo X, Sha J. In-depth proteomic analysis of the human sperm reveals complex protein compositions. J Proteomics. 2013;79:114–22.
195. Amaral A, Castillo J, Ramalho-Santos J, Oliva R. The combined human sperm proteome: cellular pathways and implications for basic and clinical science. Hum Reprod Update. 2013;20:40–62.
196. Ashrafzadeh A, Karsani SA, Nathan S. Mammalian sperm fertility related proteins. Int J Med Sci. 2013;10:1649–57.
197. Xu W, Hu H, Wang Z, Chen X, Yang F, Zhu Z, Fang P, Dai J, Wang L, Shi H, Li Z, Qiao Z. Proteomic characteristics of spermatozoa in normozoospermic patients with infertility. J Proteomics. 2012;75: 5426–36.
198. Hamada A, Sharma R, du Plessis SS, Willard B, Yadav SP, Sabanegh E, Agarwal A. Two-dimensional

differential in-gel electrophoresis-based proteomics of male gametes in relation to oxidative stress. Fertil Steril. 2013;99:1216–1226.e2. doi:10.1016/j.fertnstert.2012.11.046. pii: S0015-0282(12)02458-2.
199. Ferlin A, Raicu F, Gatta V, Zuccarello D, Palka G, Foresta C. Male infertility: role of genetic background. Reprod Biomed Online. 2007;14:734–45.
200. Reijo R, Lee TY, Salo P, Alagappan R, Brown LG, Rosenberg M, Rozen S, Jaffe T, Straus D, Hovatta O, de la Chapelle A, Silber S, Page DC. Diverse spermatogenic defects in humans caused by Y chromosome deletions encompassing a novel RNA–binding protein gene. Nat Genet. 1995;10:383–93.
201. Matzuk MM, Lamb DJ. The biology of infertility: research advances and clinical challenges. Nat Med. 2008;14:1197–213.
202. Lehmann KJ, Kovac JR, Xu J, Fischer MA. Isodicentric Yq mosaicism presenting as infertility and maturation arrest without altered SRY and AZF regions. J Assist Reprod Genet. 2012;29:939–42.
203. Park JH, Lee HC, Jeong YM, Chung TG, Kim HJ, Kim NK, Lee SH, Lee S. MTHFR C677T polymorphism associates with unexplained infertile male factors. J Assist Reprod Genet. 2005;22:361–8.
204. Lee HC, Jeong YM, Lee SH, Cha KY, Song SH, Kim NK, Lee KW, Lee S. Association study of four polymorphisms in three folate-related enzyme genes with non-obstructive male infertility. Hum Reprod. 2006;21:3162–70.
205. Ostermeier GC, Dix DJ, Miller D, Khatri P, Krawetz SA. Spermatozoal RNA profiles of normal fertile men. Lancet. 2002;360:772–7.
206. Wang H, Zhou Z, Xu LJ, Xiao J, Xu ZY, Sha J. A spermatogenesis-related gene expression profile in human spermatozoa and its potential clinical applications. J Mol Med. 2004;82:317–24.
207. Kierszenbaum AL, Tres LL. Structural and transcriptional features of the mouse spermatid genome. J Cell Biol. 1975;65:258–70.
208. Krawetz SA. Paternal contribution: new insights and future challenges. Nat Rev Genet. 2005;6:633–42.
209. Lalancette C, Miller D, Li Y, Krawetz SA. Paternal contributions: new functional insights for spermatozoa RNA. J Cell Biochem. 2008;104:1570–9.
210. Moldenhauer JS, Ostermeier GC, Johnson A, Diamond MP, Krawetz SA. Diagnosing male factor infertility using microarrays. J Androl. 2003;24:783–9.
211. Ostermeier GC, Goodrich RJ, Diamond MP, Dix DJ, Krawetz SA. Toward using stable spermatozoal RNAs for prognostic assessment of male factor fertility. Fertil Steril. 2005;83:1687–94.
212. Krawetz SA, Kruger A, Lalancette C, Tagett R, Anton E, Draghici S, Diamond MP. A survey of small RNAs in human sperm. Hum Reprod. 2011;26:3401–12.
213. Hamatani T. Human spermatozoal RNAs. Fertil Steril. 2012;97:275–81.
214. Sendler E, Johnson GD, Mao S, Goodrich RJ, Diamond MP, Hauser R, Krawetz SA. Stability, delivery and functions of human sperm RNAs at fertilization. Nucleic Acids Res. 2013;41:4104–17.
215. Jodar M, Selvaraju S, Sendler E, Diamond MP, Krawetz SA, Reproductive Medicine Network. The presence, role and clinical use of spermatozoal RNAs. Hum Reprod Update. 2013;19:604–24.
216. Montjean D, De La Grange P, Gentien D, Rapinat A, Belloc S, Cohen-Bacrie P, Menezo Y, Benkhalifa M. Sperm transcriptome profiling in oligozoospermia. J Assist Reprod Genet. 2012;29:3–10.

Sperm Selection Based on Surface Electrical Charge

Mohammad Hossein Nasr-Esfahani and Tavalaee Marziyeh

List of Abbreviations

DGC	Density gradient centrifugation
ROS	Reactive oxygen species
GPI	Glycosylphosphatidylinositol
TUNEL	Terminal deoxynucleotidyl transferase dUTP nick end labeling
AOT	Acridine orange test
PS	Phosphatidylserine
EPS	External phosphatidylserine
HA	Hyaluronic acid
MACS	Magnetic-activated cell sorting

Introduction

For assisted reproduction techniques (ART), different procedures have been developed for separating "normal" viable sperm from seminal plasma, whereas the most commonly employed procedure is density gradient centrifugation (DGC) [1]. In this respect, sperm population with normal morphology, compacted chromatin, and little residual bodies are separated. However, several studies have demonstrated that sperm processed by this procedure does not guarantee genomic integrity of separated sperm [2]. In accordance with this deduction, Avendaño et al. reported that in infertile individuals up to 50 % of sperm with normal morphology may present DNA fragmentation [3].

In vivo, sperm are separated and selected by different screening barriers such as cervical mucus, cumulus and zona pellucida to prevent insemination of defective sperm [4]. Of note, during in vitro fertilization (IVF), zona pellucida remains as the only barrier that may prevent penetration of defective sperm into oocyte, and thereby through this selection, it may increase the chance of early embryo development and pregnancy outcome [5]. However, during intracytoplasmic sperm injection (ICSI), even this barrier is bypassed and the only selection process that is implemented by the embryologist is based on sperm viability and morphology [6]. Considering the fact that selection of sperm based on morphology does not preclude the chance of insemination of defective sperm as suggested by Avendaño et al. Therefore, the role of genomic integrity, with important consequence on early development, maintenance and outcome of pregnancy, as well as future susceptibility of offspring

M.H. Nasr-Esfahani, PhD (✉)
Department of Reproductive Biotechnology at Reproductive Biomedicine Research Center, Royan Institute for Biotechnology, ACECR, Isfahan, Iran

Isfahan Fertility and Infertility Center, Isfahan, Iran
e-mail: mh.nasr-esfahani@royaninstitute.org

T. Marziyeh
Department of Reproductive Biotechnology at Reproductive Biomedicine Research Center, Royan Institute for Biotechnology, ACECR, Isfahan, Iran
e-mail: tavalaee.royan@gmail.com

to different diseases is ignored in routine sperm selection procedures [3]. To overcome the deficiencies of these procedures, like DGC, advanced strategies for sperm preparation have been proposed or implemented by different researchers.

In advanced strategies, in addition to sperm morphology and viability, sperm are separated and/or selected based on functional characteristics of sperm surface membrane (for more details see review by Said et al. [7] and Nasr-Esfahani et al. [8]). The base of these strategies is that a functional membrane may reflect a normal sperm with intact DNA. It is generally believed, factors such as reactive oxygen species (ROS), influencing integrity of spermolemma also affects the integrity of DNA. Therefore, in this chapter, we introduce two advanced sperm selection procedures based on surface electrical charge and also discuss the importance of these efficient methods in ICSI.

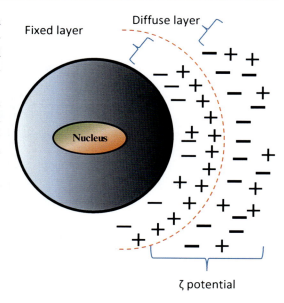

Fig. 4.1 Formation of Zeta potential (ζ potential)

Sperm Plasma Membrane

The sperm plasma membrane plays a dynamic role during sperm–oocyte cross talk and fertilization. Therefore, loss of function and integrity of the sperm plasma membrane is frequently associated with male infertility, notwithstanding normal semen parameters [9–11]. One of the elements playing a central role in this process is glycocalyx. Glycocalyx forms a "sugar coat" composed of complex array of glycans, the oligosaccharides and polysaccharides attached to glycoproteins and glycolipids. In sperm, this coat is rich in sialic acids and is liable for membrane negative charge as is called "Sias." It is intriguing to note that Sias are located in outermost layer of the sugar goat as they cap the majority of glycans at the sperm cell surface [12–14]. These sialoglycoproteins, deposited on sperm surface during spermatogenesis, pass through epididymis by means of epididymosomes and in semen through prostasomes [15]. They account for the electrical charge of the sperm plasma membrane, ranging from −16 to −20 mV, called "Zeta potential" or electrokinetic potential (Fig. 4.1) [16]. Tentative analysis of sialylated proteins responsible for conferring the Zeta potential by MALDI-TOF analysis has nominated four proteins, three of which are aminopeptidase B, fucosyltransferase, and prostatic acid phosphatase [17].

Zeta potential, in addition to preventing intracellular interaction and self-agglutination, it inhibits nonspecific binding with the genital tract epithelium during its transport and storage. It is noticeable that this negative electrical charge in other species such as chimpanzee, porcine, and bovine has been also recognized [18–23].

One of the proteins involved in creating this negative charge in sperm membrane is "CD52". CD52 is defined as a bipolar glycopeptide and a highly sialated glycosylphosphatidylinositol (GPI)-anchored protein on the sperm surface, which is acquired by sperm during epididymal transit and sperm maturation [18, 24]. The presence of high levels of sialic acid residues on the sperm membrane increases its net negative charge, and is taken as a symbol for normal spermatogenesis and sperm maturation within the testis and epididymis [24]. Therefore, transferring GPI-anchored CD52 onto the sperm surface is probably essentials for creating a membrane negative charge. This theory is in keeping with several studies in which they have demonstrated normal levels of CD52 expression are positively correlated with sperm normal morphology, capacitation, and male fertility [24, 25]. Intriguingly, following capacitation, in addition to loss of Sias including CD52, this molecule shift from a distributed surface pattern toward equatorial region, whereas any disturbance in loss and patterning of Sias is associated with male infertility [24]. This is the reason for reduced Zeta potential following capacitation [24]. Loss of Sias is accounted by their hydrolyzed through means of neuraminidase present on sperm, in the uterus and follicular fluid [12]. Loss of these Sias unmasked the proteins involved in cross talk or signaling between sperm and oocyte during fertilization and thereby allows binding of capacitated sperm with zona pellucida [26].

This "sugar coat" which provides a functional surface electrical charge or the Zeta potential has evoked the researchers in this filed to design two different sperm selection procedures based on this criterion. The procedures are (1) Zeta method and (2) electrophoretic method.

Sperm Selection Based on Zeta Method

The negative electrical charge of the sperm's membrane allows sperm to adhere to surfaces with positive charge (tube, glass slides, and ICSI needle/plate) in a protein-free medium [27]. Based on this property, for the first time, Chan et al. separated sperm based on surface electric charge. These authors showed that the selected population showed higher degree of maturity [16]. Following this report, our research group at Royan Institute and Isfahan Fertility and Infertility Center in Iran used this method for treatment of couple candidate of ICSI [8, 28–35].

Practical Approach to the Zeta Method

Zeta method is carried out according to Chan et al. [16]. Briefly, sperm is mixed with serum free basic sperm processing medium and centrifuged.

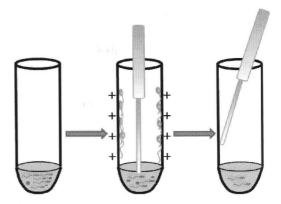

Fig. 4.2 Zeta method: sperm selection based on Zeta or electrokinetic potential

Following centrifugation, the supernatant is discarded, sperm pellet is mixed with serum free medium and sperm concentration is adjusted according to initial sperm count. The adjusted sperm solution is transferred to a new 5 ml Falcon tube which is induced to gain a positive surface charge. To induce a positive charge in lab condition, the tube is put inside a latex glove up to the cap, rotated two or three turns, and rapidly withdrawn from the latex glove. One minute is provided to allow adherence of the charged sperm to the tube wall, and then the medium containing non-adhering sperm (Fig. 4.2) is removed and discarded. Subsequently, tube surface is thoroughly washed with basic sperm processing medium containing serum to detach adhering sperm from tube wall. Subsequently, the sperm is either centrifuged or directly used for ICSI or further assessment [16].

Induction of electrostatic charge on tube surface can be confirmed using an electrostatic voltmeter (Alpha lab, Salt Lake City, USA). Another quick way to confirm the presence of electrostatic charge on tube surface is to check whether the tube will attract very small minute pieces of paper.

It is interesting to note that sperm adheres to glass surface due to their negative charge in albumin or serum-free culture medium. Following Zeta method and washing the tube surface in presence of serum or albumin, serum or albumin binds to anions and cations, so neutralizes the surface charge both on the sperm (Zeta potential) and the surface of the tube. In accordance with this hypothesis, Chan et al. reported that capacitated motile sperm when exposed to a serum free condition showed lower tendency as compared to when adhered to positive surface charge [16]. Capacitated sperm due to loss of glyocalyx on surface of sperm shows more free movement and partially sticks on the glass surface, while uncapacitated sperm is completely immobilized with occasional twitching [16].

Sperm Quality Following Zeta Method

Following selection of sperm by Zeta method, Chan et al. showed that the quality of sperm selected through this procedure, particularly in terms of morphology, DNA integrity and maturity as compared to routine sperm selection procedure (DGC), was improved. They also reported that percentage of sperm with progressive and hyperactivated motility increases following Zeta method as compared to DGC, while the percentage of total motility remains unmodified. They also postulated that these increments which are associated with increased sperm metabolic activity is likely due to brief exposure to serum free condition or manipulation from the attaching/detaching of sperm to tube surface during this process without inducing premature acrosome reaction [16]. This hypothesis was later proved by Zarei-Kheirabadi et al. [30] in our research group. Further studies in our group, included the comparison of efficiency between DGC and Zeta method for separation of mature sperm in terms of morphology, protamine content and DNA integrity. Percentage of normal sperm morphology and protamine content were significantly increased in both DGC and Zeta procedures compared to neat semen. Unlike percentage of sperm morphology, percentage of sperm protamine content was not significantly different between DGC and Zeta methods [35].

Considering the importance of separation of normal sperm with intact DNA during sperm selection procedure, especially for ICSI, our group assessed percentage of DNA fragmentation by three staining methods; Terminal deoxynucleotidyl transferase dUTP nick end labeling (TUNEL), sperm chromatin dispersion SCD and acridine orange test (AOT). The results indicated that percentage of DNA fragmentation was significantly decreased in both DGC and Zeta procedures compared to neat semen. Moreover, percentage of sperm DNA fragmentation rate was significantly decreased in Zeta methods compared to DGC [32]. It is important to note that the efficiency of Zeta and DGC methods relative to semen for DNA fragmentation were 62 % vs. 46 % for TUNEL, 42 % vs. 34 % for SCD, and 41 % vs. 34 % AO methods, respectively [32, 35].

In the above section, we provided evidence that Zeta procedure has a potential to select sperm with intact DNA, and through this procedure, it is possible to certain degree to delete defective or DNA fragmented sperm. However, in nature, the barriers which select "normal" sperm are not in physical contact with sperm nucleus. Therefore, it is the outer cellular characteristics which allow natural barrier to select the "normal" sperm with intact DNA. Therefore, assessment of sperm surface marker may provide evidence how such a sperm is selected in vivo and how these markers may be related to glycocalyx coat, playing the central role in Zeta sperm selection procedure.

Externalization of phosphatidylserine (EPS) from inner to outer layer of plasma membrane is considered as one of early markers of apoptosis in somatic and germ cells [36]. In addition, translocation of phosphatidylserine (PS) can also be considered as physiological event during the process of acquisition of capacitation [37, 38]. Another surface marker which plays a central role in redundancy of defective sperm is ubiquitination during the passage through the epididymis. Highly ubiquitinated sperm are phagocytized by epididymal epithelium [39]. Similar to EPS, it is important to bear in mind that sperm also contain ubiquitinated proteins which are destined to degradation following fertilization. These proteins are masked before capacitation, so they were become exposed to sperm surface during capacitation [40]. Therefore, it is of utmost importance that both EPS and ubiquitination act as a double-edged sword in sperm biology.

Considering important role of these markers, Zarei-Kheirabadt et al. assessed ubiquitination and external phosphatidylserine (EPS) in sperm selected by Zeta, and compared their results with DGC and neat semen. The findings of this study showed that percentage of both externalized PS, and ubiquitin positive sperm were increased in following application of Zeta method compared to DGC and control [30]. Hence, Zeta in addition to selecting sperm with reduced DNA fragmentation and normal protamine content increases the rate of ubiquitination and EPS in this population [30]. This is in agreement with pervious report of Chan et al. in which they postulated that during process of attaching and detaching, the glycocalyx might be altered, and this may induce sperm to undergo a process similar to capacitation. These results are in concordance with pervious report which suggested that increased progressive motility, hyperactivation, and ability to undergo capacitation are associated with higher fertilization rate [16]. To further add to this, Grunewald et al. reported that defective sperm is unable to undergo process of capacitation and acrosome reaction [37].

Recently, several novel sperm separation methods based on functional characteristics of sperm have been introduced [7, 8]. In this context, we compared efficiency of Zeta method with two main sperm separation procedures; HA-binding method and MACS.

Comparison of Zeta Method with Other Functional Sperm Selection Procedures

Zeta Method vs. HA-Binding

One of the sperm surface proteins which is also integral part of "sugar coat" or glycocalyx is a highly sialylated protein called PH-20. This protein has a high affinity for binding to hyaluronic acid (HA) secreted by cumulus cells and is present on Zona pellucida [41]. Therefore, based on this property, sperm has the capacity to bind to HA coated surfaces. Sperm bound to HA shows increased tail cross beat frequency without presenting forward frequency. Sperm selected based on this procedure also shows higher degree of maturity, while displaying normal morphology, low certain kinase activity, absence of cytoplasmic residues, low DNA fragmentation, normal protamine content, and low apoptosis [42].

In regard to this, Razavi et al. compared efficiency of HA-binding and Zeta methods. They reported that percentages of sperm normal morphology and protamine content have improved after HA-binding and Zeta methods compared to neat semen, while percentage of DNA damage has only been improved significantly after Zeta method, not in HA-binding method, compared to control. In addition, these authors reported that percentage of efficiency of the HA method relative to control for normal morphology, DNA integrity, and protamine content were 95 %, 5.9 %, and 19.1 %, while the efficiency of the Zeta method were 67 %, 44.6 %, and 13.1 %, respectively [29]. One of the reasons for these differences could be the fact that Zeta is accounted for all proteins present in the "sugar coat" or in the glycocalyx while HA procedure is only based on one the component of glycocalyx, the hyaluronic acid. However, HA appears to have higher superiority to recover sperm with normal morphology, and this advantage of Zeta can be overcome by selection of morphology during the process ICSI [29].

DGC-Zeta vs. MACS-DGC

Magnetic-activated cell sorting (MACS) is an efficient method for selecting functional sperm based on membrane surface markers. Therefore, different researchers have used MACS to select non-apoptotic sperm based on phosphatidylserine externalization [7]. Previous studies have shown that sperm selected based on EPS shows improved quality [7, 43]. We showed that combination of DGC followed by MACS (DGC-MACS) improved the sperm quality compared to when DGC and MACS were used independently. Furthermore, we also demonstrated that sperm selection based on EPS before the induction of capacitation during MACS-DGC procedure occurred based on EPS due to early sign apoptosis, while sperm were selected after the process of induction of capacitation by DGC followed by MACS (DGC-MACS), partially capacitated sperm may also be selected and discarded in the latter procedure [44]. It is assumed that when sperm is separated from semen in DGC procedure, the process of EPS and capacitation are initiated, and this effect is intensified when serum is used. Therefore, we strongly recommended that MACS-DGC rather than DGC-MACS method is more efficient in order to select sperm population with normal morphology, intact DNA, and low apoptosis [44].

Considering that both DGC-Zeta [32] and MACS-DGC [44] methods can improve quality of selected sperm, we compared the efficiency of two procedures in infertile population. It has been demonstrated that although both methods can select sperm with normal morphology, normal acrosome, normal protamine content, and intact DNA compared to neat semen or control, MACS-DGC method was more efficient in separation of sperm with normal acrosome and protamine content. In our study, the DGC-Zeta procedure showed a tendency toward lower DNA fragmentation rate compared to MACS-DGC [31]. However, to verify this point, further experimentation on larger population is required. It is important to remark that some studies expressed concern regarding remnant of micro beads after MACS for ICSI procedure.

Zeta Method and ART Outcome

Considering efficiency of Zeta method in separation of mature sperm population with minor DNA damage, Kheirollahi-Kouhestani et al. assessed effect of this method on ICSI outcome [32]. To initially roll out the confounding effect of female factors, they inseminated sibling oocyte using DGC and DGC-Zeta prepared sperm. They reported that percentage of fertilization (52.4 % vs. 65.4 %, $p=0.03$), percentage of pregnancy (53.57 % vs.33.4 %), and implantation rates rate (26.18 % vs.15.8 %) were increased following DGC-Zeta procedure [32]. Considering this study was performed on a small population, the study was expanded on a larger population which further confirms the outcomes of Kheirollahi-Kouhestani et al. and it was interesting to note in a couple with previous 11 IVF/ICSI failed cycle, it resulted in birth of a healthy child [34].

Advantage and Disadvantage of Zeta Method

The Zeta method is simple, low cost, and fast. It can be carried out on cryopreserved semen samples. The Zeta method has low recovery rate, but can be easily applied to ICSI cases. The procedure cannot be carried out on capacitated processed samples [8, 16, 45].

Sperm Selection Based on Electrophoresis

Similar to Zeta method, Prof. John Aitken's research group also developed a commercialized instrument called Microflow® or SpermSep® (CS-10) to select "normal" sperm. These researchers also separated sperm base on the surface electric charge using electrophoresis technology [17, 46–48].

Practical Approach to Microflow® or SpermSep

Electrophoretic device consists of two outer chambers and two inner chambers (inoculation and collection). The inner and the outer chambers are separated by polyacrylamide membranes with a typically pore sizes of 15 kDa. The inner chambers are further separated from each other by a third membrane with the pore size of 5 µM. The polyacrylamide membranes allow water and solute to flow between the chambers in the micro fluid system, while maintaining the charge on the two platinum plates at the two sides of outer chambers. Therefore, due to micro flow movement in the inner chamber (inoculation chamber), sperm with negative surface charge within the suspension is allowed to move toward the second inner chamber (collection chamber) close to the anode plate where they can be collected. The third membrane between the two inner chambers prevents movement of cells or other elements with negative surface charge and higher than 5 µM size to move toward the collection chamber close to anode plate [17, 49]. Therefore, through this procedure sperm with

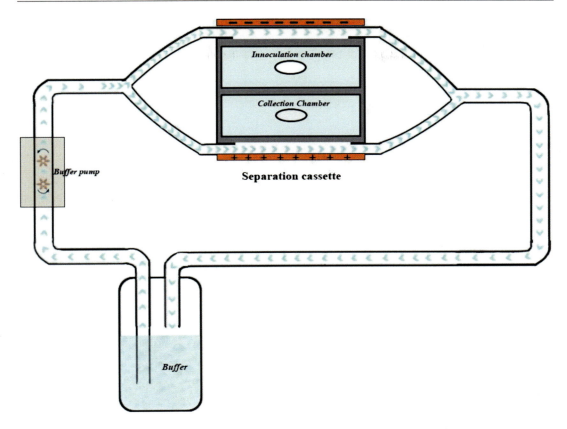

Fig. 4.3 Sperm selection based on electrophoresis

adequate cathode charge moves toward anode plate and due to fluid movement, this sperm can pass to membrane and then the selected sperm can be collected from collection chamber (Fig. 4.3).

Sperm Quality Following Electrophoresis

The research from Aitken group showed that percentages of sperm motility and viability in neat semen were similar to the sperm separated by electrophoresis, and these percentages are maintained in duration different time intervals of electrophoretic treatment. In addition, evaluation of the kinetic characteristics of sperm using CASA indicated that quality of sperm motility has not changed between semen and electrophoretically separated sperm and also during different time intervals of electrophoresis. Comparison of these parameters between sperm separated from DGC, electrophoresis, repeated centrifugation, and neat semen groups have shown that percentage of motility and viability was similar among these groups, except for DGC group in which the percentage of sperm motility were significantly higher than other groups. As a result, percentage of sperm motility has not been improved after the electrophoretic method compared to DGC and/or original ejaculation [46]. Therefore, in the light of this result, these authors have demonstrated that electrophoresis of spermatozoa can be harmful for motility and can lead to disruption of ion fluxes across the sperm plasma membrane [46]. On the other hand, Fleming et al. compared percentage of sperm motility between DGC and electrophoresis methods in infertile men underwent ICSI or IVF. This parameter was similar in DGC and electrophoresis methods in both IVF and ICSI cases. These authors explained that this difference in sperm motility is due to "differences in donor profile, nature of the gradient used (Percoll versus ISolate) and differences in the susceptibility of spermatozoa to the passage of electric current" [48].

Unlike sperm motility, percentage of sperm with DNA fragmentation was significantly reduced in sperm separated by electrophoresis compared to neat semen sample. This parameter is maintained during different time intervals of electrophoretic treatment. They also showed that percentage of DNA fragmentation significantly increases after exposure to repeated centrifugation compared to DGC and electrophoresis methods. These authors concluded that physical shearing forces associated with repeated centrifugation and cell contamination (leukocyte, senescent spermatozoa, or other cells) are involved factors in production of ROS inducing DNA fragmentation during preparation of sperm. Thereby, they showed that electrophoretic method reduces ROS production and DNA fragmentation, so they contributed these effects, absence of requirement for centrifugation and elimination of ROS, in order to produce cells such as leukocyte [46].

Percentage of sperm with normal morphology was significantly higher in sperm separated by electrophoresis compared to neat semen sample, while this parameter is maintained during different time intervals of electrophoretic treatment. In addition, percentage of morphologically normal spermatozoa was significantly higher in electrophoresis group compared to other groups [46].

These researchers also show that this method is suitable for cryostored semen, snap-frozen sperm suspension and testicular biopsies [47]; furthermore, they showed the efficiency of this procedure to recover sperm is similar to DGC and is around 20 % [46, 47]. This recovery rate also stands for testicular biopsies consisting of complex cellular mixtures [47].

Considering the role of sialic acid in Zeta and electrophoretic method, Ainsworth et al. assessed sialic acid expression in electrophoretically isolated spermatozoa, and higher levels of sialic acid residues were observed in sperm recovered in the vicinity of anode plate compared to DGC-prepared spermatozoa [17].

Electrophoretic Method and ART Outcome

Ainsworth et al. reported the first pregnancy and normal birth using electrophoresis method following ICSI technique in a couple with previous repeated failed fertilization, severe oligozoospermia and high percentage of sperm with DNA fragmentation. They suggested "the electrophoretic sperm isolation procedure could make a significant contribution to good clinical practice in this area" [47].

In the light of these considerations, Fleming and coworkers designed a prospective controlled of electrophoretic method in 28 couples underwent either ICSI or IVF and compared clinical outcome of this method with DGC following IVF and ICSI. They reported that efficiency of two sperm separation methods; electrophoresis and DGC, in terms of percentage of fertilization (62.4 % vs. 63.6 %), cleavage (99.0 % vs. 88.5 %), and high-quality embryos (27.4 % vs. 26.1 %) were similar. But since their trail was not randomized, they did not draw any conclusion regarding their clinical pregnancy outcomes [48].

Advantage and Disadvantage of Electrophoretic Method

The electrophoretic method is fast, but requires commercial instrument which may increase the cost of procedure. It can be carried out on cryopreserved semen samples with recovery of sperm count similar to DGC. But the procedure cannot be carried out on capacitated processed samples. The main advantage of this procedure is absence of centrifugation which can induce ROS and DNA fragmentation [4, 8, 17, 50].

Conclusion

It is well established that even in infertile individuals normal looking sperm might contain fragmented DNA. Therefore, novel sperm selection procedures based on different sperm functional characteristics have been designed. Among these selection procedures, sperm can be selected based on surface electric charge or the Zeta potential. Sialic acids by coating the spermolemma account for this charge. Population of sperm selected based on this characteristic has been shown to present higher normal morphology, normal protamine content, lower rate of DNA fragmentation, and higher ability to initiate capacitation. Compared to other novel sperm selection procedures, sperm selected based on Zeta potential present lower rate of DNA fragmentation. Such sperm were shown to have higher capacity to support development and lead to pregnancy. Considering that no chemical are used for selection of sperm based on Zeta potential, the data in this chapter support possible potential of both these procedures (Zeta or electrophoretic methods) for future routine clinical applications.

References

1. Henkel RR, Schill WB. Sperm preparation for ART. Reprod Biol Endocrinol. 2003;1:108.
2. Marchesi DE, Biederman H, Ferrara S, Hershlag A, Feng HL. The effect of semen processing on sperm DNA integrity: comparison of two techniques using the novel Toluidine Blue Assay. Eur J Obstet Gynecol Reprod Biol. 2010;151(2):176–80.
3. Avendaño C, Franchi A, Taylor S, Morshedi M, Bocca S, Oehninger S. Fragmentation of DNA in morphologically normal human spermatozoa. Fertil Steril. 2009;91(4):1077–84.
4. Henkel R. Sperm preparation: state-of-the-art–physiological aspects and application of advanced sperm preparation methods. Asian J Androl. 2012;14(2):260–9.
5. Liu DY, Baker HW. Disordered zona pellucida-induced acrosome reaction and failure of in vitro fertilization in patients with unexplained infertility. Fertil Steril. 2003;79(1):74–80.
6. Oehninger S, Gosden RG. Should ICSI be the treatment of choice for all cases of in-vitro conception? No, not in light of the scientific data. Hum Reprod. 2002;17(9):2237–42.
7. Said TM, Agarwal A, Zborowski M, Grunewald S, Glander HJ, Paasch U. Utility of magnetic cell separation as a molecular sperm preparation technique. J Androl. 2008;29(2):134–42.
8. Nasr-Esfahani MH, Deemeh MR, Tavalaee M. New era in sperm selection for ICSI. Int J Androl. 2012;35(4):475–84.
9. Rajeev SK, Reddy KV. Sperm membrane protein profiles of fertile and infertile men: identification and characterization of fertility-associated sperm antigen. Hum Reprod. 2004;19(2):234–42.
10. O'Rand MG. Changes in sperm surface properties correlated with capacitation. In: Fawcett DW, Bedford JM, editors. The spermatozoon. Maturation, motility, surface properties and comparative aspects. Baltimore, MD: Urban and Schwatzenberg; 1979. p. 195–204.
11. Wassarman PM. Profile of a mammalian sperm receptor. Development. 1990;108(1):1–17.
12. Ma F, Wu D, Deng L, Secrest P, Zhao J, Varki N, Lindheim S, Gagneux P. Sialidases on mammalian sperm mediate deciduous sialylation during capacitation. J Biol Chem. 2012;287(45):38073–9.
13. Varki A, Schauer R. Essentials of glycobiology. Sialic acids. Cold Spring Harbor, NY: Cold Spring Harbor Laboratory Press; 2009. p. 199–218.
14. Schröter S, Osterhoff C, McArdle W, Ivell R. The glycocalyx of the sperm surface. Hum Reprod Update. 1999;5(4):302–13.
15. Sullivan R, Frenette G, Girouard J. Epididymosomes are involved in the acquisition of new sperm proteins during epididymal transit Robert. Asian J Androl. 2007;9(4):483–91.
16. Chan PJ, Jacobson JD, Corselli JU, Patton WC. A simple zeta method for sperm selection based on membrane charge. Fertil Steril. 2006;85(2):481–6.
17. Ainsworth CJ, Nixon B, Aitken RJ. The electrophoretic separation of spermatozoa: an analysis of genotype, surface carbohydrate composition and potential for capacitation. Int J Androl. 2011;34(5 Pt 2):e422–34.
18. Kirchhoff C, Schroter S. New insights into the origin, structure and role of CD52: a major component of the mammalian sperm glycocalyx. Cells Tissues Organs. 2001;168(1–2):93–104.
19. Simon L, Ge SQ, Carrell DT. Sperm selection based on electrostatic charge. Methods Mol Biol. 2013;927:269–78.
20. Manger M, Bostedt H, Schill WB, Mileham AJ. Effect of sperm motility on separation of bovine X- and Y-bearing spermatozoa by means of free-flow electrophoresis. Andrologia. 1997;29(1):9–15.
21. Stoffel MH, Busato A, Friess AE. Density and distribution of anionic sites on boar ejaculated and epididymal spermatozoa. Histochem Cell Biol. 2002;117(5):441–5.
22. Gould KG, Young LG, Hinton BT. Alteration in surface charge of chimpanzee sperm during epididymal transit and at ejaculation. Arch Androl. 1984;2:9–17.
23. Veres I. Negative electrical charge of the surface of bull sperm. Mikroskopie. 1968;23(5):166–9.
24. Giuliani V, Pandolfi C, Santucci R, Pelliccione F, Macerola B, Focarelli R, Rosati F, Della Giovampaola C, Francavilla F, Francavilla S. Expression of gp20, a human sperm antigen of epididymal origin, is reduced in spermatozoa from subfertile men. Mol Reprod Dev. 2004;69(2):235–40.

25. Focarelli R, Rosati F, Terrana B. Sialyglycoconjugates release during in vitro capacitation of human spermatozoa. J Androl. 1990;11(2):97–104.
26. Lassalle B, Testart J. Human zona pellucida recognition associated with removal of sialic acid from human sperm surface. J Reprod Fertil. 1994;101(3):703–11.
27. Ishijima SA, Okuno M, Mohri H. Zeta potential of human X- and Y-bearing sperm. Int J Androl. 1991;14(5):340–7.
28. Deemeh MR, Nasr-Esfahani MH, Razavi SH, Nazem H, Shayeste Moghadam M, Tavalaee M. The comparison of HA binding and zeta methods efficiency in selection of sperm with normal morphology and intact chromatin. J Isf Med Sch. 2009;27(92):46–56.
29. Razavi SH, Nasr-Esfahani MH, Deemeh MR, Shayesteh M, Tavalaee M. Evaluation of zeta and HA-binding methods for selection of spermatozoa with normal morphology, protamine content and DNA integrity. Andrologia. 2010;42(1):13–9.
30. Zarei-Kheirabadi M, Shayegan Nia E, Tavalaee M, Deemeh MR, Arabi M, Forouzanfar M, Javadi GR, Nasr-Esfahani MH. Evaluation of ubiquitin and annexin V in sperm population selected based on density gradient centrifugation and zeta potential (DGC-Zeta). J Assist Reprod Genet. 2012;29(4):365–71.
31. Zahedi A, Tavalaee M, Deemeh MR, Azadi L, Fazilati M, Nasr-Esfahani MH. Zeta potential vs apoptotic marker: which is more suitable for ICSI sperm selection? J Assist Reprod Genet. 2013;30(9):1181–6.
32. Kheirollahi-Kouhestani M, Razavi S, Tavalaee M, Deemeh MR, Mardani M, Moshtaghian J, Nasr-Esfahani MH. Selection of sperm based on combined density gradient and Zeta method may improve ICSI outcome. Hum Reprod. 2009;24(10):2409–16.
33. Khajavi NA, Razavi S, Mardani M, Tavalaee M, Deemeh MR, Nasr-Esfahani MH. Can Zeta sperm selection method, recover sperm with higher DNA integrity compare to density gradient centrifugation? Iran J Reprod Med. 2009;7(2):73–7.
34. Deemeh MR, Tavalaee M, Ahmadi M, Kalantari A, Alavi Nasab V, Najafi MH, Nasr-Esfahani MH. The first report of successfully pregnancy after ICSI with combined DGC/zeta sperm selection procedure in a couple with eleven repeated fail IVF/ICSI cycles. IJFS. 2010;4(1):41–3.
35. Nasr-Esfahani MH, Razavi S, Mardani M, Khajavi NA, Deemeh MR, Tavalaee M. The comparison of efficiency of density gradient centrifugation and zeta methods in separation of mature sperm with normal chromatin structure. Yakhteh. 2009;11(2):168–75.
36. Almeida C, Sousa M, Barros A. Phosphatidylserine translocation in human spermatozoa from impaired spermatogenesis. Reprod Biomed Online. 2009;19(6):770–7.
37. Grunewald S, Baumann T, Paasch U, Glander HJ. Capacitation and acrosome reaction in nonapoptotic human spermatozoa. Ann N Y Acad Sci. 2006;1090:138–46.
38. Grunewald S, Kriegel C, Baumann T, Glander HJ, Paasch U. Interactions between apoptotic signal transduction and capacitation in human spermatozoa. Hum Reprod. 2009;24:2071–8.
39. Sutovsky P, Moreno R, Ramalho-Santos J, Dominko T, Thompson WE, Schatten G. A putative, ubiquitin-dependent mechanism for the recognition and elimination of defective spermatozoa in the mammalian epididymis. J Cell Sci. 2001;114(9):1665–75.
40. Wang HM, Song CC, Duan CW, Shi WX, Li CX, Chen DY, Wang YC. Effects of ubiquitin-proteasome pathway on mouse sperm capacitation, acrosome reaction and in vitro fertilization. Chin Sci Bull. 2002;47:127–32.
41. Hunnicutt GR, Primakoff P, Myles DG. Sperm surface protein PH-20 is bifunctional: one activity is a hyaluronidase and a second, distinct activity is required in secondary sperm-zona binding. Biol Reprod. 1996;55(1):80–6.
42. Huszar G, Jakab A, Sakkas D, Ozenci CC, Cayli S, Delpiano E, Ozkavukcu S. Fertility testing and ICSI sperm selection by hyaluronic acid binding: clinical and genetic aspects. Reprod Biomed Online. 2007;14(5):650–63. Review.
43. Said T, Agarwal A, Grunewald S, Rasch M, Baumann T, Kriegel C, Li L, Glander HJ, Thomas Jr AJ, Paasch U. Selection of nonapoptotic spermatozoa as a new tool for enhancing assisted reproduction outcomes: an in vitro model. Biol Reprod. 2006;74(3):530–7.
44. Tavalaee M, Deemeh MR, Arbabian M, Nasr-Esfahani MH. Density gradient centrifugation before or after magnetic-activated cell sorting: which technique is more useful for clinical sperm selection? J Assist Reprod Genet. 2012;29(1):31–8.
45. Kam TL, Jacobson JD, Patton WC, Corselli JU, Chan PJ. Retention of membrane charge attributes by cryopreserved-thawed sperm and zeta selection. J Assist Reprod Genet. 2007;24(9):429–34.
46. Ainsworth C, Nixon B, Aitken RJ. Development of a novel electrophoretic system for the isolation of human spermatozoa. Hum Reprod. 2005;20(8):2261–70.
47. Ainsworth C, Nixon B, Jansen RP, Aitken RJ. First recorded pregnancy and normal birth after ICSI using electrophoretically isolated spermatozoa. Hum Reprod. 2007;22(1):197–200.
48. Fleming SD, Ilad RS, Griffin AM, Wu Y, Ong KJ, Smith HC, Aitken RJ. Prospective controlled trial of an electrophoretic method of sperm preparation for assisted reproduction: comparison with density gradient centrifugation. Hum Reprod. 2008;23(12):2646–51.
49. Ortega NM, Bosch P. In vitro fertilization - innovative clinical and laboratory aspects. In: Friedler S, editor. Methods for sperm selection for in vitro fertilization. Rijeka, Croatia: InTechOpen; 2012. under CC BY 3.0 license. ISBN 978-953-51-0503-9.
50. Said TM, Land JA. Effects of advanced selection methods on sperm quality and ART outcome: a systematic review. Hum Reprod Update. 2011;17(6):719–33.

Microfluidics for Sperm Selection

Gary D. Smith, André Monteiro da Rocha, and Laura Keller

Introduction

Sperm preparation was described and recognized as an essential step in human in vitro fertilization (IVF) before IVF was demonstrated to be a realistic therapeutic option for female infertility [1, 2]. In the early days of IVF, semen samples were prepared by a simple wash, meaning that samples were diluted with culture medium and the cellular components were separated by centrifugation [1, 3–5]. As the use of IVF progressed, it was also recognized as an effective treatment for mild cases of male infertility [6, 7], and thus sperm preparation evolved to a series of procedures ensuring the selection of competent sperm for oocyte insemination [8–10].

The most common methods currently used for sperm selection, swim-up and isopycnic (density gradient) centrifugation were described in the early 1980s [8–10]. Subsequently, studies sought to determine which method of sperm preparation would yield the highest quality sample [11–16]. While some studies pointed superiority of isopycnic centrifugation for preparation of semen samples; swim-up technique continues to be an option due to its ease of preparation and extremely low cost.

Swim-up and isopycnic centrifugation have been used for decades with few modifications and revisions. However, recently it has been found that long periods of incubation and centrifugation of sperm increases accumulation and/or production of reactive oxygen species which impacts sperm chromatin integrity [17–21]. Sperm chromatin damage has been associated with infertility and poor IVF outcomes [22–29] and therefore new methods for sperm selection avoiding production/accumulation of reactive oxygen species and DNA damage are being explored.

New concepts and techniques for noninvasive selection of sperm for IVF have been emerging in the past decade and include: selection based on

G.D. Smith, PhD (✉)
Department of Obstetrics and Gynecology,
Medical School, University of Michigan,
6422 Medical Sciences Building I,
1301 E. Catherine Street1301 E. Catherine Street,
Ann Arbor, MI 48109, USA

Department of Urology, University of Michigan
Medical School, 6422 Medical Sciences Building I,
1137 E Catherine St, Ann Arbor,
MI 48109, USA

Department of Molecular and Integrative Physiology,
Medical School, University of Michigan,
6422 Medical Sciences Building I, 1137 E Catherine St,
Ann Arbor, MI 48109, USA

Reproductive Sciences Program, Medical School,
University of Michigan, 6422 Medical Sciences
Building I, 1137 E Catherine St, Ann Arbor,
MI 48109, USA
e-mail: smithgd@umich.edu

A.M. da Rocha, DVM, PhD • L. Keller, AASc
Department of Obstetrics and Gynecology,
Medical School, University of Michigan,
6422 Medical Sciences Building I,
1137 E Catherine St, Ann Arbor, MI 48109, USA
e-mail: moandre@umich.edu; andmontr@gmail.com;
lmkeller@med.umich.edu

motile sperm organelle morphology examination (MSOME), sperm surface charge, hyaluronic acid or zona pellucida binding ability, non-apoptotic sperm selection, and microfluidic-assisted sperm selection. This chapter reviews the use of microfluidics devices and microfluidic devices associated to chemotaxis in sperm selection for in vitro fertilization.

Microfluidic Devices for Sperm Selection

Microfluidics is a discipline that studies the mechanics of fluids in micro-scale and facilitates engineering of devices or assemblies to manipulate very small volumes of fluid and or cells [30]. Microfluidics has several applications from inkjet droplet generators in printers to microarray chips for assessment of gene expression and other lab-on-a-chip uses [30, 31]. Uses of microfluidics in assisted reproduction technologies was proposed over a decade ago for sperm selection, fertilization, embryo culture, and integration of IVF procedures on a chip [32, 33]. These proposals were shortly followed by reports on the creation and use of a passively driven microfluidic device for separation of motile sperm [34, 35].

The challenge of creating a microfluidic sperm sorter that was easy to produce, simple to operate, and self-powered was accomplished with soft lithography [34] that entails easy and inexpensive microfabrication techniques used to mold elastomers and shape microchannels [36]. Polydimethylsiloxane (PDMS) was chosen for the fabrication of the microfluidic sperm sorter prototypes because it is a polymer commonly used in soft lithography, has moderate stiffness, hydrophobic characteristics, optical transparency and commercial availability [34–36].

Toxicity of PDMS to human sperm was analyzed with exposure of sperm to PDMS for 30 min followed by overnight incubation. Motility of human sperm exposed to PDMS (64 ± 4 %) was similar to the motility observed in control samples incubated overnight without exposure to PDMS (69 ± 4 %) [35].

A prototype PDMS microfluidic sperm sorter was manufactured for proof-of-concept studies. The sperm sorter was comprised of four wells interlinked by microscopic channels for the production of an area where fluids coming together would display laminar flow, with a slight meniscus between the two fluids, and with negligible mixing by turbulence (Fig. 5.1) [34]. The operator would load the semen sample in one well to generate a stream by gravity pumping and the ipsilateral chamber would be filled with fresh media to produce another stream. With the mechanics of fluids on a micro-scale, the two streams would run in parallel at different speeds without turbulent mixing [34]. The PDMS prototype microfluidic sperm sorter allowed motile sperm to cross the interface between the laminar flows and be collected into a specific well, while the dead/low motile sperm, other semen cellular components, and seminal plasma would be directed to a discard well [34].

Preparation of semen with the microfluidic sperm sorter increased the percentage of motile sperm in comparison to unprocessed semen (98 % vs. 44 %, respectively). Moreover, the percentage of sperm with normal Kruger strict morphology was significantly improved after preparation with the microfluidic sperm-sorting device (22 %) in comparison to unprocessed semen (10 %) [35]. This microfluidics sperm sorter was also able to select sperm from samples with 5×10^6 sperm/mL that were spiked with 50×10^6 round immature germ cells/mL (1:10 ratio). The ratio of sperm to round immature germ cells after selection with this microfluidic sperm sorter was 33:1 [35], illustrating that even samples with a high concentration of round cells can be successfully prepared with this device.

In comparison to other methods of sperm preparation previously mentioned, such as serial centrifugation, density gradient, and swim-up; microfluidics separation of sperm increased the percentage of motile sperm (microfluidics sperm selection: 96.2 %; serial centrifugation: 50.1 %, density gradient: 73.4 %; and swim-up: 85.8 %) and reduced the percentages of sperm with DNA fragmentation [unpublished data].

5 Microfluidics for Sperm Selection

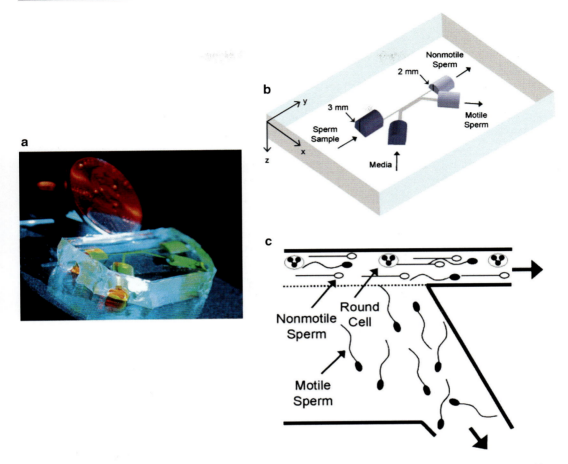

Fig. 5.1 Polydimethylsiloxane was used for the production of a microfluidic sperm sorter device (**a**). This device comprising four wells interlinked by microscopic channels (**b**) is operated by gravity; specifically, different volumes of semen and media loaded to the wells create pressure gradients and displace fluids through the microchannels. Round cells, motile and immotile sperm are dragged with the semen sample flow; however, only motile sperm are able to cross the fluid interface and to be sorted to the motile sperm outlet (**c**). Reprinted (adapted) with permission from Cho, B. S., Schuster, T. G., Zhu, X., Chang, D., Smith, G. D. & Takayama, S. 2003. Passively driven integrated microfluidic system for separation of motile sperm. *Anal Chem*, 75, 1671–5. Copyright 2003 American Chemical Society

The prototype PDMS microfluidic sperm-sorting device provided simplicity and ease of use with a sufficient yield of high quality motile sperm for conventional in vitro fertilization and fertilization with intracytoplasmic sperm injection. Absence of centrifugation steps or prolonged periods of incubation in microfluidics sperm sorting suggests it to be a beneficial technique; however, positive effects of sperm selection with this microfluidic sperm sorter on fertilization rates, embryo development, and pregnancy rates remain to be confirmed by randomized clinical trials.

Recently, a microfluidic device for fast selection of sperm for ICSI has been described using porcine sperm [37]. Production of this device used cyclic olefin polymer. The channels and chambers were microdrilled and laminated with cling wrap of polyvinylidenechloride forming three chambers linked by channels [37]. This device was filled with medium through a lateral loading chamber and diluted semen was loaded through the same port. Sperm migrated into the large mid chamber, were collected through a puncture made in the resin cover, and transferred to an ICSI droplet [37].

Time required for preparation of samples with low concentration (10^4 sperm/mL) with this microfluidic device (265 ± 15 s) was decreased in comparison to traditional sperm preparation (347 ± 19 s); however, the use of this mode of sperm selection for ICSI did not improve cleavage or blastocyst formation rates in this animal model [37]. Studies exploring the effects of this device for preparation of sperm for ICSI need to be replicated with human samples to determine the clinical impacts of this type of sperm selection for ICSI.

In the future, use of new microfluidic technologies for sperm preparation might provide a simple non-subjective sperm selection and automation within the IVF laboratories. Proof of concept devices that are still undergoing evaluation served as a basis for considering supplementary methods of sperm selection using microfluidics linked with other principles and technologies, such as chemotaxis. The following section describes the integration of chemotaxis into microfluidics devices for sperm selection.

Integration of Chemotaxis into Microfluidics Devices for Sperm Selection

Chemotaxis of animal sperm was described over 100 years ago, but was considered controversial until the 1960s [38]. Follicular fluid was demonstrated to carry soluble factors promoting migration and accumulation of sperm in vitro [39–41]. Initially, screening of candidate compounds of sperm chemoattractants produced vague results [41, 42], except for evidence suggesting that progesterone was a major chemoattractant candidate [43].

Sperm are attracted by oocyte and cumulus cell conditioned media [44]. Cumulus cells secrete progesterone after ovulation, and human sperm respond to picomolar concentrations of this hormone [45]. These responses include redirection of sperm movement in vitro if the progesterone source is repositioned in the culture dish [46], and migration through microchannels towards the source of progesterone and accumulation in the vessels containing progesterone [47].

Chemotaxis was first integrated in a microfluidic sperm sorter as a tool to investigate the role of the extracellular peptide coating of sea urchin eggs (*Arbacia punctulata*) in sperm migration during fertilization [48]. This device had a simple design based on the previous human sperm sorter [34]. Composed in PDMS and produced with soft lithography, this device comprised one sperm reservoir linked to a chemo-reservoir through a microchannel where chemoattractant gradient takes place [48]. This microfluidic chemoattractant gradient generator was used to understand sperm diffusion and migration towards the gradients. Accumulation of sperm for functional studies was not attempted [48]; nevertheless, this device is simple and it might be used as a microfluidic/chemotaxis based method for selection of human sperm.

More recently, a microfluidics device created to combine sperm motility and chemotaxis screening has been tested with a mouse model [49]. In comparison to the microfluidic chemoattractant gradient generator previously described [48], integration of chemotaxis into this device was accomplished with a more complex design: four chambers in a "Y" array to imitate the female reproductive tract outline (Fig. 5.2) [37]. Photolithography was used to mold wells and channels in PDMS. An inlet well for sperm sample loading was linked to a diffusion chamber by a motility-screening channel. Two other channels starting in larger wells (pools A and B) located in opposite sides of the diffusion chamber [49].

Sperm swimming from the inlet through the motility-screening channel reached the diffusion chamber in 5–10 min and started to migrate into the channels leading to the larger wells. In order to determine if chemotaxis influenced sperm migration to pool A and B, three conditions were used: (a) pools A and B were not coated with live cumulus cells, (b) pools A and B were coated with live cumulus cells. (c) only pool A or B was coated with live cumulus cells. Outcome of this test was

5 Microfluidics for Sperm Selection

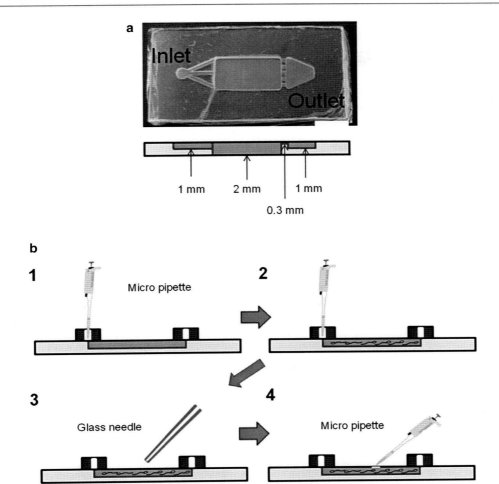

Fig. 5.2 Experimental device for preparation of semen for ICSI microdrilled in polyvinylidenechloride) (**a**). Operation of this device is simple and comprises four steps (**b**). Sperm sample is loaded in the inlet well (*1*) and sperm defuses/swims to the larger chamber (*2*) towards the outlet well. Sperm retrieval takes place after puncture of membrane covering the central well (*3*) and aspiration of sperm from the surface of the opening with a regular pipette (*4*). Reprinted with permission from Matsuura, K., Uozumi, T., Furuichi, T., Sugimoto, I., Kodama, M. & Funahashi, H. 2013. A microfluidic device to reduce treatment time of intracytoplasmic sperm injection. *Fertility and sterility*, 99, 400–7. Copyright 2013 Elsevier

sperm migration index, which measures the ratio between sperm migrating to pools A and B in a given amount of time (number of sperm migrating to pool A/number of sperm migrating to pool B). Sperm migration index was approximately 1 when both wells were not coated with cumulus cells (condition a), as well as when both of them were coated with cumulus cells (conditions b); however, sperm migration index was skewed to pool A or B when only one of these wells were coated with cumulus cells (condition c) [49].

Results obtained by the integration of motility and chemotaxis selection in a microfluidic device are promising; however, studies focusing on the validation of these results with human samples and optimization of conditions for maximal sperm accumulation are required. Additionally, replacement of live cells by a controlled-release source of a chemotaxis factor, like progesterone, would increase the ease of use and make this type of device ready for clinical trials as a noninvasive sperm selection method for human in vitro fertilization.

Concluding Remarks

Applications of microfluidics to human assisted reproduction envisioned a decade ago have been developed. Soft lithography and molding of PDMS have been used to produce most of the microfluidic devices for sperm sorting already described, and the complexity of design might vary; however, simple designs allying ease of fabrication, elementary use, and self-powering are desired for sperm selection. Microfluidic devices with these characteristics exist and are wanting for validation with human samples or clinical trials to determine their utility and impact on IVF outcomes.

Chemotaxis can be integrated with microfluidics, offering additional scrutiny with selection based on sperm competence; however, microfluidic devices with chemotaxis components are more recent and need further investigation to establish their use in assisted reproduction. Adaptability of microfluidics or integration with to other modes of sperm selection other than chemotaxis (i.e., selection based on electric charge) is possible and might increase the utility of devices available in the future. Microfluidic applications to human assisted reproduction are nascent technologies and represent a field open for innovation.

References

1. Edwards RG, Bavister BD, Steptoe PC. Early stages of fertilization in vitro of human oocytes matured in vitro. Nature. 1969;221:632–5.
2. Steptoe PC, Edwards RG. Birth after the reimplantation of a human embryo. Lancet. 1978;2:366.
3. Bavister BD, Edwards RG, Steptoe PC. Identification of the midpiece and tail of the spermatozoon during fertilization of human eggs in vitro. J Reprod Fertil. 1969;20:159–60.
4. Edwards RG, Steptoe PC, Purdy JM. Fertilization and cleavage in vitro of preovulator human oocytes. Nature. 1970;227:1307–9.
5. Steptoe PC, Edwards RG, Purdy JM. Human blastocysts grown in culture. Nature. 1971;229:132–3.
6. Cohen J, Edwards RG, Fehilly CB, Fishel SB, Hewitt J, Rowland G, Steptoe PC, Webster J. Treatment of male infertility by in vitro fertilization: factors affecting fertilization and pregnancy. Acta Eur Fertil. 1984;15:455–65.
7. Cohen J, Edwards R, Fehilly C, Fishel S, Hewitt J, Purdy J, Rowland G, Steptoe P, Webster J. In vitro fertilization: a treatment for male infertility. Fertil Steril. 1985;43:422–32.
8. Makler A, Murillo O, Huszar G, Tarlatzis B, Decherney A, Naftolin F. Improved techniques for collecting motile spermatozoa from human semen. I. A self-migratory method. Int J Androl. 1984;7:61–70.
9. Bolton VN, Braude PR. Preparation of human spermatozoa for in vitro fertilization by isopycnic centrifugation on self-generating density gradients. Arch Androl. 1984;13:167–76.
10. Mathieu C, Guerin JF, Gille Y, Pinatel MC, Lornage J, Boulieu D. Separation of spermatozoa using Percoll gradients: value for in vitro fertilization. J Gynecol Obstet Biol Reprod (Paris). 1988;17:237–41.
11. Berger T, Marrs RP, Moyer DL. Comparison of techniques for selection of motile spermatozoa. Fertil Steril. 1985;43:268–73.
12. Pousette A, Akerlof E, Rosenborg L, Fredricsson B. Increase in progressive motility and improved morphology of human spermatozoa following their migration through Percoll gradients. Int J Androl. 1986;9:1–13.
13. Hyne RV, Stojanoff A, Clarke GN, Lopata A, Johnston WI. Pregnancy from in vitro fertilization of human eggs after separation of motile spermatozoa by density gradient centrifugation. Fertil Steril. 1986;45:93–6.
14. Le Lannou D, Blanchard Y. Nuclear maturity and morphology of human spermatozoa selected by Percoll density gradient centrifugation or swim-up procedure. J Reprod Fertil. 1988;84:551–6.
15. Van Der Zwalmen P, Bertin-Segal G, Geerts L, Debauche C, Schoysman R. Sperm morphology and IVF pregnancy rate: comparison between Percoll gradient centrifugation and swim-up procedures. Hum Reprod. 1991;6:581–8.
16. Englert Y, Van Den Bergh M, Rodesch C, Bertrand E, Biramane J, Legreve A. Comparative auto-controlled study between swim-up and Percoll preparation of fresh semen samples for in-vitro fertilization. Hum Reprod. 1992;7:399–402.
17. Muratori M, Maggi M, Spinelli S, Filimberti E, Forti G, Baldi E. Spontaneous DNA fragmentation in swim-up selected human spermatozoa during long term incubation. J Androl. 2003;24:253–62.
18. Piomboni P, Bruni E, Capitani S, Gambera L, Moretti E, La Marca A, De Leo V, Baccetti B. Ultrastructural and DNA fragmentation analyses in swim-up selected human sperm. Arch Androl. 2006;52:51–9.
19. Viloria T, Garrido N, Fernandez JL, Remohi J, Pellicer A, Meseguer M. Sperm selection by swim-up in terms of deoxyribonucleic acid fragmentation as measured by the sperm chromatin dispersion test is altered in heavy smokers. Fertil Steril. 2007;88:523–5.

20. Matsuura R, Takeuchi T, Yoshida A. Preparation and incubation conditions affect the DNA integrity of ejaculated human spermatozoa. Asian J Androl. 2010;12:753–9.
21. Jackson RE, Bormann CL, Hassun PA, Rocha AM, Motta EL, Serafini PC, Smith GD. Effects of semen storage and separation techniques on sperm DNA fragmentation. Fertil Steril. 2010;94:2626–30.
22. Saleh RA, Agarwal A, Nada EA, El-Tonsy MH, Sharma RK, Meyer A, Nelson DR, Thomas AJ. Negative effects of increased sperm DNA damage in relation to seminal oxidative stress in men with idiopathic and male factor infertility. Fertil Steril. 2003;79(3):1597–605.
23. Varghese AC, Bragais FM, Mukhopadhyay D, Kundu S, Pal M, Bhattacharyya AK, Agarwal A. Human sperm DNA integrity in normal and abnormal semen samples and its correlation with sperm characteristics. Andrologia. 2009;41(4):207–15. doi:10.1111/j.1439-0272.2009.00917.x.
24. Bungum M, Humaidan P, Spano M, Jepson K, Bungum L, Giwercman A. The predictive value of sperm chromatin structure assay (SCSA) parameters for the outcome of intrauterine insemination, IVF and ICSI. Hum Reprod. 2004;19:1401–8.
25. Zini A, Meriano J, Kader K, Jarvi K, Laskin CA, Cadesky K. Potential adverse effect of sperm DNA damage on embryo quality after ICSI. Hum Reprod. 2005;20:3476–80.
26. Bungum M, Humaidan P, Axmon A, Spano M, Bungum L, Erenpreiss J, Giwercman A. Sperm DNA integrity assessment in prediction of assisted reproduction technology outcome. Hum Reprod. 2007;22:174–9.
27. Velez De La Calle JF, Muller A, Walschaerts M, Clavere JL, Jimenez C, Wittemer C, Thonneau P. Sperm deoxyribonucleic acid fragmentation as assessed by the sperm chromatin dispersion test in assisted reproductive technology programs: results of a large prospective multicenter study. Fertil Steril. 2008;90:1792–9.
28. Simon L, Lutton D, Mcmanus J, Lewis SE. Sperm DNA damage measured by the alkaline Comet assay as an independent predictor of male infertility and in vitro fertilization success. Fertil Steril. 2011;95:652–7.
29. Simon L, Proutski I, Stevenson M, Jennings D, Mcmanus J, Lutton D, Lewis SE. Sperm DNA damage has a negative association with live-birth rates after IVF. Reprod Biomed Online. 2013;26:68–78.
30. Nguyen N-T, Wereley ST, Ebrary I. Fundamentals and applications of microfluidics. Boston, MA: Artech House; 2006.
31. Tabeling P, Ebrary I. Introduction to microfluidics. Oxford, U.K.: Oxford University Press; 2005.
32. Beebe D, Wheeler M, Zeringue H, Walters E, Raty S. Microfluidic technology for assisted reproduction. Theriogenology. 2002;57:125–35.
33. Suh RS, Phadke N, Ohl DA, Takayama S, Smith GD. Rethinking gamete/embryo isolation and culture with microfluidics. Hum Reprod Update. 2003;9:451–61.
34. Cho BS, Schuster TG, Zhu X, Chang D, Smith GD, Takayama S. Passively driven integrated microfluidic system for separation of motile sperm. Anal Chem. 2003;75:1671–5.
35. Schuster TG, Cho B, Keller LM, Takayama S, Smith GD. Isolation of motile spermatozoa from semen samples using microfluidics. Reprod Biomed Online. 2003;7:75–81.
36. Whitesides GM, Ostuni E, Takayama S, Jiang X, Ingber DE. Soft lithography in biology and biochemistry. Annu Rev Biomed Eng. 2001;3:335–73.
37. Matsuura K, Uozumi T, Furuichi T, Sugimoto I, Kodama M, Funahashi H. A microfluidic device to reduce treatment time of intracytoplasmic sperm injection. Fertil Steril. 2013;99:400–7.
38. Kaupp UB. 100 years of sperm chemotaxis. J Gen Physiol. 2012;140:583–6.
39. Villanueva-Diaz C, Vadillo-Ortega F, Kably-Ambe A, Diaz-Perez MA, Krivitzky SK. Evidence that human follicular fluid contains a chemoattractant for spermatozoa. Fertil Steril. 1990;54:1180–2.
40. Ralt D, Goldenberg M, Fetterolf P, Thompson D, Dor J, Mashiach S, Garbers DL, Eisenbach M. Sperm attraction to a follicular factor(s) correlates with human egg fertilizability. Proc Natl Acad Sci U S A. 1991;88:2840–4.
41. Ralt D, Manor M, Cohen-Dayag A, Tur-Kaspa I, Ben-Shlomo I, Makler A, Yuli I, Dor J, Blumberg S, Mashiach S, et al. Chemotaxis and chemokinesis of human spermatozoa to follicular factors. Biol Reprod. 1994;50:774–85.
42. Zamir N, Riven-Kreitman R, Manor M, Makler A, Blumberg S, Ralt D, Eisenbach M. Atrial natriuretic peptide attracts human spermatozoa in vitro. Biochem Biophys Res Commun. 1993;197:116–22.
43. Villanueva-Diaz C, Arias-Martinez J, Bermejo-Martinez L, Vadillo-Ortega F. Progesterone induces human sperm chemotaxis. Fertil Steril. 1995;64:1183–8.
44. Sun F, Bahat A, Gakamsky A, Girsh E, Katz N, Giojalas LC, Tur-Kaspa I, Eisenbach M. Human sperm chemotaxis: both the oocyte and its surrounding cumulus cells secrete sperm chemoattractants. Hum Reprod. 2005;20:761–7.
45. Teves ME, Guidobaldi HA, Unates DR, Sanchez R, Miska W, Publicover SJ, Morales Garcia AA, Giojalas LC. Molecular mechanism for human sperm chemotaxis mediated by progesterone. PLoS One. 2009;4:e8211.
46. Blengini CS, Teves ME, Unates DR, Guidobaldi HA, Gatica LV, Giojalas LC. Human sperm pattern of movement during chemotactic re-orientation towards a progesterone source. Asian J Androl. 2011;13:769–73.
47. Gatica LV, Guidobaldi HA, Montesinos MM, Teves ME, Moreno AI, Unates DR, Molina RI, Giojalas LC. Picomolar gradients of progesterone select functional human sperm even in subfertile samples. Mol Hum Reprod. 2013;19(9):559–69.

48. Inamdar MV, Kim T, Chung YK, Was AM, Xiang X, Wang CW, Takayama S, Lastoskie CM, Thomas FI, Sastry AM. Assessment of sperm chemokinesis with exposure to jelly coats of sea urchin eggs and resact: a microfluidic experiment and numerical study. J Exp Biol. 2007;210:3805–20.

49. Xie L, Ma R, Han C, Su K, Zhang Q, Qiu T, Wang L, Huang G, Qiao J, Wang J, Cheng J. Integration of sperm motility and chemotaxis screening with a microchannel-based device. Clin Chem. 2010;56:1270–8.

Sperm Binding to the Zona Pellucida, Hyaluronic Acid Binding Assay, and PICSI

Sergio C. Oehninger and Dirk Kotze

Introduction

Current it is estimated that male contributions area causative factors in as many as half of infertile couples. Unequivocal evidence from the IVF setting has shown that sperm quality influences fertilization and cleavage rates, embryo morphology, blastocyst formation, and implantation rates. Currently, the routine semen analysis remains the most common way to evaluate for male factor infertility. Such evaluation typically includes: seminal volume and other semen physical-chemical characteristics, sperm concentration, progressive motility, and strict morphology. However, up to 15 % of patients with male factor infertility have a "normal" semen analysis and a definitive diagnosis of male infertility cannot be made purely based on the results of a routine semen analysis [1]. Furthermore, it was demonstrated that the basic semen parameters of the unprocessed ejaculate or even after separation of the fraction with highest motility had no impact on the outcome of ICSI [2, 3].

Over the last decade a whole body of circumstantial evidence has linked nuclear/DNA damage in human spermatozoa with adverse reproductive outcomes during *IVF* augmentation with *ICSI*. Sperm nuclear factors that may have implications on reproductive outcome include chromatin anomalies, different forms of DNA damage including strand breaks (evidence have been presented that spermatozoa with damaged DNA are more prevalent in infertile versus fertile men), numerical and structural chromosomal abnormalities, Y chromosome micro-deletions, and alterations in the epigenetic regulation of the paternal genome as reviewed in [1, 4]. Currently, there has been no consensus reached as to which test better identifies ejaculated sperm of poor quality. Although nuclear damage in sperm is poorly characterized, it is believed to involve multiple potential pathophysiological mechanisms including: (1) chromatin abnormalities associated with alteration of protamine/histone ratios, (2) hypo-methylation of certain genes and DNA, (3) oxidative base damage, (4) endonuclease-mediated cleavage, and (5) the formation of adducts as a results of xenobiotics and the products of lipid peroxidation [4].

The number of de novo structural chromosome aberrations of male descent appears to be increased among children born after ICSI. Although the exact etiology of structural chromosomal aberrations is unknown, miss-repair of double-strand DNA breaks appears to be a prerequisite. Structural chromosomal aberrations such as dysenteric chromosomes, reciprocal translocations, and eccentric fragments represent failure of the oocyte's repair mechanisms that may be overwhelmed by the

S.C. Oehninger, MD, PhD (✉) • D. Kotze, PhD
Department of Obstetrics and Gynecology, The Jones Institute for Reproductive Medicine, Eastern Virginia Medical School, Norfolk, VA 23507, USA
e-mail: Oehninsc@evms.edu; kotzedj@evms.edu

degree of nuclear/DNA damage carried by the fertilizing spermatozoon [1, 4].

The risk of transmitting a genetic or epigenetic lesion to the offspring as a consequence of a combination of such factors is significant. It is believed that nuclear/DNA damage in the male germ-line can be associated with defective pre-implantation embryonic development, high rates of miscarriage, and increased rates of morbidity in the offspring, including childhood cancer [4]. The chance of generating a visibly abnormal phenotype is low, but this does not mean that the lesions are not there and will not emerge in future generations. In light of such considerations; it would seem rational (1) to determine the causes of nuclear/DNA damage in the male germ line, (2) to develop efficient systemic preventive and/or therapeutic measures, and (3) to use sperm isolation techniques that will select for gametes possessing minimal-to-none levels of nuclear/DNA damage in assisted conception.

The ICSI technique bypasses multiple steps of the natural fertilization process by introducing a selected and apparently intact spermatozoon into the ooplasm. The utilization of ICSI has become the most common oocyte fertilization method (as compared with standard IVF insemination), being performed in 64 % of IVF cases in the USA, and with an increased worldwide application including Europe that reported 63 % ICSI usage [5, 6]. This strongly suggests that ICSI is being performed for other indications in addition to male factors, for which there is questionable support for their use based on available evidence. It has been reported that the increase in the proportion of ICSI cycles observed in the last decade seems primarily due to an increased use in couples classified as having mixed causes of infertility, unexplained infertility, and advanced age. As a more rare indication, the use of ICSI may represent the solution for oocyte pathology in cases of zona pellucida anomalies, deficiency of the oolemma fusion ability or absence of cortical reaction [1]. These facts stress even further the need for a prioritized examination of sperm-selection techniques for ICSI, and performing long-term follow-up studies on the children born [7].

Additionally, information gathered from in vitro fertilization (IVF) and embryo transfer data has demonstrated that an abnormal sperm–zona pellucida interaction is frequently observed in infertile men. Impaired sperm–zona pellucida interaction can result in failure of fertilization and can be observed in the presence of normal or abnormal "basic" sperm parameters, resulting in decreasing chances of pregnancy when couples are being subjected to intrauterine insemination (IUI) or IVF therapies when conventional in vitro insemination is performed. Sperm–zona pellucida binding assays were consequently developed to assess sperm functionality and competence in the "extended" evaluation of the infertility work-up [8–10]. The latest World Health Organization (WHO) manual depicts sperm–zona pellucida binding assays as research tests [11]. Furthermore, these bio-assays provide valuable information to the clinician in order to direct clinical management to low complexity alternatives such as IUI or to proceed directly to IVF augmented with assisted microfertilization applying ICSI [1, 10, 12, 13].

Sperm morphology grading is more universally based on WHO or Kruger on stained slides to determine the percentage of 'normal" sperm present. This criterion is also applied by the embryologist when selecting the "best sperm" to inject during ICSI. Semen preparation for IUI and for /IVF/ICSI can be anywhere from a simple "wash" or a more complex series of gradient layers—followed or not by a "swim-up" procedure. Zona-binding assays can be prospectively performed which will provide a binding score for each sample aiding the clinical decision of IUI, IVF, or ICSI [1, 10, 12, 13]. Others have introduced the hyaluronic acid binding assay (HBA) in a commercially available hyaluronic acid-coated plate (PICSI dish) [14, 15]. The objective of this chapter is to critically describe the application of the hemizona assay (HZA), a well characterized sperm–zona pellucida binding assay, and the HBA-PICSI assays, as noninvasive sperm tests used in the ART clinical scenario.

The Hemizona Assay

The HZA has been extensively validated as a diagnostic test for the binding of human spermatozoa to human zona pellucida to predict fertilization potential [8, 10]. In the HZA, each of the two matching zona hemispheres created by microbisection of a human oocyte provide three main advantages: (1) the two halves (hemizonae) have functionally equal surfaces allowing controlled comparison of binding and reproducible measurements of sperm binding from a single egg, (2) the limited number of available human oocytes is amplified because an internally controlled test can be performed on a single oocyte, and (3) because the oocyte is split microsurgically, even fresh oocytes cannot lead to inadvertent fertilization and pre-embryo formation. A highly specific type of binding is essential for fertilization to proceed and therefore, the HZA provides a unique homologous (human) bioassay to assess sperm functionality at the fertilization level [8, 10].

Oocytes recovered from surgically removed ovaries or post-mortem ovarian tissue, and/or surplus oocytes from an IVF program, can be used for this assay. This need for scarce human material makes the test less available and more cumbersome. Since fresh oocytes are not always available to perform this assay, different alternatives for preservation have been implemented. The storage methods of human oocytes include using ultra low temperatures with dimethylsulfoxide (DMSO) as cryoprotectant [16]. Additionally, Yanagimachi et al., showed that high concentrations of salt solutions provided effective storage of hamster and human oocytes and the sperm-binding characteristics of the zona pellucida were preserved [17]. During the developing of the HZA, the binding ability of fresh versus DMSO and salt-stored (under controlled pH conditions) human oocytes were examined and it was concluded that the sperm binding ability of the zona remains intact under all these conditions. Subsequently, the kinetics of sperm binding to the zona was assessed and showed that the maximum binding was at 4–5 h post gamete co-incubation. Interestingly, the binding curves were similar for both fertile and infertile semen samples [18].

This assay has been validated by specifically defining the factors affecting data interpretation; such as, kinetics of binding, egg sources, variability and maturation status, intra-assay variation, and influence of sperm concentration morphology, motility, and acrosome reaction status. Over a period of 90 days' evaluation, spermatozoa from fertile men do not exhibit a time-dependent change in zona binding potential, therefore, reassuring their utilization as controls in this bioassay. Within each pool of donors utilized in the assay, a cut-off value or minimal threshold of binding has to be established in order to validate each assay. The purpose is to identify a poor semen specimen and/or a poor zona control. In the control population, this cut-off value should be approximately 20 sperm tightly bound to the control hemizona (fertile donor). Therefore, it is important that each laboratory statistically assess its own control data in order to establish a reasonable lower limit for assay acceptance. If the control hemizona (matching hemizona exposed to fertile sperm) has a good binding capability, that is, tightly binding of at least 20 spermatozoa after a 4 h incubation period is confirmed (information derived from a statistical evaluation of a pool of fertile donors), then a single oocyte will give reliable information about the fertilizing ability of the tested spermatozoa specimen [18–20].

The variability between eggs is high for oocytes representing different stages of maturation (immature versus mature eggs), as well as within a certain population of eggs at the same maturational stage as well as cohort variations. However, this factor is internally controlled (eliminated as a variable) in the assay by the use of matching hemizonae from the same egg. This allows a comparison of fertile versus an infertile semen sample binding in the same assay under the same oocyte quality conditions. Incubating matching hemizona from eggs at the same maturational stage with homologous spermatozoa from the same fertile ejaculate, established a low (<10 %) intra-egg (intra-assay) viability both for human and monkey (cynomolgus) oocytes [21–23].

Importantly, it has been shown that sperm with full meiotic competence were associated with an increased zona pellucida binding potential to human and monkey oocytes. Furthermore, the specificity of the interaction between human spermatozoa and the human zona pellucida under HZA conditions is strengthened by the fact that the sperm tightly bound to the zona are acrosome reacted. Moreover, results of interspecies experimented performed with human, cynomolgus monkey, and hamster gametes have demonstrated a high species specificity of human sperm/zona pellucida functions under HZA conditions, thus providing further support for the use of this bioassay for infertility testing [24, 25].

Prospective blinded studies have reported a robust statistical association between sperm binding to the hemizona and conventional IVF. These studies suggest that the HZA can successfully be used to differentiate between the populations of male-factor patients that are at risk for failed or poor fertilization with high predictive value. Using a cut-off value of fertilization rate of 65 ± 2 % of the overall fertilization rates for non-male-factor patients, or distinguishing between failed (0 %) versus successful fertilization (1–100 %) the hemizona assay results expressed as a Hemi-zona-Index (HZI) can provide a valuable tool to distinguish between different categories of patients. The HZI is calculated as the number of bound sperm from the test sample/number of bound sperm from the control sample × 100. Interpretation: a HZI >30–35 is associated with successful fertilization in IVF and with pregnancy in IUI and IVF. A powerful statistical analysis (logistical regression), provides strong support to the clinical the application of the HZA in the prediction of fertilization and provides a robust HZI range predictive of an oocyte's potential to be fertilized [24–27].

It has been reported by Liu [28] that embryo quality and implantation rates were significantly improved and resulted into more pregnancies when zona pellucida-bound sperm ICSI were used as compared to a conventional ICSI; however the difference in fetal heart pregnancy rate was not significant. In another study by Casciani et al. [29] also evaluated whether zona binding sperm selection could be utilized to select superior spermatozoa for ICSI. Spermatozoa that were tightly bound to the zona pellucida were used for micro-injection (ZP-ICSI) versus the conventional method of sperm selection for ICSI. Results showed no significant difference in fertilization, pregnancy, implantation, and take-home-baby-rates. Interestingly, the authors confirmed previous reports by Oehninger et al. [12] that higher sperm concentration and morphology correlated with higher zona pellucida-sperm binding. Additionally, patients with higher zona binding seemed to have improved pregnancy and take-home-baby rates. It was concluded that ZP-ICSI is not superior compared to conventional ICSI, but that some clinical ICSI outcomes were improved in the presence of adequate sperm–zona pellucida binding.

A meta-analytical approach to examine the predictive value of four categories of sperm functional assays and for predicting fertilization outcome have been reported by Oehninger et al. [30]: computer-aided sperm motion analysis (CASA); induced-acrosome reaction testing; heterologous hamster oocyte-sperm penetration assay (SPA); and sperm–zona pellucida binding assays (including the HZA). Subsequent studies have been reported by Arslan et al. [13] that investigated the predictive value of the HZA assay for pregnancy outcome in patients undergoing intrauterine insemination (IUI) with controlled ovarian hyperstimulation (COH). The European Society of Human Reproduction and Embryology (ESHRE) and the World Health Organization (WHO) have recognized the value of sperm binding assays as research tests [10, 11]. In addition, results of the HZA function test can be effectively applied to counseling couples before allocating them into COH/IUI, IVF, or ICSI therapies.

The Hyaluronic Acid Binding Assay

The sperm Hyaluronic Binding Acid (HBA) assay can be applied to select sperm for ICSI. It has been proposed that the results of the test indicate that the selected spermatozoa have undergone normal spermatogenesis [14, 15]. The rationale is that during the events of human spermiogenesis, spermatids undergo alterations in their plasma membranes that involve formation of HA-binding sites. Original studies by Huszar et al. [14] reported on the effect that HA had on the stimulation of sperm motility and by later Slotte et al. [31] on the acrosome reaction.

Later, Huszar et al. [15, 32] reported a correlation between the percentage of HA-bound sperm and their maturation and functional status. It was suggested that this observation could be used for fertility diagnosis as well as for the selection of functional spermatozoa for ICSI.

Hyaluronic acid (HA) is an integral component of the extracellular matrix of the cumulus oophorus [33] and is composed of alternating repeats of D-glucuronic and N-acetyl-D-glucosamine residues [34]. In humans, oocytes are naturally surrounded by HA during the fertilization process and it is also the environment where natural sperm selection takes place. It has been proposed that such spermatozoa are mature and have the best chance penetrating the oocyte and subsequently fertilizing it, by forming a complex with a glycodelin-interacting protein which retains and concentrates glycodelin-C, a component that is crucial for sperm–zona binding as reported by Chung et al. [35]. In the human, final maturation steps of spermatogenesis involve plasma membrane modifications that prepare the male germ cell for binding to hyaluronan and subsequently to the zona pellucida [36]. Furthermore, HA receptors are present in mature human spermatozoa and at least three hyaluronan-binding proteins are involved in sperm maturation, acrosome reaction, motility, hyaluronidase activity, and sperm-zona binding [37–40].

The application of HA as a "physiologic selector" in vitro has been acknowledged: reports have demonstrated that the spermatozoa that were immobilized and bound to HA in vitro had also completed their plasma membrane remodeling, cytoplasmic extrusion, and nuclear maturation. These spermatozoa are also believed to have a reduced risk of chromosomal imbalance or chromatin anomalies [41, 42]. It could be argued that the above consequences of selection of spermatozoa by HA-binding prior to ICSI, might contribute in optimizing ART outcome.

According to Jakab et al. [41] HA-bound sperm have completed the process of spermiogenesis with cytoplasmic extrusion and demonstrate enhanced levels of the testis-expressed HspA2 chaperone protein. Furthermore, Cayli et al. [43] reported that HA-bound sperm are devoid of DNA fragmentation and the apoptotic marker, caspase-3. Most significantly, sperm bound to hyaluronan display a reduced frequency of chromosomal aneuploidies in comparison to their nonbinding counterparts. Each of these biochemical and molecular parameters of developmental maturity play a critical role in the paternal contribution to successful preimplantation embryogenesis.

Recent studies have provided data that indicated that HA-bound sperm that were selected for ICSI lead to increased implantation rates. In one such study, Parmegiani et al. [44] reported that in 293 couples treated with HA-ICSI compared with 86 couples treated with conventional ICSI, all outcome measures (fertilization, embryo quality, and implantation and pregnancy rates) were at least similar or improved in the HA-bound sperm group. Furthermore, the implantation rate was increased from 10.3 % in conventional ICSI to 17.1 % in the HA-bound group. Studies by Worrilow et al. [45, 46] reported improved clinical pregnancy rates when using HA-selected sperm were compared with conventional sperm selection criteria for ICSI. These authors also showed that in patients with a prescreened binding efficiency of <65 % HA-binding efficiency before ICSI, the rates of pregnancy loss were slightly higher. In patients with a HA-binding score of 65 % or greater, an implantation rate of 37.4 % compared with 30.7 % for control subjects ($P>0.05$) was reported. Additionally, they reported a 50.8 % clinical pregnancy rate in patients randomized to the HA-binding group of compared with 37.9 % for those randomized to the control group ($P>0.05$). Importantly, for patients with HA binding score of higher that 65 %, there was a significant reduction in their pregnancy loss rate from 15.1 % in the control group down to 3.3 % in HA group ($P=0.021$). In contrast, Tarozzi et al. [47] reported that the application of HA was not useful in the context of the limited use of oocytes under Italian law.

ICSI performed with HA-bound spermatozoa has been defined as "physiologic ICSI" and currently, two systems, specially designed for sperm-HA binding selection are available. Due to the different design of these systems, mature HA-bound spermatozoa behave different in each.

Firstly: a special culture dish with microdots circling the area of attached HA hydrogel to the bottom of the dish (PICSI Sperm Selection Device; MidAtlantic Diagnostic–Origio) [48]. In the PICSI-dish sperm are bound by the head to the bottom of the dish, and the tail depicts vigorous spinning (in circles) around their bound head. Secondly: a viscous medium containing HA (Sperm Slow; MediCult–Origio) [49] is available. In the viscous HA containing Sperm Slow medium, HA-bound sperm exhibits very low progression and are therefore easier to be morphologically evaluated. The above described technical differences makes selection and recovery with both these HA systems difficult, therefore the embryologist should be able to choose the system most suitable to their own ability.

There are other some reports comparing conventional ICSI with "physiologic"HA-ICSI. HA represents also a more natural alternative for handling spermatozoa before ICSI than the potentially toxic PVP used in conventional ICSI [45, 50–54].

On the other hand, Ye at al. [55] and Nijs et al. [56] reported that even though spermatozoa bound to HA had inferior DNA damage and improved chromatin condensation as compared to the control group, the HB-assay failed to predict fertilization, pregnancy, and baby take-home rate after IVF and ICSI and concluded that it has no predictive value as a clinical test. Similarly, Petersen et al. [57], reported no differences in the percentages of normal spermatozoa in the HA-bound and nonbound fractions. Van den Bergh et al. [50], also found no significant differences in fertilization rates and zygote score. HA-binding did not predict spontaneous fertilization in patients with unexplained infertility undergoing IVF/ICSI treatment. When it was used for "screening" it did not help to select the method of fertilization [58]. Therefore, the true benefit/advantage of HB-bound sperm selection needs to be confirmed in larger-scale studies.

HA-containing products have no known negative effects on post-injection zygote development and can be metabolized by the oocyte [50–52]. The failure of the HBA binding test to predict fertility may indicate only the partial role of isolated hyaluronan in sperm selection. Sperm function and the spermatozoa's ability to penetrate the cumulus depend on a combination of components from the cumulus (extracellular matrix containing hyaluronan) and the cumulus cells (converting glycodelin-A and -F into glycodelin-C) [59, 60].

Summary and Conclusions

There is unequivocal evidence to support the use of sperm–zona binding bioassays, including the HZA, in the clinical setting. Results obtained from these prospectively performed assays assist in the clinician's direct management towards IUI, IVF, or ICSI. Unfortunately, the need for human material (eggs) makes the assay cumbersome and difficult to be performed by most laboratories. Efforts to use recombinant zona pellucida proteins in soluble or solid-phase assays have not been successful [7, 61]. On the other hand, the HBA test is easier to perform, but contradictory clinical results have limited its value.

The use of alternative molecular binding methods for sperm selection for ICSI needs to be further explored to be able to drawn firm conclusions about their clinical value [62]. These methods include the use of annexin V microbeads which are based on the identification of apoptotic markers such as the presence of externalized phosphatidylserine on the surface membrane of spermatozoa [63]. Flow cytometric cell sorting technique—a procedure that utilizes fluorescence labeled Annexin V to mark phosphatidylserine positive spermatozoa, is highly effective in separating a subpopulation of spermatozoa with normal morphology, as developed by Hoogendijk et al. [64]. Other methods of sperm selection for ICSI have been introduced such as the (1) zeta potential based on sperm membrane charge [65] and (2) an electrophoretic technique where functional sperm penetrates through a polycarbonate membrane and separates highly motile sperm with good DNA integrity and morphology [66].

Sperm selection can also be attempted though microscopic methods. It remains to be established whether any of these molecular binding assays is superior, or can be additive to morphological evaluations using motile sperm organelle morphological examination (MSOME) or ICSI using morphologically selected sperm injection (IMSI) [67–72]. With this technique, selection of sperm cells is performed using an inverted microscope equipped with Nomarski optics coupled with a digital system to reach a final magnification of >×6,000. Other novel methods are also being investigated. Huser et al. [73] reported that Raman spectroscopy of DNA packaging in individual human spermatozoa cells distinguishes normal from abnormal cells. Gianaroli et al. [74] used polarized light that permitted microscopic analysis of the pattern of birefringence in the human sperm head to examine the impact of acrosomal status on ICSI outcome. We estimate that novel and emergent noninvasive technologies should take into consideration the morphological normalcy of the spermatozoa, because such spermatozoa are the ones typically selected for ICSI, and may have "hidden" DNA as described by Avendaño et al. [75, 76].

We conclude that more well-designed studies are needed to confirm the clinical utility, cost-efficiency, and temporal aspects of application (learning curves and real time needed to complete sperm selection in the laboratory) of all these tests, in order to determine accuracy for sperm selection and safe use in the IVF setting.

References

1. Oehninger S. Clinical management of male infertility in assisted reproduction: ICSI and beyond. Int J Androl. 2011;34(5 Pt 2):e319–29.
2. Nagy ZP, Liu J, Joris H, Verheyen G, Tournaye H, Camus M, Derde MC, Devroey P, Van Steirteghem AC. The result of intracytoplasmic sperm injection is not related to any of the three basic sperm parameters. Hum Reprod. 1995;10(5):1123–9.
3. Oehninger S, Veeck L, Lanzendorf S, Maloney M, Toner J, Muasher S. Intracytoplasmic sperm injection: achievement of high pregnancy rates in couples with severe male factor infertility is dependent primarily upon female and not male factors. Fertil Steril. 1995;64(5):977–81.
4. Aitken RJ, De Iuliis GN. Origins and consequences of DNA damage in male germ cells. Reprod Biomed Online. 2007;14(6):727–33.
5. Centers for Disease Control (CDC), American Society for Reproductive Medicine & Society for Assisted Reproductive Technology. 2007 Assisted Reproductive Technology Success Rates. Atlanta, GA: US Department of Health and Human Services, CDC; 2009.
6. Nyboe Andersen A, Goossens V, Bhattacharya S, Ferraretti AP, Kupka MS, de Mouzon J, Nygren KG. European IVF-monitoring (EIM) Consortium, for the European Society of Human Reproduction and Embryology (ESHRE). Assisted reproductive technology and intrauterine inseminations in Europe, 2005: results generated from European registers by ESHRE: ESHRE. The European IVF Monitoring Programme (EIM), for the European Society of Human Reproduction and Embryology (ESHRE). Hum Reprod. 2009;24(6):1267–87.
7. Barroso G, Valdespin C, Vega E, Kershenovich R, Avila R, Avendaño C, Oehninger S. Developmental sperm contributions: fertilization and beyond. Fertil Steril. 2009;92(3):835–48.
8. Burkman LJ, Coddington CC, Franken DR, Krugen TF, Rosenwaks Z, Hogen GD. The hemizona assay: development of a diagnostic test for the binding of human spermatozoa to the human zona pellucida to predict fertilization potential. Fertil Steril. 1988;49(4):688–97.
9. Liu DY, Lopata A, Johnston WI, Baker HW. A human sperm-zona pellucida binding test using oocytes that failed to fertilize in vitro. Fertil Steril. 1988;50(5):782–8.
10. ESHRE Andrology Special Interest Group. Consensus workshop on advanced diagnostic andrology techniques. Hum Reprod. 1996;11(7):1463–79.
11. World Health Organization (WHO). WHO laboratory manual for the examination of human semen and sperm-cervical mucus interaction. 5th ed. UK: WHO Cambridge University Press; 2010. p. 31–3.
12. Oehninger S, Franken D, Kruger T. Approaching the next millennium: how should we manage andrology diagnosis in the intracytoplasmic sperm injection era? Fertil Steril. 1997;67(3):434–6.
13. Arslan M, Morshedi M, Arslan EO, Taylor S, Kanik A, Duran HE, Oehninger S. Predictive value of the hemizona assay for pregnancy outcome in patients undergoing controlled ovarian hyperstimulation with intrauterine insemination. Fertil Steril. 2006; 85(6):1697–707.
14. Huszar G, Willetts M, Corrales M. Hyaluronic acid (Sperm Select) improves retention of sperm motility and velocity in normospermic and oligospermic specimens. Fertil Steril. 1990;54(6):1127–34.
15. Huszar G, Jakab A, Sakkas D, Ozenci CC, Cayli S, Delpiano E, Ozkavukcu S. Fertility testing and ICSI sperm selection by hyaluronic acid binding: clinical and genetic aspects. Reprod Biomed Online. 2007; 14(5):650–63.
16. Overstreet JW, Hembree WC. Penetration of the zona pellucida of nonliving human oocytes by human spermatozoa in vitro. Reprod Biomed Online. 2007;14(5): 650–63.
17. Yanagimachi R, Lopata A, Odom CB, Bronson RA, Mahi CA, Nicolson GL. Retention of biologic characteristics of zona pellucida in highly concentrated salt

solution: the use of salt-stored eggs for assessing the fertilizing capacity of spermatozoa. Fertil Steril. 1979;31(5):562–74.
18. Oehninger S, Morshedi M, Franken D. The hemizona assay for assessment of sperm function. Methods Mol Biol. 2013;927:91–102.
19. Oehninger S, Franken D, Alexander N, Hodgen GD. Hemizona assay and its impact on the identification and treatment of human sperm dysfunctions. Andrologia. 1992;24(6):307–21.
20. Oehninger S, Mahony M, Ozgur K, Kolm P, Kruger T, Franken D. Clinical significance of human sperm-zona pellucida binding. Fertil Steril. 1997;67(6): 1121–7.
21. Franken DR, Kruger TF, Oehninger S, Coddington CC, Lombard C, Smith K, Hodgen GD. The ability of the hemizona assay to predict human fertilization in different and consecutive in-vitro fertilization cycles. Hum Reprod. 1993;8(8):1240–4.
22. Oehninger S, Scott RT, Coddington CC, Franken DR, Acosta AA, Hodgen GD. Validation of the hemizona assay in a monkey model: influence of oocyte maturational stages. Fertil Steril. 1989;51(5):881–5.
23. Oehninger S, Morshedi M, Ertunc H, Philput C, Bocca SM, Acosta AA, Hodgen GD. Validation of the hemizona assay (HZA) in a monkey model. II Kinetics of binding and influence of cryopreserved-thawed spermatozoa. J Assist Reprod Genet. 1993;10(4): 292–301.
24. Franken DR, Oosthuizen WT, Cooper S, Kruger TF, Burkman LJ, Coddington CC, Hodgen GD. Electron microscopic evidence on the acrosomal status of bound sperm and their penetration into human hemizonae pellucida after storage in a buffered salt solution. Andrologia. 1991;23(3):205–8.
25. Oehninger S, Coddington CC, Scott R, Franken DA, Burkman LJ, Acosta AA, Hodgen GD. Hemizona assay: assessment of sperm dysfunction and prediction of in vitro fertilization outcome. Fertil Steril. 1989;51(4):665–70.
26. Franken DR, Oehninger S, Burkman LJ, Coddington CC, Kruger TF, Rosenwaks Z, Acosta AA, Hodgen GD. The hemizona assay (HZA): a predictor of human sperm fertilizing potential in in vitro fertilization (IVF) treatment. J In Vitro Fertil Embryo Transf. 1989;6(1):44–50.
27. Oehninger S, Franken D, Kruger T, Toner JP, Acosta AA, Hodgen GD. Hemizona assay: sperm defect analysis, a diagnostic method for assessment of human sperm-oocyte interactions, and predictive value for fertilization outcome. Ann N Y Acad Sci. 1991;626: 111–24.
28. Liu DY. Could using the zona pellucida bound sperm for intracytoplasmic sperm injection (ICSI) enhance the outcome of ICSI? Asian J Androl. 2011;13(2): 197–8.
29. Casciani V, Minasi MG, Fabozzi G, Scarselli F, Colasante A, Lobascio AM, Greco E. Traditional intracytoplasmic sperm injection provides equivalent outcomes compared with human zona pellucida-bound selected sperm injection. Zygote. 2013;9:1–6.
30. Oehninger S, Franken DR, Sayed E, Barroso G, Kolm P. Sperm function assays and their predictive value for fertilization outcome in IVF therapy: a meta-analysis. Hum Reprod Update. 2000;6(2):160–8.
31. Slotte H, Akerlof E, Pousette A. Separation of human spermatozoa with hyaluronic acid induces, and Percoll inhibits, the acrosome reaction. Int J Androl. 1993;16(6):349–54.
32. Huszar G, Ozenci CC, Cayli S, Zavaczki Z, Hansch E, Vigue L. Hyaluronic acid binding by human sperm indicates cellular maturity, viability, and unreacted acrosomal status. Fertil Steril. 2003;79 Suppl 3:1616–24.
33. Russell DL, Salustri A. Extracellular matrix of the cumulus-oocyte complex. Semin Reprod Med. 2006; 24(4):217–27.
34. Kogan G, Soltes L, Stern R, Gemeiner P. Hyaluronic acid: a natural biopolymer with a broad range of biomedical and industrial applications. Biotechnol Lett. 2007;29(1):17–25.
35. Chung MK, Chiu PC, Lee CL, Pang RT, Ng EH, Lee KF, Koistinen R, Koistinen H, Seppala M, Yeung WS. Cumulus-associated alpha2-macroglobulin derivative retains proconceptive glycodelin-C in the human cumulus matrix. Hum Reprod. 2009;24(11):2856–67.
36. Ranganathan S, Ganguly AK, Datta K. Evidence for presence of hyaluronan binding protein on spermatozoa and its possible involvement in sperm function. Mol Reprod Dev. 1994;38(1):69–76.
37. Hunnicutt GR, Primakoff P, Myles DG. Sperm surface protein PH-20 is bifunctional: one activity is a hyaluronidase and a second, distinct activity is required in secondary sperm-zona binding. Biol Reprod. 1996;55(1):80–6.
38. Hunnicutt GR, Mahan K, Lathrop WF, Ramarao CS, Myles DG, Primakoff P. Structural relationship of sperm soluble hyaluronidase to the sperm membrane protein PH-20. Biol Reprod. 1996;54(6):1343–9.
39. Sabeur K, Cherr GN, Yudin AI, Overstreet JW. Hyaluronic acid enhances induction of the acrosome reaction of human sperm through interaction with the PH-20 protein. Zygote. 1998;6(2):103–11.
40. Ghosh I, Chattopadhaya R, Kumar V, Chakravarty BN, Datta K. Hyaluronan binding protein-1: a modulator of sperm-oocyte interaction. Soc Reprod Fertil Suppl. 2007;63:539–43.
41. Jakab A, Sakkas D, Delpiano E, Cayli S, Kovanci E, Ward D, Revelli A, Huszar G. Intracytoplasmic sperm injection: a novel selection method for sperm with normal frequency of chromosomal aneuploidies. Fertil Steril. 2005;84(6):1665–73.
42. Cayli S, Jakab A, Ovari L, Delpiano E, Celik-Ozenci C, Sakkas D, Ward D, Huszar G. Biochemical markers of sperm function: male fertility and sperm selection for ICSI. Reprod Biomed Online. 2003;7(4):462–8.
43. Cayli S, Sakkas D, Vigue L, Demir R, Huszar G. Cellular maturity and apoptosis in human sperm: creatine kinase, caspase-3 and Bcl-XL levels in

mature and diminished maturity sperm. Mol Hum Reprod. 2004;10(5):365–72.
44. Parmegiani L, Cognigni GE, Bernardi S, Troilo E, Ciampaglia W, Filicori M. "Physiologic ICSI": hyaluronic acid (HA) favors selection of spermatozoa without DNA fragmentation and with normal nucleus, resulting in improvement of embryo quality. Fertil Steril. 2010;93(2):598–604.
45. Worrilow KC, Eid S, Matthews J, Pelts E, Khoury C, Liebermann J. Multi-site clinical trial evaluating PICSI, a method for selection of hyaluronan bound sperm (HBS) for use in ICSI: improved clinical outcomes. Hum Reprod. 2010;25 Suppl 1:6–9.
46. Worrilow KC, Eid S, Woodhouse D, Perloe M, Smith S, Witmyer J, Ivani K, Khoury C, Ball GD, Elliot T, Lieberman J. Use of hyaluronan in the selection of sperm for intracytoplasmic sperm injection (ICSI): significant improvement in clinical outcomes–multicenter, double-blinded and randomized controlled trial. Hum Reprod. 2013;28(2):306–14.
47. Tarozzi N, Nadalini M, Bizzaro D, Serrao L, Fava L, Scaravelli G, Borini A. Sperm-hyaluronan-binding assay: clinical value in conventional IVF under Italian law. Reprod Biomed Online. 2009;19 Suppl 3:35–43.
48. Origio I. PICSIw sperm selection device: instructions for use. http://www.origio.com/download%20center/quality%20and%20regulatory%20documents/instructions%20for%20use/~/media/files_to_download/IFU/MAD/PICSI%20US%20ONLY%20IFU%20283200%20Rev%20A%20LM%2020110819.ashx (2012). Accessed 21 Nov 2012.
49. Origio I. Instructions for use: HBAw sperm hyaluronan bindingassay. http://www.origio.com/download%20center/quality%20and%20regulatory%20documents/instructions%20for%20use/~/media/files_to_download/IFU/MAD/HBA%20IFU%20For%20US%20Distribution%20Only%202352%20Rev%20A%20LM%20201108.19.ashx (2011). Accessed 21 Nov 2012.
50. Van Den Bergh MJ, F-DM HMK. Pronuclear zygote score following intracytoplasmic injection of hyaluronan-bound spermatozoa: a prospective randomized study. Reprod Biomed Online. 2009;19(6):796–801.
51. Menezo Y, Junca A, Dumont-Hassan M, De Mouzon J, Cohen-Bacrie P, Ben KM. "Physiologic" (hyaluronic acid-carried) ICSI results in the same embryo quality and pregnancy rates as with the use of potentially toxic polyvinylpyrrolidone (PVP). Fertil Steril. 2010;93(5):S232.
52. Menezo Y, Nicollet B. Replacement of PVP by hyaluronate (SpermSlow) in ICSI—impact on outcome. IFFS Abstract of 18th World Congress on Fertilityand Sterility 2004. 23–28 May 2004, Montreal, Canada.
53. Nasr-Esfahani MH, Razavi S, Vahdati AA, Fathi F, Tavalaee M. Evaluation of sperm selection procedure based on hyaluronic acid binding ability on ICSI outcome. J Assist Reprod Genet. 2008;25(5):197–203.
54. Strehler E, Baccetti B, Sterzik K, Capitani S, Collodel G, De Santo M, et al. Detrimental effects of polyvinylpyrrolidone on the ultrastructure of spermatozoa (Notulae seminologicae 13). Hum Reprod. 1998;13(1):120–3.
55. Ye H, Huang GN, Gao Y, de Liu Y. Relationship between human sperm-hyaluronan binding assay and fertilization rate in conventional in vitro fertilization. Hum Reprod. 2006;21(6):1545–50.
56. Nijs M, Creemers E, Cox A, Franssen K, Janssen M, Vanheusden E, De Jonge C, Ombelet W. Chromomycin A3 staining, sperm chromatin structure assay and hyaluronic acid binding assay as predictors for assisted reproductive outcome. Reprod Biomed Online. 2009;19(5):671–6984.
57. Petersen CG, Massaro FC, Mauri AL, Oliveira JB, Baruffi RL, Franco Jr JG. Efficacy of hyaluronic acid binding assay in selecting motile spermatozoa with normal morphology at high magnification. Reprod Biol Endocrinol. 2010;8:149.
58. Kovacs P, Kovats T, Sajgo A, Szollosi J, Matyas S, Kaali SG. The role of hyaluronic acid binding assay in choosing the fertilization method for patients undergoing IVF for unexplained infertility. J Assist Reprod Genet. 2011;28(1):49–54.
59. Yeung WS, Lee KF, Koistinen R, Koistinen H, Seppala M, Ho PC, Chiu PC. Roles of glycodelin in modulating sperm function. Mol Cell Endocrinol. 2006;250(1–2):149–56.
60. Yeung WS, Lee KF, Koistinen R, Koistinen H, Seppala M, Chiu PC. Effects of glycodelins on functional competence of spermatozoa. J Reprod Immunol. 2009;83(1–2):26–30.
61. Dong KW, Chi TF, Juan YW, Chen CW, Lin Z, Xiang XQ, Mahony M, Gibbons WE, Oehninger S. Characterization of the biologic activities of a recombinant human zona pellucida protein 3 expressed in human ovarian teratocarcinoma (PA-1) cells. Am J Obstet Gynecol. 2001;184(5):835–43.
62. Henkel R. Sperm preparation: state-of-the-art—physiological aspects and application of advanced sperm preparation methods. Asian J Androl. 2012;14(2):260–9.
63. Gronwald W, Huber F, Grünewald P, Spörner M, Wohlgemuth S, Herrmann C, Kalbitzer HR. Solution structure of the Ras binding domain of the protein kinase Byr2 from Schizosaccharomyces pombe. Structure. 2001;9(11):1029–41.
64. Hoogendijk CF, Kruger TF, Bouic PJ, Henkel RR. A novel approach for the selection of human sperm using annexin V-binding and flow cytometry. Fertil Steril. 2009;91(4):1285–92.
65. Chan PJ, Jacobson JD, Corselli JU, Patton WC. A simple zeta method for sperm selection based on membrane charge. Fertil Steril. 2006;85(2):481–6.
66. Ainsworth C, Nixon B, Aitken RJ. Development of a novel electrophoretic system for the isolation of human spermatozoa. Hum Reprod. 2005;20(8):2261–70.
67. Bartoov B, Berkovitz A, Eltes F. Selection of spermatozoa with normal nuclei to improve the pregnancy rate with intracytoplasmic sperm injection. N Engl J Med. 2001;345(14):1067–8.

68. Bartoov B, Berkovitz A, Eltes F, Kogosovsky A, Yagoda A, Lederman H, Artzi S, Gross M, Barak Y. Pregnancy rates are higher with intracytoplasmic morphologically selected sperm injection than with conventional intracytoplasmic injection. Fertil Steril. 2003;80(6):1413–9.
69. Berkovitz A, Eltes F, Ellenbogen A, Peer S, Feldberg D, Bartoov B. Does the presence of nuclear vacuoles in human sperm selected for ICSI affect pregnancy outcome? Hum Reprod. 2006;21(7):1787–90.
70. Berkovitz A, Eltes F, Lederman H, Peer S, Ellenbogen A, Feldberg B, Bartoov B. How to improve IVF-ICSI outcome by sperm selection. Reprod Biomed Online. 2006;12(5):634–8.
71. Klement AH, Koren-Morag N, Itsykson P, Berkovitz A. Intracytoplasmic morphologically selected sperm injection versus intracytoplasmic sperm injection: a step toward a clinical algorithm. Fertil Steril. 2013; 99(5):1290–3.
72. Garolla A, Fortini D, Menegazzo M, De Toni L, Nicoletti V, Moretti A, Selice R, Engl B, Foresta C. High-power microscopy for selecting spermatozoa for ICSI by physiological status. Reprod Biomed Online. 2008;17(5):610–6.
73. Huser T, Orme CA, Hollars CW, Corzett MH, Balhorn R. Raman spectroscopy of DNA packaging in individual human sperm cells distinguishes normal from abnormal cells. J Biophotonics. 2009; 2(5):322–32.
74. Gianaroli L, Magli MC, Ferraretti AP, Crippa A, Lappi M, Capitani S, Baccetti B. Birefringence characteristics in sperm heads allow for the selection of reacted spermatozoa for intracytoplasmic sperm injection. Fertil Steril. 2010;93(3):807–13.
75. Avendaño C, Oehninger S. DNA fragmentation in morphologically normal spermatozoa: how much should we be concerned in the ICSI era? J Androl. 2011;32(4):356–63.
76. Avendaño C, Franchi A, Duran H, Oehninger S. DNA fragmentation of normal spermatozoa negatively impacts embryo quality and intracytoplasmic sperm injection outcome. Fertil Steril. 2010;94(2):549–57.

Non-apoptotic Sperm Selection

Tamer Said, Reda Z. Mahfouz, Iryna Kuznyetsova, and Alfonso P. Del Valle

Apoptosis in Human Spermatozoa

Programmed cell death (apoptosis) is a cascade of cellular events that are genetically controlled and lead to a series of cellular, morphological, and biochemical changes away from healthy homeostasis culminating into cellular suicide [1] (Fig. 7.1a–c). Mature human spermatozoa result from unique differentiation/maturation processes of germ cell progenitors. Germ cell progenitors are supported and nourished by Sertoli cells. Testicular blood barrier protects early germ cell progenitors from being attacked from external injurious agents or their own immune system [2]. Disruption of this barrier by trauma, surgery or infection may induce germ cell stresses [3]. Depending upon the repair capacity and severity of injurious factors will be the affection level on spermatogenesis. Figure 7.1a shows testis, anatomical sections with germinal epithelium differentiation in normal conditions. Figure 7.1b represents morphological changes in damaged sperm progenitors. The most common pathways which may be activated in germinal epithelium in response to injuries are demonstrated in Fig. 7.1c.

Apoptotic pathways in mature spermatozoa remain not fully understood due to almost absence of cytoplasm and reduced nuclear functional activities. The most accepted theory is "abortive apoptosis" by Sakkas [4]. Other possible ones include oxidative stress sperm damage [5] or activation of endonucleases by external DNA [6].

T. Said, MD, PhD, HCLD/CC (✉)
Andrology Laboratory & Reproductive Tissue Bank,
The Toronto Institute for Reproductive Medicine –
ReproMed, 56 Aberfoyle Crescent, Toronto,
ON, Canada M8X-2W4
e-mail: tsaid@repromed.ca

R.Z. Mahfouz, MD, PhD
Translational Haematology/Oncology,
Taussig Cancer Institute, Cleveland Clinic,
Euclid Avenue, Desk R-40, Rm:R04-35,
Cleveland, OH 44195, USA
e-mail: mahfour@ccf.org

I. Kuznyetsova, PhD, HCLD
Embryology Laboratory, The Toronto Institute
for Reproductive Medicine – ReproMed,
56 Aberfoyle Cres, Toronto, ON, Canada M8X 2W4
e-mail: ikuznyetsova@repromed.ca

A.P. Del Valle, MD, FRCS(C)
The Toronto Institute for Reproductive Medicine –
ReproMed, 56 Aberfoyle Cres, Toronto, ON,
Canada M8X 2W4
e-mail: adelvalle@repromed.ca

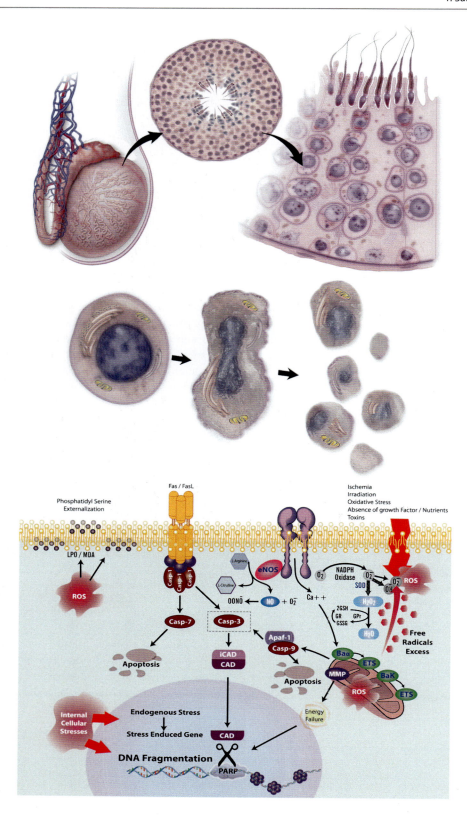

Apoptotic Changes in Sperm

Apoptosis-related features, reported in human spermatozoa, may indicate anomalies in the regulation of apoptosis in the testis [7]. Depending upon the degree of damage, plasma membrane insults occur early before apoptosis becomes irreversible following extensive or nuclear damage [8, 9]. The most common apoptotic biomarkers are as follows:

Plasma Membrane Changes (Phosphatidylserine Externalization)

Phosphatidylserine (PS) is a phospholipid located on the inner leaflet of the plasma membrane. Externalization of PS from the inner leaflet, (its normal location) in the sperm plasma membrane to its outer surface, is one of early reversible changes observed in human spermatozoa which becomes irreversible when it is accompanied with extensive DNA damage [10]. PS has a high and selective affinity for annexin V, a 35–36 kDa phospholipid binding protein. Annexin-PS binding occurs after translocation of PS from inner to outer leaflets of plasma membrane resulting in externalization of PS (EPS) on the surface. EPS negatively correlates with the sperm quality [11]. Reduced integrity of sperm membrane is more frequently seen in spermatozoa from infertile men that contributes to infertility [12].

Mitochondrial Changes

Sperm mitochondria are susceptible to injurious agents' apoptotic stimuli due to their compartmentalization within the midpiece region. Intact mitochondrial membrane potential (MMP) is determined to be essential for sperm motility [13]. MMP disruption is considered as a key for apoptosis signaling cascade which is observed in human spermatozoa. A strong correlation could be found between MMP and DNA fragmentation levels in human spermatozoa [14].

Cytoplasmic Changes: Caspase(s) Activation

Caspase (CP) activation is believed to be a well-defined point of no return for apoptosis progression, and a number of apoptotic events downstream of caspase activation have been characterized among which DNA fragmentation stands as a critical apoptotic event [15, 16]. Activated CP-3 induces activation of caspase-activated deoxyribonuclease (CAD; also called caspase-activated nuclease), which is integrally involved in degrading DNA. Therefore, CP-3 executes the final disassembly of the cell by generating DNA strand breaks [17] (Fig. 7.1c).

Semen from infertile men are characterized by increased percentage of cells positive for activated caspases, especially in those with cytoplasmic

Fig. 7.1 (a) Gross structure of testis shows distribution of the seminiferous tubules collecting together to end in the epididymis, then vas deferens. Spermatic vessels plexus forms the main components of spermatic cord. Tortuous spermatic venous plexus observed in infertile men and is considered the most common pathologies in male infertility. Magnified cross section in a seminiferous tubule is to show the diameter and its lining of the anatomical unit of spermatogenesis. Seminiferous tubules as further studied longitudinally to show its lining layer of Sertoli cells with differentiating germ cells maturation stages (b). Morphological changes of germ cells which occur in response to injurious agents such as apoptosis. (c) Activation of the most common pathways for oxidative stress (OS) and apoptosis which may get activated in response to external or internal cellular injurious stimuli. There may be activation of interacting pathways which favor OS induced damage with apoptotic machinery activation. These interactions cause energy failure and augment DNA fragmentations and suppression of DNA repair (*ETS* electron transfer system, *MMP* mitochondrial membrane potential, *GR* glutathione reductase, *GPx* glutathione peroxidase, *SOD* superoxide dismutase, *Bax/Bak* proapoptotic proteins essentials for mitochondrial induced apoptosis, *eNOS* endothelial nitric oxide synthase, *CAD* caspase activated DNase, *ApoF1* apoptosis inducing factor, *PARP* poly (ADP)-ribose polymerase, *Cas* caspase). Reprinted with permission, Cleveland Clinic Center for Medical Art and Photography © 2013. All rights reserved

droplets, with positive correlation to EPS [18]. The presence of precursors and activated forms of CP-8 and CP-9 in conjunction with aCP-3 in human spermatozoa has also been confirmed [19].

Nuclear Changes: DNA fragmentation

Sperm DNA fragmentation may be a result of activation of one or more pathways shown in Fig. 7.1c, which occur late due to extensive cellular damage. In addition, DNA damage seems to be correlated with abnormal sperm morphology and low motility [20].

Impact of Sperm Apoptosis on ART Clinical Outcomes

Assisted reproductive techniques (ART) have offered the possibility of treating in many infertile couples with male factor infertility. However, success is not guaranteed and success rates for ART procedures still remain suboptimal [21]. Reports link the presence of apoptotic markers in human sperm with the failure of in vivo as well as in vitro fertilization [22–24].

The use of spermatozoa from ejaculates with poor quality or from non-physiological sources such as the epididymis and testis raises a number of concerns. It is for instance possible that some sperm selected for ART will display features of damage at the molecular levels despite they appear normal, which may be partially responsible for low blastocyst development rates (BDR), pregnancy rates (PR), and recurrent pregnancy loss (RPL) [22, 25]. The negative effects of sperm damage, specifically DNA fragmentation appear during genome activation after fertilization [26].

In support of the implication of apoptosis in human reproduction, EPS, mitochondrial dysfunction, and nuclear DNA damage were detected in significantly higher levels in infertile men and those with varicoceles [27]. The use of these damaged spermatozoa may not only compromise the fertilization potential, but also affecting the clinical pregnancy outcome [26, 28].

Rationale for Selection of Non-apoptotic Spermatozoa

Sperm apoptosis and apoptosis-like manifestations are associated with decreased male fertility potential [29]. Evidence shows that ART success rates are diminished in cases where a significant portion of the sperm population presents with apoptosis manifestations [22, 30–32]. Specifically, the impact of sperm DNA damage as one of the manifestations of apoptosis on determining ART success rates was extensively studied. There is ample evidence documenting that sperm with high DNA fragmentation will result in poor ART outcomes [33–36]. However, this was contradicted by evidence showing that no such correlation exists [37–40]. In 2008, a meta-analysis of 13 studies found only small but statistically significant impact of sperm DNA fragmentation on IVF/ICSI outcome. This ill defined relationship maybe due to different methodologies used (SCSA and TUNEL), different ART end points, which will always be a challenge in similar types of studies [41].

While the relationship between sperm DNA damage and IVF/ICSI outcomes remains controversial, evidence demonstrating the impact of sperm DNA damage on pregnancy loss following IVF/ICSI is very consistent. A recent meta-analysis which included 16 studies and around 3,000 couples evaluated the effects of sperm DNA fragmentation on miscarriage rates following IVF/ICSI. The analysis showed significant increase in the rate of miscarriage in cases with high sperm DNA damage [42]. Based on this finding, the notion of selecting sperm without DNA fragmentation for inclusion in ART presents as a valid hypothesis. It is important to note that sperm selection in routine IVF/ICSI is mainly based on motility and morphology assessment at 400× inverted phase contrast microscopy. The same sperm that appears normal at this magnification may have fragmented DNA, one of the late manifestations of apoptosis using the TUNEL assay [43]. Therefore, apoptotic sperm may be used in ART since it appears morphologically normal and motile leading to poor outcomes.

Characteristics of the selected spermatozoa are influenced by semen preparation techniques, and in turn these characteristics will influence the odds for success [44, 45]. Thus, the targeted exclusion of apoptotic spermatozoa by negative selection prior to ART is recommended to ensure that only sperm with the highest fertilization potential is being used. While semen preparation techniques that are routinely used such as density gradient centrifugation and swim-up are capable of selecting motile, morphologically normal sperm [46], they lack the ability to specifically target non-apoptotic spermatozoa. Also, research applications used to identify sperm apoptosis and DNA damage are invasive in nature and rely on sperm fixation and staining leading to sperm damage to the extent that they cannot be used in ART. Alternatively, a noninvasive approach is needed as a feasible approach to select non-apoptotic spermatozoa.

Magnetic Activated Cell Sorting (MACS) for Selection of Non-apoptotic Spermatozoa

Magnetic Activated Cell Sorting (MACS) was proposed as a sperm selection method for isolation of non-apoptotic spermatozoa [47]. The principle of this method depends on labeling the cells that display one of the early markers of apoptosis, externalized phosphatidylserine, with paramagnetic microbeads (~50 nm) conjugated with annexin V. The externalized phosphatidylserine bound to annexin V paramagnetic beads can be separated using a magnetic activated cell sorting system (MACS, Miltenyi Biotec GmbH, Bergisch Gladbach, Germany) [48]. When sperm/bead cell suspension is placed in a column containing iron balls inside a strong magnet, the apoptotic sperm labeled with microbeads will be retained. As the column is rinsed, all the unlabeled sperm will be washed out thoroughly (Fig. 7.2). These unlabeled spermatozoa represent the non-apoptotic fraction which could be used for fertilization in vitro.

MACS as a technique is effective in the removal of apoptotic sperm but lacks the ability to remove white blood cells, immature germ cells, seminal plasma, and other extraneous components of the seminal fluid. Therefore, we proposed to use a combination of 2-layer density gradient centrifugation (DGC) and MACS. The gradient will yield a clean sperm suspension and thereafter MACS will separate non-apoptotic sperm [47]. The average duration for the combined protocol is 50 min including all processing, incubation, and centrifugation steps, which renders this approach simple and fast [49].

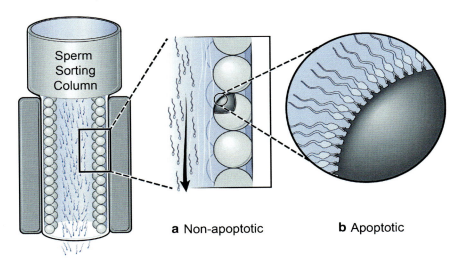

Fig. 7.2 Schematic diagram of magnetic cell separation column. The column which contains steel spheres is placed inside an external magnet. (**a**) The non-labeled cells flow through the column to be collected. (**b**) The immuno-magnetically labeled cells remain attached to the magnetized spheres and are retained inside the column. Reprinted with permission, Cleveland Clinic Center for Medical Art and Photography © 2013. All rights reserved

MACS as a Sperm Selection Method: Proof of Principle

We described the clinical utility of using MACS as a sperm selection method. The proof of principle was documented in a study that showed significantly higher motility and viability in non-apoptotic sperm separated by DGC/MACS combination compared to those prepared by DGC only [47]. As regards sperm morphology, we found no significant difference between non-apoptotic sperm and controls prepared by DGC using the strict morphology criteria; however, there was significant difference in the sperm deformity index (calculated by looking at the percentage of anomalies over the number of sperm evaluated). There was also significant difference as regards the percentage of acrosomal damage and also interestingly as regards the percentage of sperm with cytoplasmic droplets [50].

In support of the proof principle for using MACS, annexin-negative sperm separated by DGC/MACS combination had less apoptosis markers, specifically less expression of caspase-3 and higher mitochondrial membrane potential compared to controls prepared by DGC only. On the other hand, the annexin positive sperm had the highest percentage of expressing apoptosis markers. These findings were consistently reported in fresh and cryopreserved-thawed samples of healthy donors and patients with infertility [51–54]. Similarly, lower values of sperm DNA damage were seen in annexin-negative sperm of healthy donors as well as patients with unexplained infertility [53, 55]. Consistently, the MACS application was capable of enriching samples from men undergoing fertility evaluation with a higher percentage of spermatozoa with intact DNA regardless of sperm concentration, motility and morphology (normozoospermic vs. asthenoteratozoospermic vs. teratozoospermic) [56]. Compared to Zeta potential sperm selection which is based on membrane surface charge, MACS more efficiently selects of sperm with normal acrosome and protamine content [57]. These findings support considering MACS in cases where high sperm DNA fragmentation is suspected.

The benefits of integrating MACS in cryopreservation protocols were also assessed. Non-apoptotic sperm selected by DGC and MACS had the highest motility values before and after cryopreservation compared to samples prepared by DGC only, which was reflected by displaying the highest cryosurvival rates. This could possibly be due to the elimination of apoptotic sperm and sperm with cytoplasmic droplets which would generate reactive oxygen species [54].

In vitro models were used to evaluate the potential benefits of using DGC/MACS in clinical ART. Using the sperm penetration assay, the fertilization potential of sperm separated by MACS was assessed. The percentage of oocytes that showed sperm penetration and the sperm capacitation index were significantly higher in the annexin-negative sperm compared to the annexin-positive and compared to the control fractions prepared by DGC only. To emphasize the impact of apoptosis, the sperm motility and the percentage of intact mitochondria showed significant positive correlation with the number of oocytes penetrated during the sperm penetration assay, while the percentage of activated caspase-3 and externalized phosphatidylserine showed a significant negative correlation [53]. These findings document that spermatozoa with the highest motility and the lowest expression of apoptosis markers will have the highest oocyte penetration.

Sperm chromatin decondensation following hamster oocyte ICSI was also used to evaluate sperm selected by DGC/MACS. In healthy donors, no benefits were observed [53]. However, in infertile men with abnormal sperm parameters, sperm chromatin decondensation after 18 h of hamster oocyte ICSI was significantly higher using sperm selected by DGC/MACS compared to sperm selected by DGC [58]. Thus, it is clearly evident that integrating MACS in sperm selection protocols will yield higher quality spermatozoa in terms of motility, morphology, viability, cryosurvival rates, lesser expression of apoptosis markers including DNA damage, and higher fertilization potential (Table 7.1).

7 Non-apoptotic Sperm Selection

Table 7.1 Summary of studies describing effects of magnetic cell selection of non-apoptotic sperm on sperm parameters

Author, year	Study design	Study population	Outcomes reported
Said et al., 2005 [47]	Prospective, controlled	Healthy donors ($n=15$)	Motility (S) Morphology (NS) Viability (S) Apoptosis markers (MMP, CP-3, EPS) (S)
Said et al., 2005 [54]	Prospective, controlled	Healthy donors ($n=10$)	Motility (S) Sperm cryosurvival rate (NS)
Said et al., 2006 [53]	Prospective, controlled	Healthy donors ($n=35$)	Motility (S) Apoptosis markers (MMP, CP-3, EPS) (S) DNA integrity (S) Oocyte penetration (S) Chromatin decondensation after HICSI (NS)
Said et al., 2006 [72]	Prospective, controlled	Healthy donors ($n=19$)	Motility (S) Sperm recovery rate (NS)
Grunewald et al., 2006 [52]	Prospective, controlled	Healthy donors ($n=10$)	Apoptosis marker (MMP) following cryopreservation (S)
Aziz et al., 2007 [50]	Prospective, controlled	Healthy donors ($n=50$)	Motility (S) Morphology, SDI (S) Apoptosis markers (MMP, CP-3) (S)
Grunewald et al., 2007 [74]	Prospective, controlled	Healthy donors ($n=42$)	Apoptosis markers (MMP, CP-3, EPS) (S)
Grunewald et al., 2008 [75]	Prospective, controlled	Healthy donors ($n=76$)	Apoptosis markers (MMP, CP-3, EPS) (S) Oocyte penetration (S)
Grunewald et al., 2009 [58]	Prospective, controlled	Infertile men with abnormal sperm parameters ($n=21$)	Motility (S) Apoptosis markers (MMP, CP-3) (S) Chromatin decondensation after HICSI (S)
de Vantéry Arrighi et al., 2009 [51]	Prospective, controlled	Men undergoing fertility evaluation ($n=17$)	Apoptosis markers (EPS, MMP) (S)
Lee et al., 2010 [55]	Prospective, controlled	Men from couple with unexplained infertility and 2 failed IUI ($n=60$)	Apoptosis markers (EPS, MMP) (S) DNA integrity (S) IAR (S)
Delbes et al., 2013 [56]	Prospective, controlled	Men undergoing fertility evaluation: Normozoospermic ($n=13$) Asthenozoospermic ($n=17$) Teratozoospermic ($n=12$)	Sperm DNA integrity by SCSA and TUNEL (S in all groups)

ART = assisted reproductive techniques, Bcl = B cell lymphoma protein, CK = creatine kinase, CP-3 = caspase-3, DGC = density gradient centrifugation, EPS = externalized phosphatidylserine, HA = hyaluronic acid, HICSI = hamster oocyte ICSI, HspA2 = heat shock protein, IAR = induced acrosome reaction, ICSI = intracytoplasmic sperm injection, IUI = intrauterine insemination, IVF = in vitro fertilization, MACS = magnetic activated cell sorting, MSOME = motile sperm organelle morphology examination, MMP = mitochondrial membrane potential, NS = no statistically significant difference, S = statistically significant difference, SDI = sperm deformity index, SCSA = sperm chromatin structure assay, TUNEL = terminal deoxynucleotidyl transferase dUTP nick end labeling

MACS as a Sperm Selection Method: Effects on Clinical ART

As regards the effect of MACS sperm selection on ART outcomes, there are reports for improvement of pregnancy rates after IUI in humans and mice [59, 60]. Improvements were also reported after ICSI; however, it is not clear which parameter would benefit the most. One study reported improvement in fertilization rate [61], while another contradicted this finding [62]. Alternatively it showed that the embryo cleavage rates and the pregnancy rates are the parameters that increase the most following MACS [62]. The difference in the quality of patients' sample (normozoospermia vs. abnormal parameters) between these studies could be the reason for the discrepancy. Nevertheless, it is assuring that healthy live births were reported after the use of MACS for sperm selection before ICSI [63, 64].

In an effort to reach a consensus, the current knowledge about the impact of MACS on ART outcomes was defined in a recent meta-analysis. The analysis included five prospective controlled studies that encompassed 499 patients. The findings showed a significantly higher pregnancy rate following MACS, but the same positive effect was not detected for implantation or miscarriage rates [65]. When it comes to which patients would benefit the most from MACS, a large ($n = 172$) case series reported that those with levels of caspase-3 or DNA fragmentation are the ones who highest increase in pregnancy and implantation rates [66]. Similarly, it has been reported that the benefits of using MACS would be mostly recognized in patients with failed IVF/ICSI cycles associated high levels of sperm DNA fragmentation and apoptosis [64, 67]. In support, the potential of MACS technique to improve pregnancy rates in ICSI cycles using sperm samples from patients with high level of sperm DNA fragmentation was recently studied. It was consistently demonstrated that sperm DNA fragmentation was notably lower after MACS technique (13.2 %) than in neat samples (22.6 %). Pregnancy rate in control cycles was 36.6 %, whereas in MACS cycles the pregnancy rate significantly increases to 64.9 % [68].

Future Directions

Although sperm selection using MACS is technically simple and quick, the proposed protocol includes a combination with DGC, which will result in additional technical steps and added processing times. In turn, iatrogenic damage should be ruled out to exclude the occurrence of sperm DNA damage, impaired embryo development and offspring disorders [69–71]. The proposed combined protocol may also result in additional sperm loss and limited recovery of motile sperm. It is estimated that samples processed by DGC and MACS will experience an additional 15 % loss of recovered spermatozoa compared to samples prepared by DGC only [72]. Therefore, samples with limited sperm counts are not the best candidates for this approach of sperm selection. The exact minimum cutoff value remains to be identified.

The integration of MACS as a clinical utility in Andrology Laboratories warrants careful examination of some safety aspects such as unwanted sperm sex selection. Another concern would be the presence of paramagnetic beads in the annexin negative sperm fraction which is used for oocyte fertilization. Although MACS microbeads are biodegradable and do not affect cell viability [73], it is imperative to ensure that no paramagnetic beads will be carried into oocytes during ART. One approach would be to eliminate the possibility of freely floating paramagnetic beads by coating glass wool separation columns with annexin V leading to the retention of apoptotic sperm [74].

In conclusion, isolation of non-apoptotic spermatozoa using MACS has been established in combination with DGC as an effective sperm selection method. The proposed protocol has showed definitive positive outcomes in terms of selecting spermatozoa with higher quality (motility, viability, and morphology), lesser apoptosis manifestations, and higher fertilization potential. The initial results following IVF/ICSI are also very encouraging regarding the beneficial impact of MACS on clinical human ART outcomes. While healthy live births have been reported following MACS application, it is important to note that the technique's safety is not fully established. Also, further confirmation of target cases that would stand to benefit the most is still needed.

References

1. Vaux D, Korsmeyer S. Cell death in development. Cell. 1999;96:245–54.
2. Morrow CM, Hostetler CE, Griswold MD, Hofmann MC, Murphy KM, Cooke PS, Hess RA. ETV5 is required for continuous spermatogenesis in adult mice and may mediate blood testes barrier function and testicular immune privilege. Ann N Y Acad Sci. 2007;1120:144–51.

3. Koksal IT, Ishak Y, Usta M, Danisman A, Guntekin E, Bassorgun IC, Ciftcioglu A. Varicocele-induced testicular dysfunction may be associated with disruption of blood-testis barrier. Arch Androl. 2007;53:43–8.
4. Sakkas D, Moffatt O, Manicardi GC, Mariethoz E, Tarozzi N, Bizzaro D. Nature of DNA damage in ejaculated human spermatozoa and the possible involvement of apoptosis. Biol Reprod. 2002;66:1061–7.
5. Mahfouz RZ, du Plessis SS, Aziz N, Sharma R, Sabanegh E, Agarwal A. Sperm viability, apoptosis, and intracellular reactive oxygen species levels in human spermatozoa before and after induction of oxidative stress. Fertil Steril. 2010;93:814–21.
6. Maione B, Pittoggi C, Achene L, Lorenzini R, Spadafora C. Activation of endogenous nucleases in mature sperm cells upon interaction with exogenous DNA. DNA Cell Biol. 1997;16:1087–97.
7. Taylor SL, Weng SL, Fox P, Duran EH, Morshedi MS, Oehninger S, Beebe SJ. Somatic cell apoptosis markers and pathways in human ejaculated sperm: potential utility as indicators of sperm quality. Mol Hum Reprod. 2004;10:825–34.
8. Scabini M, Stellari F, Cappella P, Rizzitano S, Texido G, Pesenti E. In vivo imaging of early stage apoptosis by measuring real-time caspase-3/7 activation. Apoptosis. 2011;16:198–207.
9. Martinez MM, Reif RD, Pappas D. Early detection of apoptosis in living cells by fluorescence correlation spectroscopy. Anal Bioanal Chem. 2010;396:1177–85.
10. Oosterhuis GJ, Mulder AB, Kalsbeek-Batenburg E, Lambalk CB, Schoemaker J, Vermes I. Measuring apoptosis in human spermatozoa: a biological assay for semen quality? Fertil Steril. 2000;74:245–50.
11. Zhang HB, Lu SM, Ma CY, Wang L, Li X, Chen ZJ. Early apoptotic changes in human spermatozoa and their relationships with conventional semen parameters and sperm DNA fragmentation. Asian J Androl. 2008;10:227–35.
12. Moskovtsev SI, Willis J, Azad A, Mullen JB. Sperm DNA integrity: correlation with sperm plasma membrane integrity in semen evaluated for male infertility. Arch Androl. 2005;51:33–40.
13. Evenson DP, Darzynkiewicz Z, Melamed MR. Simultaneous measurement by flow cytometry of sperm cell viability and mitochondrial membrane potential related to cell motility. J Histochem Cytochem. 1982;30:279–80.
14. Troiano L, Granata AR, Cossarizza A, Kalashnikova G, Bianchi R, Pini G, Tropea F, Carani C, Franceschi C. Mitochondrial membrane potential and DNA stainability in human sperm cells: a flow cytometry analysis with implications for male infertility. Exp Cell Res. 1998;241:384–93.
15. Thornberry N. Caspases: key mediators of apoptosis. Chem Biol. 1998;5:R97–103.
16. Thornberry NA, Lazebnik Y. Caspases: enemies within. Science. 1998;281:1312–6.
17. Paasch U, Grunewald S, Fitzl G, Glander H. Deterioration of plasma membrane is associated with activated caspases in human spermatozoa. J Androl. 2003;24:246–52.
18. Paasch U, Grunewald S, Wuendrich K, Glander HJ. Caspases are associated with apoptosis in human ejaculated spermatozoa and in spermatogenesis. J Androl. 2001;22:91.
19. Paasch U, Grunewald S, Glander H. Presence of up- and downstream caspases in relation to impairment of human spermatogenesis. Andrologia. 2002;34:279.
20. Almeida C, Cardoso MF, Sousa M, Viana P, Goncalves A, Silva J, Barros A. Quantitative study of caspase-3 activity in semen and after swim-up preparation in relation to sperm quality. Hum Reprod. 2005;20:1307–13.
21. Wright VC, Chang J, Jeng G, Macaluso M. Assisted reproductive technology surveillance–United States, 2005. MMWR Surveill Summ. 2008;57:1–23.
22. Seli E, Gardner DK, Schoolcraft WB, Moffatt O, Sakkas D. Extent of nuclear DNA damage in ejaculated spermatozoa impacts on blastocyst development after in vitro fertilization. Fertil Steril. 2004;82:378–83.
23. Barroso G, Taylor S, Morshedi M, Manzur F, Gavino F, Oehninger S. Mitochondrial membrane potential integrity and plasma membrane translocation of phosphatidylserine as early apoptotic markers: a comparison of two different sperm subpopulations. Fertil Steril. 2006;85:149–54.
24. Chen Z, Hauser R, Trbovich AM, Shifren JL, Dorer DJ, Godfrey-Bailey L, Singh NP. The relationship between human semen characteristics and sperm apoptosis: a pilot study. J Androl. 2006;27:112–20.
25. Carrell D, Wilcox A, Lowy L, Peterson C, Jones K, Erickson L, Campbell B, Branch D, Hatasaka H. Elevated sperm chromosome aneuploidy and apoptosis in patients with unexplained recurrent pregnancy loss. Obstet Gynecol. 2003;101:1229–35.
26. Tesarik J, Greco E, Mendoza C. Late, but not early, paternal effect on human embryo development is related to sperm DNA fragmentation. Hum Reprod. 2004;19:611–5.
27. Wu GJ, Chang FW, Lee SS, Cheng YY, Chen CH, Chen IC. Apoptosis-related phenotype of ejaculated spermatozoa in patients with varicocele. Fertil Steril. 2008;91(3):831–7.
28. Tavares RS, Silva AF, Lourenco B, Almeida-Santos T, Sousa AP, Ramalho-Santos J. Evaluation of human sperm chromatin status after selection using a modified Diff-Quik stain indicates embryo quality and pregnancy outcomes following in vitro fertilization. Andrology. 2013;1:830–7.
29. Zorn B, Golob B, Ihan A, Kopitar A, Kolbezen M. Apoptotic sperm biomarkers and their correlation with conventional sperm parameters and male fertility potential. J Assist Reprod Genet. 2012;29:357–64.
30. Host E, Lindenberg S, Smidt-Jensen S. DNA strand breaks in human spermatozoa: correlation with fertilization in vitro in oligozoospermic men and in men with unexplained infertility. Acta Obstet Gynecol Scand. 2000;79:189–93.
31. Host E, Lindenberg S, Smidt-Jensen S. The role of DNA strand breaks in human spermatozoa used for IVF and ICSI. Acta Obstet Gynecol Scand. 2000;79:559–63.

32. Sharbatoghli M, Valojerdi MR, Amanlou M, Khosravi F, Jafar-abadi MA. Relationship of sperm DNA fragmentation, apoptosis and dysfunction of mitochondrial membrane potential with semen parameters and ART outcome after intracytoplasmic sperm injection. Arch Gynecol Obstet. 2012;286:1315–22.
33. Benchaib M, Lornage J, Mazoyer C, Lejeune H, Salle B, Francois Guerin J. Sperm deoxyribonucleic acid fragmentation as a prognostic indicator of assisted reproductive technology outcome. Fertil Steril. 2007;87:93–100.
34. Frydman N, Prisant N, Hesters L, Frydman R, Tachdjian G, Cohen-Bacrie P, Fanchin R. Adequate ovarian follicular status does not prevent the decrease in pregnancy rates associated with high sperm DNA fragmentation. Fertil Steril. 2008;89:92–7.
35. Simon L, Castillo J, Oliva R, Lewis SE. Relationships between human sperm protamines, DNA damage and assisted reproduction outcomes. Reprod Biomed Online. 2011;23:724–34.
36. Virro MR, Larson-Cook KL, Evenson DP. Sperm chromatin structure assay (SCSA) parameters are related to fertilization, blastocyst development, and ongoing pregnancy in in vitro fertilization and intracytoplasmic sperm injection cycles. Fertil Steril. 2004;81:1289–95.
37. Bungum M, Spano M, Humaidan P, Eleuteri P, Rescia M, Giwercman A. Sperm chromatin structure assay parameters measured after density gradient centrifugation are not predictive for the outcome of ART. Hum Reprod. 2008;23:4–10.
38. Gandini L, Lombardo F, Paoli D, Caruso F, Eleuteri P, Leter G, Ciriminna R, Culasso F, Dondero F, Lenzi A, Spano M. Full-term pregnancies achieved with ICSI despite high levels of sperm chromatin damage. Hum Reprod. 2004;19:1409–17.
39. Lin MH, Kuo-Kuang Lee R, Li SH, Lu CH, Sun FJ, Hwu YM. Sperm chromatin structure assay parameters are not related to fertilization rates, embryo quality, and pregnancy rates in in vitro fertilization and intracytoplasmic sperm injection, but might be related to spontaneous abortion rates. Fertil Steril. 2008;90:352–9.
40. Payne JF, Raburn DJ, Couchman GM, Price TM, Jamison MG, Walmer DK. Redefining the relationship between sperm deoxyribonucleic acid fragmentation as measured by the sperm chromatin structure assay and outcomes of assisted reproductive techniques. Fertil Steril. 2005;84:356–64.
41. Collins JA, Barnhart KT, Schlegel PN. Do sperm DNA integrity tests predict pregnancy with in vitro fertilization? Fertil Steril. 2008;89:823–31.
42. Robinson L, Gallos ID, Conner SJ, Rajkhowa M, Miller D, Lewis S, Kirkman-Brown J, Coomarasamy A. The effect of sperm DNA fragmentation on miscarriage rates: a systematic review and meta-analysis. Hum Reprod. 2012;27:2908–17.
43. Barroso G, Valdespin C, Vega E, Kershenovich R, Avila R, Avendano C, Oehninger S. Developmental sperm contributions: fertilization and beyond. Fertil Steril. 2009;92:835–48.
44. Greco E, Scarselli F, Iacobelli M, Rienzi L, Ubaldi F, Ferrero S, Franco G, Anniballo N, Mendoza C, Tesarik J. Efficient treatment of infertility due to sperm DNA damage by ICSI with testicular spermatozoa. Hum Reprod. 2005;20:226–30.
45. Moskovtsev SI, Jarvi K, Mullen JB, Cadesky KI, Hannam T, Lo KC. Testicular spermatozoa have statistically significantly lower DNA damage compared with ejaculated spermatozoa in patients with unsuccessful oral antioxidant treatment. Fertil Steril. 2010;93:1142–6.
46. Le Lannou D, Blanchard Y. Nuclear maturity and morphology of human spermatozoa selected by Percoll density gradient centrifugation or swim-up procedure. J Reprod Fertil. 1988;84:551–6.
47. Said TM, Grunewald S, Paasch U, Glander H-J, Baumann T, Kriegel C, Li L, Agarwal A. Advantage of combining magnetic cell separation with sperm preparation techniques. RBM Online. 2005;10:740–6.
48. Grunewald S, Paasch U, Glander HJ. Enrichment of non-apoptotic human spermatozoa after cryopreservation by immunomagnetic cell sorting. Cell Tissue Bank. 2001;2:127–33.
49. Said TM, Agarwal A, Zborowski M, Grunewald S, Glander HJ, Paasch U. Utility of magnetic cell separation as a molecular sperm preparation technique. J Androl. 2008;29:134–42.
50. Aziz N, Said T, Paasch U, Agarwal A. The relationship between human sperm apoptosis, morphology and the sperm deformity index. Hum Reprod. 2007;22:1413–9.
51. de Vantery Arrighi C, Lucas H, Chardonnens D, de Agostini A. Removal of spermatozoa with externalized phosphatidylserine from sperm preparation in human assisted medical procreation: effects on viability, motility and mitochondrial membrane potential. Reprod Biol Endocrinol. 2009;7:1.
52. Grunewald S, Paasch U, Said TM, Rasch M, Agarwal A, Glander HJ. Magnetic-activated cell sorting before cryopreservation preserves mitochondrial integrity in human spermatozoa. Cell Tissue Bank. 2006;7:99–104.
53. Said TM, Agarwal A, Grunewald S, Rasch M, Baumann T, Kriegel C, Li L, Glander H-J, Thomas Jr A, Paasch U. Selection of non-apoptotic spermatozoa as a new tool for enhancing assisted reproduction outcomes: an in-vitro model. Biol Reprod. 2006;74:530–7.
54. Said TM, Grunewald S, Paasch U, Rasch M, Agarwal A, Glander HJ. Effects of magnetic-activated cell sorting on sperm motility and cryosurvival rates. Fertil Steril. 2005;83:1442–6.
55. Lee TH, Liu CH, Shih YT, Tsao HM, Huang CC, Chen HH, Lee MS. Magnetic-activated cell sorting for sperm preparation reduces spermatozoa with apoptotic markers and improves the acrosome reaction in couples with unexplained infertility. Hum Reprod. 2010;25:839–46.
56. Delbes G, Herrero MB, Troeung ET, Chan PT. The use of complimentary assays to evaluate the enrichment of human sperm quality in asthenoteratozoospermic and teratozoospermic samples processed with Annexin-V magnetic activated cell sorting. Andrology. 2013;1:698–706.

57. Zahedi A, Tavalaee M, Deemeh MR, Azadi L, Fazilati M, Nasr-Esfahani MH. Zeta potential vs apoptotic marker: which is more suitable for ICSI sperm selection? J Assist Reprod Genet. 2013;30:1181–6.
58. Grunewald S, Reinhardt M, Blumenauer V, Said TM, Agarwal A, Abu Hmeidan F, Glander HJ, Paasch U. Increased sperm chromatin decondensation in selected nonapoptotic spermatozoa of patients with male infertility. Fertil Steril. 2009;92:572–7.
59. Khalid SN, Qureshi IZ. Impact of apoptotic sperm population in semen samples on the outcome of pregnancy. Fertil Steril. 2011;96:S59–60.
60. Romany L, Meseguer M, Garcia-Herrero S, Pellicer A, Garrido N. Magnetic activated sorting selection (MACS) of non-apoptotic sperm (NAS) improves pregnancy rates in homologous intrauterine insemination (IUI). preliminary data. Fertil Steril. 2010;94:S14.
61. Arnanz A, Quintana F, Peñalva I, Aspichueta F, Ferrando M, Larreategui Z. Does the use of magnetic activated cell sorting of non-apoptotic spermatozoa improve the fertilization rates in patients with second IVF cycles? Fertil Steril. 2012;98:S106.
62. Dirican EK, Ozgun OD, Akarsu S, Akin KO, Ercan O, Ugurlu M, Camsari C, Kanyilmaz O, Kaya A, Unsal A. Clinical outcome of magnetic activated cell sorting of non-apoptotic spermatozoa before density gradient centrifugation for assisted reproduction. J Assist Reprod Genet. 2008;25:375–81.
63. Polak de Fried E, Denaday F. Single and twin ongoing pregnancies in two cases of previous ART failure after ICSI performed with sperm sorted using annexin V microbeads. Fertil Steril. 2010;94:351.e315–358.
64. Rawe VY, Boudri HU, Sedo CA, Carro M, Papier S, Nodar F. Healthy baby born after reduction of sperm DNA fragmentation using cell sorting before ICSI. Reprod Biomed Online. 2010;20:320–3.
65. Gil M, Sar-Shalom V, Melendez Sivira Y, Carreras R, Checa MA. Sperm selection using magnetic activated cell sorting (MACS) in assisted reproduction: a systematic review and meta-analysis. J Assist Reprod Genet. 2013;30:479–85.
66. Alvarez Sedo C, Uriondo H, Lavolpe M, Noblia F, Papier S, Nodar F. Clinical outcome using non-apoptotic sperm selection for ICSI procedures: report of 1 year experience. Fertil Steril. 2010;94:S232.
67. Herrero MB, Delbes G, Chung JT, Son WY, Holzer H, Buckett W, Chan P. Case report: the use of annexin V coupled with magnetic activated cell sorting in cryopreserved spermatozoa from a male cancer survivor: healthy twin newborns after two previous ICSI failures. J Assist Reprod Genet. 2013;30(11):1415–9.
68. Carchenilla MSC, Agudo D, Rubio S, Becerra D, Bronet F, Garcia-Velasco JA, Pacheco A. Magnetic Activated Cell Sorting (MACS) is a useful technique to improved pregnancy rate in patients with high level of sperm DNA fragmentation. Hum Reprod. 2013;28:i118–37.
69. Marchetti F, Wyrobek AJ. Mechanisms and consequences of paternally-transmitted chromosomal abnormalities. Birth Defects Res C Embryo Today. 2005;75:112–29.
70. Twigg J, Irvine DS, Houston P, Fulton N, Michael L, Aitken RJ. Iatrogenic DNA damage induced in human spermatozoa during sperm preparation: protective significance of seminal plasma. Mol Hum Reprod. 1998;4:439–45.
71. Verhofstad N, Linschooten JO, van Benthem J, Dubrova YE, van Steeg H, van Schooten FJ, Godschalk RW. New methods for assessing male germ line mutations in humans and genetic risks in their offspring. Mutagenesis. 2008;23:241–7.
72. Said TM, Agarwal A, Grunewald S, Rasch M, Glander HJ, Paasch U. Evaluation of sperm recovery following annexin V magnetic-activated cell sorting separation. Reprod Biomed Online. 2006;13:336–9.
73. Miltenyi S, Muller W, Weichel W, Radbruch A. High gradient magnetic cell separation with MACS. Cytometry. 1990;11:231–8.
74. Grunewald S, Miska W, Miska G, Rasch M, Reinhardt M, Glander HJ, Paasch U. Molecular glass wool filtration as a new tool for sperm preparation. Hum Reprod. 2007;22:1405–12.
75. Grunewald S, Said TM, Paasch U, Glander HJ, Agarwal A. Relationship between sperm apoptosis signalling and oocyte penetration capacity. Int J Androl. 2008;31:325–30.

Motile Sperm Organelle Morphology Examination (MSOME)

José Gonçalves Franco Jr.

Introduction

The application of assisted reproduction techniques has provided help to many men seeking to father a child, although the current success of these procedures remains suboptimal. For many years the sperm selection methods were based on washing procedures with subsequent resuspension of the male germ cells. Double density gradient centrifugation and the swim-up procedure were used as standard preparations. Today some protocols allow sperm to be selected according to their ultrastructural morphology.

On the other hand, successful human reproduction relies partly on the inherent integrity of sperm DNA. Clinical evidence has shown that sperm nuclear DNA damage is closely related to male-derived repeated failure of ICSI attempts [1, 2]. It was also noted that the late paternal effect, but not the early one, is associated with increased sperm DNA fragmentation [2]. Sperm DNA damage is associated with a significantly increased risk of pregnancy loss after IVF and ICSI [3, 4].

Therefore, it is now necessary to improve the safety of the sperm selection method. It is urgent to optimize procedures to isolate spermatozoa for ICSI with low risk of DNA damage. In recent years, one technology has attracted the attention of specialists as a method capable of identifying a spermatozoon with low risk of DNA damage: ultrastructural morphology sperm selection at high magnification [5, 6].

Motile Sperm Organelle Morphology Examination (MSOME)

The accuracy with which morphological normality of spermatozoa for ICSI can be assessed depends on the resolution power of the optical magnification system. Conventionally, ICSI is performed with a ×20/×40 objective, resulting in an overall optical magnification of 200–400× [7, 8] (Fig. 8.1). At this magnification, only major sperm morphological defects can be observed, whereas it is more difficult to identify subtle sperm organelle malformations that seem to be related to the ICSI outcome. To test this latter hypothesis, in 2001, Bartoov's group developed a new method of unstained, real-time, high-magnification motile sperm organellar morphology examination called MSOME. High magnification is made possible by the use of an inverted light microscope equipped with high-power Nomarski differential interference contrast optics enhanced by digital imaging to achieve a

J.G. Franco Jr, MD, PhD (✉)
Centre for Human Reproduction 'Professor Franco Jr',
Avenida Joao Fiusa 689, Ribeirão Preto, Sao Paulo, Brazil
e-mail: crh@crh.com.br

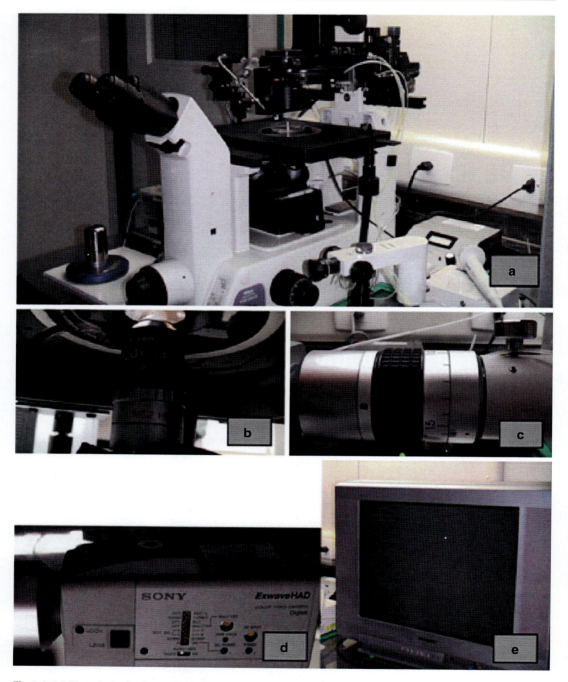

Fig. 8.1 (**a**) The polarization inverted microscope (TE 300 Nikon, Japan) equipped with Hoffman contrast and polarizing lens; (**b**) Hoffman objective of 20×; (**c**) C-mount; (**d**) Camera; and (**e**) 21-inch monitor

magnification of up to 6,600× [5, 6]. Inclusion of MSOME, together with a micromanipulation system, enables the retrieval of a single motile spermatozoon with strictly defined morphologically normal nucleus to be injected into the retrieved oocytes. Bartoov and his group named this modified IVF procedure intracytoplasmic morphologically selected sperm injection (IMSI) [5].

Furthermore, spermatozoa appearing morphologically normal at this magnification (×400) may in fact carry various structural abnormalities that can only be detected at higher optical magnification. The spermatozoa with vacuoles would not be detected in conventional ICSI [7]. This is a serious disadvantage, because microinjection of spermatozoa with vacuolated nuclei has been shown to be associated with low implantation and pregnancy rates, and with early miscarriage [9, 10].

Sperm Preparation and Microscopy Equipment for MSOME

In our laboratory, a 1 µl aliquot of sperm cell suspension was transferred to a 5 µl microdroplet of modified HTF medium containing 7 % polyvinylpyrrolidone solution (PVP medium; Irvine Scientific). This microdroplet was placed in a sterile glass dish (FluoroDish; Word Precision Instrument, USA) under sterile paraffin oil (Ovoil-100; VitroLife, Goteborg, Sweden). The sperm cells, suspended in the microdroplet, were placed on a microscope stage above an Uplan Apo ×100 oil/1.35 objective lens previously covered by a droplet of immersion oil. In this manner, suspended motile sperm cells in the observation droplet could be examined at high magnification by an inverted microscope (Eclipse TE 2000 U; Nikon, Japan) equipped with high-power differential interference contrast optics (DIC/Nomarski). The images were captured by a color video camera containing effective picture elements (pixel) for high-quality image production, and a color video monitor (Fig. 8.2). Morphological evaluation was accomplished on a monitor screen and the total calculated magnification 8,400× (total magnification: objective magnification = 100 × magnification selector = 1.0 × video coupler magnification = 1.0 × calculated video magnification = 84.50) [11, 12].

MSOME Criteria for Selected Sperm Cells

Normal Spermatozoa

A spermatozoon was classified as morphologically normal (Fig. 8.3a) when it exhibited a normal nucleus as well as acrosome, post-acrosomal

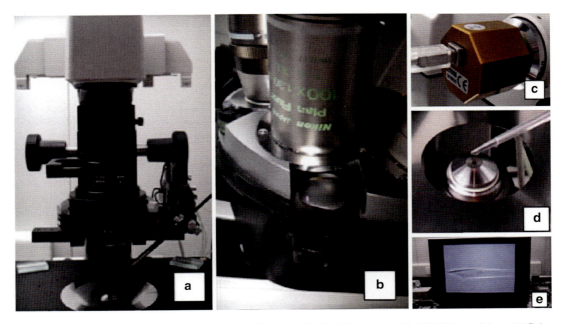

Fig. 8.2 Microscope equipment for MSOME: (**a**) DIC system; (**b**) Plan Fluor Apo ×100 oil/1.35 lens + Prism; (**c**) Color video camera; (**d**) Immersion oil on objective; (**e**) Video monitor 21″

Fig. 8.3 (a) Normal spermatozoa, (b, c); Abnormality of nuclear form: spermatozoa with small or large oval nuclear forms (b); spermatozoa with wide or narrow nuclear forms (c); (d–f) Abnormalities in nuclear chromatin: spermatozoa with regional shape abnormality of nuclear form (d), spermatozoa with vacuoles occupying 5–50 % of the nuclear area (e), spermatozoa with large nuclear vacuoles (>50 % of the nuclear area) (f)

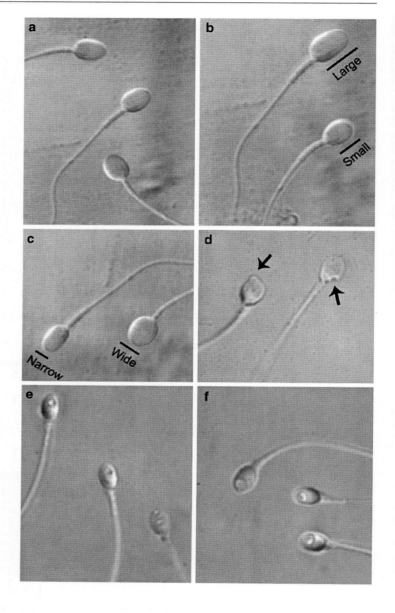

lamina, neck, and tail, besides not presenting a cytoplasmic droplet or cytoplasm around the head [5, 6]. For the nucleus, the morphological state was defined by the form and content of the chromatin. The criterion for normality of nuclear form was a smooth, symmetric, and oval configuration. Normal means for length and width were estimated as 4.75 ± 2.8 and 3.28 ± 0.20 μm, respectively, whereas the form classified as abnormal presented variation of 2SD in at least one of the axes (length: ≥5.31 or ≤4.19 μm, width: >3.7 or <2.9 mm). For rapid evaluation of nuclear form, a fixed, transparent, celluloid form of sperm nucleus fitting the criteria should be superimposed on examined cell (chablon construction based on ASTM E 1951-2). In the same manner, the form of the nucleus was considered normal if no extrusion or invagination of the nuclear chromatin mass had been detected (regional abnormality of nuclear form). Chromatin content was considered normal if the total vacuole area was found to occupy less than 4 % of the nuclear area. A nucleus was considered normal if both nuclear form and chromatin content were normal.

Abnormalities of Nuclear Form

(a) Spermatozoa with small or large oval nuclear forms (Fig. 8.3b). Sperm cells exhibiting an abnormal but oval nuclear shape and a morphologically normal nucleus, content length ≤4.19 or ≥5.31 μm.
(b) Spermatozoa with wide or narrow nuclear forms (Fig. 8.3c). Sperm cells with non-oval, abnormal nuclear shapes, but with normal nuclear content, width: >3.7 or <2.9 mm.
(c) Spermatozoa with regional shape abnormality of nuclear form (Fig. 8.3d). Sperm cells with an extrusion or invagination of the nuclear mass.

Abnormalities of Nuclear Chromatin Content

(a) Spermatozoa with vacuoles occupying >4–50 % of the nuclear area (Fig. 8.3e).
(b) Spermatozoa with large nuclear vacuoles (Fig. 8.3f). sperm cells with vacuoles occupying >50 % of the nuclear area.

Sperm cells with a severe abnormality (such as pin, amorphous, tapered, round, multinucleated head, double tail) easily identified at low magnification (200–400×) were not assessed. The abnormalities observed at high magnification, in both form and nuclear content, also presented normal acrosome, post-acrosomal lamina, neck, and tail, and did not show a cytoplasmic droplet or cytoplasm around the head. Spermatozoids that presented more than one alteration were classified as having the most severe alteration (small/large < wide/narrow < regional shape abnormality < with vacuoles occupying >4–50 % < with vacuoles occupying >50 % of the nuclear area).

MSOME and Sperm Nuclear Vacuoles

One specific sperm malformation, which has been negatively associated with natural male fertility potential, is the presence of large nuclear vacuoles. In 2006, Berkovitz et al. [9] carried out a more specific analysis on the impact of sperm cells with normal nuclear shape but large vacuoles, identified by MSOME, on ICSI pregnancy outcome. They performed a comparative study testing the outcomes of two matched IMSI groups: an experimental group ($n=28$), where spermatozoa with strictly defined normal nuclear shape but large vacuoles were available for oocyte microinjection, and a control group ($n=28$), where strictly defined morphologically normal spermatozoa (including nuclear shape and content) were retrieved for microinjection into the oocytes. Both groups satisfied the following selection criteria: maternal age <40 years and three or more retrieved metaphase II oocytes in the present cycle. As a result, the groups showed no differences as to fertilization, implantation rates, or development of top quality embryos, whereas the pregnancy rate per cycle in the experimental IMSI groups was significantly lower, and the early miscarriage rate per pregnancy was significantly higher than that of the control group (18 % versus 50 %, $p<0.01$, and 80 % versus 7 %, respectively, $p<0.01$). In this work, therefore, retrieval of spermatozoa with strictly normal nuclear shape but large vacuoles appeared to reduce ICSI pregnancy outcome and to be associated with early miscarriage. In fact, embryo development seemed normal at the early stages (no differences in top quality embryos, normal fertilization, or implantation), whereas it seemed impaired at the later ones (low pregnancy and high miscarriage rates).

On the other hand, the rate of vacuolated spermatozoa increases with the patient's age, regardless of vacuole size (occupying less or more than 4 % of the sperm head area) [13]. The rate of spermatozoa containing large vacuoles (≥50 % of sperm head area) also increases with patient's age [14]. The vacuole area increased significantly when semen parameters were impaired. These impairments included a decrease in sperm concentration, altered vitality, and a reduced number of spermatozoa with normal morphology [15].

There is evidence that DNA damage may derive from abnormal chromatin packaging due to underprotamination, which induces DNA strand breaks [16, 17]. In the same way, Franco Jr et al. [18] showed that the presence of large nuclear vacuoles reflects the presence of abnormal chromatin packaging, which may facilitate sperm DNA damage.

At the level of the sperm cell, the presence of large sperm head vacuoles can be considered a potential indicator of sperm nuclear abnormalities (chromatin descondensation). At the level of the male population, these vacuoles relate particular male infertility factors (age, abnormal chromatin compaction, increased DNA fragmentation, and abnormal conventional semen parameters). However, the evaluation of sperm head vacuoles in daily practice remains nondefinitely standardized, with varying methods being used [15, 19].

In addition, according to Berkovitz et al. [20] sperm nucleus morphological normality, assessed at high magnification, could decrease the prevalence of major fetal malformations in ICSI offspring. Recently, Cassuto et al. [21] compared the risk of major malformations of children born after standard ICSI and after IMSI, a prospective population-based study was conducted from 2005 to 2010. ICSI and IMSI were performed in only one assisted reproduction unit. Medical data and follow up during 2 years of 1028 infants were collected. Major malformations were identified and classified by an external independent physician. The two groups were similar concerning the parent's age, treatment, number of oocytes recovered, days of transfer, gestational age, and birthweight. However, major malformations were significantly lower with IMSI (4/450, 1.33 %) versus ICSI (22.578, 3.80 %) (adjusted odds ratio 2.84, 95 % confidential interval 0.14–0.87, $p = 0.014$).

MSOME and Embryo Development

Recently, it has been demonstrated that IMSI has no significant effect on embryo quality at day 2 in relation to the conventional ICSI procedure [22]. In addition, a relationship has been shown between defective spermatozoa and higher early miscarriage rates, despite the apparent lack of decrease in embryo quality on day 3 [10]. Based on the hypothesis that the employment of spermatozoa with large nuclear vacuoles would not produce any early paternal effects on embryo development (up to day 3), Vanderzwalmen and his group [23] investigated the possible influence of such nuclear vacuoles on the embryo's competence to develop to the blastocyst stage; according to the researchers this may suggest a late paternal influence on embryo development after paternal DNA content begins to contribute to such advancement at around day 3 after fertilization. The outcome of embryo development (until day 5) was assessed in a group of 25 patients who underwent sibling oocyte microinjection with four different grades of sperm cells: (1) grade I (absence of vacuoles); (2) grade II (≤ 2 small vacuoles); (3) grade III (>2 small vacuoles or ≥ 1 large vacuole); and (4) grade IV (large vacuoles with abnormal head shape or other abnormalities). Small (<4 % of the head volume) and large vacuoles were defined according the classification of Bartoov [5, 6], while grading was performed between 6,000× and 12,000× high magnification. To reduce the influence of female factor infertility, the inclusion criteria were female age less than 40 years and availability of at least eight oocytes at retrieval. As a whole, the four groups did not differ significantly as to the number of zygotes and embryo development up to day 3, including the subgroup analysis; on the contrary, the data showed highly significant differences in the development to blastocysts and the blastocyst quality among the four grades ($p < 0.001$). On the other hand, comparing the groups one by one with regard to development to blastocysts, statistically significant differences were found between groups I (56.3 %) and II (61.4 %) and between groups III (5.1 %) and IV (0 %). Even when combining the groups into pairs, no significant difference in terms of embryo development to day 3 was seen (group I/II: 87.1 % versus group III/IV: 66.7 %), whereas the incidence of blastocyst and good quality blastocyst formation was significantly different between combined grades I/II and grades III/IV spermatozoa (43.5 and 19.1 % versus 10.1 and 2.9 % respectively, $p < 0.001$). Based on these results, the researchers postulated that the size and number of sperm nuclear vacuoles, identified accurately at high magnification, negatively affected blastocyst development, especially after a day-3 embryo transfer, and reinforced previous studies suggesting the paternal effects on initial embryonic development [23, 24].

MSOME for Routine Laboratory Semen Analysis

Although MSOME was initially developed by its creator only as a selection criterion [5], its application as a morphological semen classification method could represent an improvement in routine laboratory sperm analysis, with potential clinical implications, especially in the field of medically assisted reproduction. In the past, only one study [6] has examined the relationship between normal spermatozoa obtained by the WHO routine method [25] and by MSOME in 20 patients. As a result, no significant correlation was found between the incidence of morphologically normal spermatozoa as defined by the WHO and by MSOME. Nevertheless, routine analysis reported a significantly higher percentage of sperm normality in relation to MSOME. However, Oliveira et al. [26] adopted a similar approach, evaluating the correlation between MSOME classification and a highly diffuse sperm morphology classification (Tygerberg criteria) [27], in order to better understand the potential diagnostic/prognostic value of the MSOME method. The study design included 97 randomly selected semen samples. Regression analysis showed a significant positive correlation between the incidence of normal sperm forms by Tygerberg criteria and that obtained by MSOME ($r=0.83$; 95 % CI: 0.75–0.88; $p<0.0001$). Similarly to the work presented by Bartoov et al. [6], the MSOME criteria appear to be much more restrictive, presenting significantly lower sperm normality percentages for the semen samples in comparison to those found after routine analysis by the Tygerberg classification (3.3±3.2 %, range 0–18 %; and 9.4±4.8 %, range 2–23 % respectively, $p<0.0001$). Based on these results, the researchers postulated that despite the high positive correlation, MSOME represented a much stricter evaluation criterion for sperm morphology, since its resolution power ($\geq 6,000\times$) enabled the identification of vacuoles and chromatin abnormalities that could not be described with the same accuracy by a Tygerberg method analysis. In addition, its focus on motile sperm fractions could only represent an additional advantage for MSOME by providing information on the fertilization and development potential of the sample fraction referred for assisted reproduction treatment. Therefore, our group stressed the importance of not only including MSOME among the criteria for routine laboratory semen analysis, but of performing this step prior to the conventional ICSI procedure [26].

In 2006, Hazout et al. [10] reported a positive association between high-magnification selection of sperm cells with normal nuclear shape and pregnancy outcome in patients with repeated conventional ICSI failures; in a subgroup of patients ($n=72$) involved in the study, the level of sperm DNA integrity (by TUNEL assay) was assessed, and the outcomes of IMSI could be compared in patients with several degrees of sperm DNA damage. The improvement of clinical ICSI outcomes was evident both in patients with an elevated degree of sperm DNA fragmentation and in those with normal sperm DNA status.

In 2008, Franco et al. [11] compared the amount of DNA fragmentation (by TUNEL assay) and the incidence of denatured single-stranded or normal double-stranded DNA (by acridine orange fluorescence method) in sperm cells characterized by the presence of large nuclear vacuoles (LNV group) and in strictly morphologically normal spermatozoa (NN group), both selected at high magnification ($8,400\times$). The analyses were carried out on fresh semen samples of 30 unselected patients. The authors reported a significantly higher level of DNA fragmentation in LNV sperm cells than in NN spermatozoa (29.1 % versus 15.9 %, $p<0.0001$). In addition, the LNV group also showed a significantly increased amount of single-stranded denatured DNA with respect to the NN sperm cells (67.9 % versus 33.1 %, $p<0.0001$). Thus, we postulated that the high levels of denatured DNA in LNV sperm cells pointed to early decondensation and disaggregation of sperm chromatin fibers: an unwanted high degree of sperm decondensation could result in asynchronous chromosome decondensation, and may lead to cytoplasmic fragments in the embryo [28]. Therefore, the data presented stressed the link between the presence of large nuclear vacuoles and increased DNA damage in sperm cells and supported the routine selection of morphologically motile spermatozoa at high magnification (by MSOME) before conventional ICSI. A similar approach was adopted by Garolla et al. [29] in particular, after observation via a high magnification system ($\times 13{,}000$), 20 strictly morphologically normal sperm cells (for acrosome, head, neck, and tail, including those cells which had large nuclear vacuoles, but were otherwise normal) were selected from each semen sample of ten patients with severe testicular alteration and absent sperm motility: ten with normal morphology and no vacuoles (group A) and ten with normal morphology and at least one large head vacuole (group B), for a total of 200 sperm cells. Each spermatozoon was studied for mitochondrial membrane potential, DNA integrity (by acridine orange staining), DNA fragmentation (by TUNEL assay), and sperm aneuploidies (by FISH analysis). The data showed that single cells from group A exhibited a significantly better physiological status than cells from group B with regard to mitochondrial function, DNA integrity, and DNA fragmentation (13.3 ± 4.9 % versus 52.2 ± 14.7 %, 5.3 ± 3.0 % versus 71.9 ± 11.1 %, and 9.3 ± 4.8 % versus 40.1 ± 11.6 % respectively, all $p<0.001$). No chromosomal alteration was present in cells from group A. Therefore, although the study was conducted on a highly restricted number of cells, the results strengthened the concept of an association between the incidence of sperm DNA damage and the presence of nuclear vacuoles and stressed the importance of a morphological selection by high-magnification microscopy [24].

In conclusion, all the publications [7, 9, 10, 30–32] about IMSI reported not only better results as to implantation and clinical pregnancy rates but also a reduction in the miscarriage rates in couples whose sperm cells were strictly morphologically selected at high magnification (MSOME). In addition, the IMSI procedure improved the clinical ICSI outcome in patients with several degrees of sperm DNA damage.

It has been reported that the presence of vacuoles could reflect molecular anomalies responsible for abnormal chromatin remodeling during the sperm maturation process and may contribute to making the spermatozoa more susceptible to sperm DNA impairment. The current results establish a crucial association between normal blastocyst development and both the number and size of vacuoles, indicating that routine morphological analysis of sperm cells, performed at high magnification ($6{,}000\times$), is of fundamental importance to improving the embryo implantation potential. In addition, the presence of vacuoles in the nuclei of spermatozoa is also associated with reduced pregnancy and with a high level of DNA damage.

Conclusions

Spermatozoa appearing morphologically normal at a magnification of $\times 400$ may in fact carry various structural abnormalities. With the advent of MSOME it is now possible to analyze the spermatozoa under high-magnification, which allows the detection of nuclear vacuoles that may affect the ICSI outcomes. In light of the findings, the MSOME method seems to be a powerful tool for selecting strictly morphologically normal spermatozoa, with a lower incidence of DNA defects that cannot be detected at routine ICSI magnification.

References

1. Tesarik J. Paternal effects on cell division in the human preimplantation embryo. Reprod Biomed Online. 2005;10(3):370–5.
2. Tesarik J, Greco E, Mendoza C. Late, but not early, paternal effect on human embryo development is related to sperm DNA fragmentation. Hum Reprod. 2004;19(3):611–5.

3. Robinson L, Gallos ID, Conner SJ, Rajkhowa M, Miller D, Lewis S, et al. The effect of sperm DNA fragmentation on miscarriage rates: a systematic review and meta-analysis. Hum Reprod. 2012;27(10):2908–17.
4. Zini A, Boman JM, Belzile E, Ciampi A. Sperm DNA damage is associated with an increased risk of pregnancy loss after IVF and ICSI: systematic review and meta-analysis. Hum Reprod. 2008;23(12):2663–8.
5. Bartoov B, Berkovitz A, Eltes F. Selection of spermatozoa with normal nuclei to improve the pregnancy rate with intracytoplasmic sperm injection. N Engl J Med. 2001;345(14):1067–8.
6. Bartoov B, Berkovitz A, Eltes F, Kogosowski A, Menezo Y, Barak Y. Real-time fine morphology of motile human sperm cells is associated with IVF-ICSI outcome. J Androl. 2002;23(1):1–8.
7. Bartoov B, Berkovitz A, Eltes F, Kogosovsky A, Yagoda A, Lederman H, et al. Pregnancy rates are higher with intracytoplasmic morphologically selected sperm injection than with conventional intracytoplasmic injection. Fertil Steril. 2003;80(6):1413–9.
8. De Vos A, Van De Velde H, Joris H, Verheyen G, Devroey P, Van Steirteghem A. Influence of individual sperm morphology on fertilization, embryo morphology, and pregnancy outcome of intracytoplasmic sperm injection. Fertil Steril. 2003;79(1):42–8.
9. Berkovitz A, Eltes F, Ellenbogen A, Peer S, Feldberg D, Bartoov B. Does the presence of nuclear vacuoles in human sperm selected for ICSI affect pregnancy outcome? Hum Reprod. 2006;21(7):1787–90.
10. Hazout A, Dumont-Hassan M, Junca AM, Cohen Bacrie P, Tesarik J. High-magnification ICSI overcomes paternal effect resistant to conventional ICSI. Reprod Biomed Online. 2006;12(1):19–25.
11. Franco Jr JG, Baruffi RL, Mauri AL, Petersen CG, Oliveira JB, Vagnini L. Significance of large nuclear vacuoles in human spermatozoa: implications for ICSI. Reprod Biomed Online. 2008;17(1):42–5.
12. Mauri AL, Oliveira JB, Baruffi RL, Petersen CG, Vagnini LD, Massaro FC, et al. Significance of extruded nuclear chromatin (regional nuclear shape malformation) in human spermatozoa: implications for ICSI. Int J Androl. 2011;34(6 Pt 1):594–9.
13. de Almeida Ferreira Braga DP, Setti AS, Figueira RC, Nichi M, Martinhago CD, Iaconelli Jr A, et al. Sperm organelle morphologic abnormalities: contributing factors and effects on intracytoplasmic sperm injection cycles outcomes. Urology. 2011;78(4):786–91.
14. Silva LF, Oliveira JB, Petersen CG, Mauri AL, Massaro FC, Cavagna M, et al. The effects of male age on sperm analysis by motile sperm organelle morphology examination (MSOME). Reprod Biol Endocrinol. 2012;10:19.
15. Perdrix A, Saidi R, Menard JF, Gruel E, Milazzo JP, Mace B, et al. Relationship between conventional sperm parameters and motile sperm organelle morphology examination (MSOME). Int J Androl. 2012; 35(4):491–8.
16. Sakkas D, Urner F, Bizzaro D, Manicardi G, Bianchi PG, Shoukir Y, et al. Sperm nuclear DNA damage and altered chromatin structure: effect on fertilization and embryo development. Hum Reprod. 1998;13 Suppl 4:11–9.
17. Plastira K, Msaouel P, Angelopoulou R, Zanioti K, Plastiras A, Pothos A, et al. The effects of age on DNA fragmentation, chromatin packaging and conventional semen parameters in spermatozoa of oligoasthenoteratozoospermic patients. J Assist Reprod Genet. 2007;24(10):437–43.
18. Franco Jr JG, Mauri AL, Petersen CG, Massaro FC, Silva LF, Felipe V, et al. Large nuclear vacuoles are indicative of abnormal chromatin packaging in human spermatozoa. Int J Androl. 2012;35(1):46–51.
19. Perdrix A, Rives N. Motile sperm organelle morphology examination (MSOME) and sperm head vacuoles: state of the art in 2013. Hum Reprod Update. 2013;19(5):527–41.
20. Berkovitz A, Eltes F, Paul M, Adrian E, Bartoov B. The chance of having a healthy normal child following intracytoplasmic morphologically-selected sperm injection (IMSI) treatment is higher compared to conventional IVF-ICSI treatment. Fertil Steril. 2007;88:S20.
21. Cassuto NG, Hazout A, Bouret D, Balet R, Larue L, Benifla JL, et al. Low birth defects by deselecting abnormal spermatozoa before ICSI. Reprod Biomed Online. 2013;28(1):47–53.
22. Mauri AL, Petersen CG, Oliveira JB, Massaro FC, Baruffi RL, Franco Jr JG. Comparison of day 2 embryo quality after conventional ICSI versus intracytoplasmic morphologically selected sperm injection (IMSI) using sibling oocytes. Eur J Obstet Gynecol Reprod Biol. 2010;150(1):42–6.
23. Vanderzwalmen P, Hiemer A, Rubner P, Bach M, Neyer A, Stecher A, et al. Blastocyst development after sperm selection at high magnification is associated with size and number of nuclear vacuoles. Reprod Biomed Online. 2008;17(5):617–27.
24. Nadalini M, Tarozzi N, Distratis V, Scaravelli G, Borini A. Impact of intracytoplasmic morphologically selected sperm injection on assisted reproduction outcome: a review. Reprod Biomed Online. 2009;19 Suppl 3:45–55.
25. WHO. WHO laboratory manual for the examination of human semen and sperm-cervical mucus interaction. 4th ed. Cambridge: Published on behalf of the World Health Organization by Cambridge University Press; 1999. p. 128.
26. Oliveira JB, Massaro FC, Mauri AL, Petersen CG, Nicoletti AP, Baruffi RL, et al. Motile sperm organelle morphology examination is stricter than Tygerberg criteria. Reprod Biomed Online. 2009;18(3):320–6.
27. Menkveld R, Stander FS, Kotze TJ, Kruger TF, van Zyl JA. The evaluation of morphological characteristics of human spermatozoa according to stricter criteria. Hum Reprod. 1990;5(5):586–92.
28. Menezo YJ, Hazout A, Panteix G, Robert F, Rollet J, Cohen-Bacrie P, et al. Antioxidants to reduce sperm DNA fragmentation: an unexpected adverse effect. Reprod Biomed Online. 2007;14(4):418–21.

29. Garolla A, Fortini D, Menegazzo M, De Toni L, Nicoletti V, Moretti A, et al. High-power microscopy for selecting spermatozoa for ICSI by physiological status. Reprod Biomed Online. 2008;17(5):610–6.
30. Antinori M, Licata E, Dani G, Cerusico F, Versaci C, d'Angelo D, et al. Intracytoplasmic morphologically selected sperm injection: a prospective randomized trial. Reprod Biomed Online. 2008;16(6):835–41.
31. Wilding M, Coppola G, di Matteo L, Palagiano A, Fusco E, Dale B. Intracytoplasmic injection of morphologically selected spermatozoa (IMSI) improves outcome after assisted reproduction by deselecting physiologically poor quality spermatozoa. J Assist Reprod Genet. 2011;28(3):253–62.
32. Knez K, Tomazevic T, Zorn B, Vrtacnik-Bokal E, Virant-Klun I. Intracytoplasmic morphologically selected sperm injection improves development and quality of preimplantation embryos in teratozoospermia patients. Reprod Biomed Online. 2012;25(2): 168–79.

Setup of Micromanipulator for Sperm Selection and Injection for IMSI: Configuring the Microscope for Intracytoplasmic Morphology-Selected Sperm Injection (IMSI)

Lynne Chang and Joseph G. LoBiondo

Introduction

Sperm morphology is an important prognostic factor in the diagnosis of male fertility and has been shown to influence in vitro pregnancy outcomes [1–3]. Intracytoplasmic sperm injection (ICSI) is a technique that was introduced in 1992 and involves the selection of morphologically normal and motile sperm under a ~200–400× magnification for microinjection into the oocyte [4]. This type of sperm selection has been reported to improve assisted treatment outcomes [5, 6] and has become a common procedure in the in vitro fertilization (IVF) process.

Sperm quality may be evaluated through a number of criteria such as maturity, sperm count, motility, and morphology. For example, sperm with severely abnormal head shape such as pin, amorphous, tapered, round, and multinucleated have been shown to reduce implantation and reproduction rates and are rejected during selection for ICSI. These defects can be identified using microscopic observation at relatively low magnifications. However, even sperm that appear normal at low magnifications may have subtle organelle defects in the sperm head or sperm surface that prevent fertilization.

Since the introduction of ICSI, a higher magnification examination method of sperm morphology called MSOME, for motile sperm organelle morphology examination, was developed [7]. MSOME utilizes high-power light microscopy coupled with digital magnification to examine sperm morphology at ~6,000 times magnification. At these higher magnifications, it is possible to identify sperm whose nuclei have abnormal shapes or contents and are less likely to produce a healthy embryo [8]. The MSOME criteria are based on the morphological status of six subcellular organelles comprising the acrosome, post-acrosomal lamina, neck, mitochondria, tail, and nucleus. Studies have shown that nuclear shape and the state of chromatin condensation as determined by the number and size of vacuoles present in the nucleus appear to be the most important parameters in influencing fertilization and pregnancy rates [7] (Fig. 9.1). The MSOME approach was subsequently adopted for the sperm selection process that precedes micro-injection, leading to the development of an advanced form of ICSI called IMSI, or intracytoplasmic morphologically selected sperm injection [9]. In IMSI, sperm morphology is examined and selected at high magnification prior to microinjection into the oocyte.

L. Chang, PhD (✉) • J.G. LoBiondo
Microscopy Product & Marketing,
Nikon Instruments, Inc., 1300 Walt Whitman Road,
Melville, NY 11747, USA
e-mail: lchang@nikon.net; jlobiondo@nikon.net

Fig. 9.1 Images of sperm generated by DIC microscopy. Panel (**a**) shows sperm visualized with a 60× oil immersion objective. Panel (**b**) shows abnormal sperm containing nuclear vacuoles, visualized with a 100× oil immersion lens

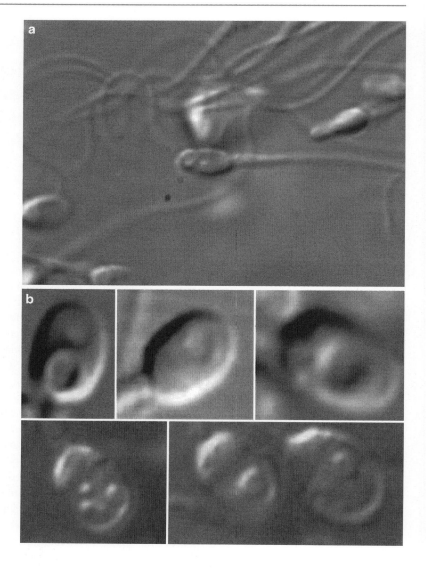

In the following sections, we will provide an overview of the techniques used for generating high-contrast, high-magnification images and microscope instrumentation and accessories required for performing IMSI.

Hoffman Modulation Contrast in ICSI

Most living cells including spermatozoa and oocytes appear transparent when observed by brightfield illumination as differences in light absorption between the cell and its surrounding medium, as well as between subcellular components are almost negligible. Therefore, various types of contrasting methods have been developed for the light microscope to amplify minute differences and generate contrast in unstained biological specimens. In ICSI, a simple contrasting method originally developed by Robert Hoffman in 1975 termed Hoffman Modulation Contrast (HMC) is typically used to generate the contrast necessary to visualize sperm morphology at low magnifications and to perform microinjection of selected sperm cells into oocytes.

9 Setup of Micromanipulator for Sperm Selection and Injection for IMSI...

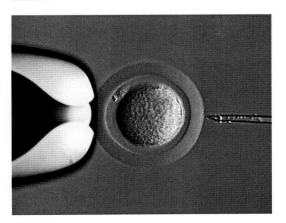

Fig. 9.2 An image of an oocyte being microinjected acquired using a Nikon Advanced Modulation Contrast imaging system. Note the shadowed pseudo relief effect and level of detail present in the image

Since the advent of HMC, various manufacturers have introduced variants of this technique including the Nikon Advanced Modulation Contrast (NAMC) system.

The HMC method and its variants detect and convert phase gradients present in the sample into variations in light intensity to generate a pseudo three-dimensional image (see Fig. 9.2). The basic microscope configuration for HMC is a brightfield microscope with two additional components, a slit aperture inserted at the front focal plane of the condenser and a HMC objective lens which contains a modulator or optical amplitude filter installed at its back focal plane. The modulator in the objective lens contains dark, gray, and clear zones, each of which transmit light to different extents. In this basic HMC configuration, the slit aperture is positioned within the gray area of the modulator. Zero order light, or undeflected light from the background or flat areas of the specimen, are thereby assigned a neutral gray intensity. As light passes through a specimen containing phase gradients, these gradients will deflect light into either the dark or clear zones of the modulator in the objective lens depending on the direction of the gradient present in the sample, resulting in generation of contrast dictated by the position and slope of the phase gradients in the specimen. In more modern advanced modulation contrast systems, both the condenser slit aperture and the modulator at the back focal plane of the objective lens are offset from the optical axis of the microscope, resulting in improved spatial resolution and detail (Fig. 9.3). In addition, the slit aperture is partially covered by a small piece of polarizer and a circular polarizer is inserted between the illumination light source and the slit aperture (Fig. 9.3). By rotating the circular polarizer and its vibration direction relative to the fixed polarizer in the slit aperture, one can effectively change the width of the slit and consequently the amount of contrast in the image. "Narrowing" the slit by rotating the circular polarizer such that its vibration direction is 90° to that of the polarizer in the slit aperture, results in increased contrast and improved optical sectioning. When the circular polarizer is oriented such that its vibration direction is parallel to that of the polarizer in the slit, the effective width of the slit is at its maximum and this configuration results in reduced contrast. However, the "wider" slit aperture improves images of thicker objects where large differences in refractive index exist.

Nikon's NAMC system consists of a brightfield microscope equipped with NAMC objective lenses, matching condenser slit apertures, and a rotatable polarizer between the light source and the condenser slit aperture to vary the width of the slit aperture and the resulting degree of contrast (Fig. 9.3a). As the slit aperture is different for each objective of different magnification, most modern modulation contrast microscope systems also utilize a condenser "turret" that can hold multiple slit apertures to match a variety of objective lenses (Figs. 9.3a and 9.4). In the NAMC system, both the condenser slit modules and the modulators inside the objective lenses can be individually rotated to achieve the same directionality in the pseudo shadow-cast appearance for different objective lenses. By positioning the modulator/slit aperture combination in a perpendicular orientation to the microinjector pipettes, the contrast produced by the highly refractive glass can be minimized and the contrast at the tip of the pipette maximized. Further, by orienting the modulator/slit aperture combination in the same direction for all magnification objectives, quick magnification changes can be

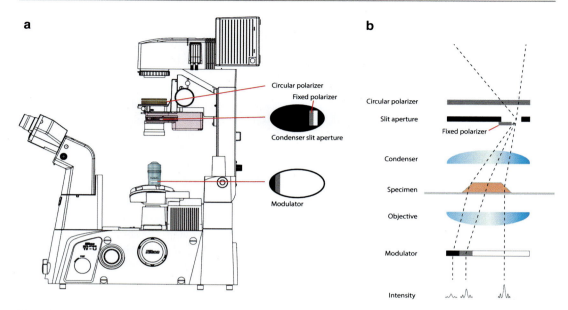

Fig. 9.3 Hoffman Modulation Contrast (and NAMC) system. Panel (**a**) shows the Hoffman modulation contrast components in a typical inverted microscope setup. The first polarizer is highlighted in *yellow*; the condenser slit aperture is housed in a turret (*pink*) between the polarizer and the condenser lens. The modulator or optical amplitude filter is housed inside a Hoffman or NAMC objective lens (*blue*), at the back aperture plane of the objective. Panel (**b**) shows the deflection of oblique light rays by phase gradients in the sample, resulting in differential modulation of amplitudes

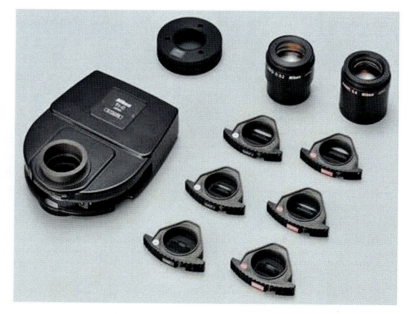

Fig. 9.4 NAMC components. A condenser turret is shown on the *left*, an NAMC polarizer on *top*, two types of condensers to its right and six different condenser slit apertures

made without the need to re-position the contrast control polarizer.

The majority of modulation contrast objective lenses are achromats and planachromats. These types of lenses are designed with a minimal level of correction for optical aberrations but provide high transmission of light. When using achromats or planachromats for modulation contrast, using a green filter placed between the illumination light source and the polarizer can significantly improve image quality as these lenses have been corrected for spherical aberration in the color green. Spherical aberration, when present, leads to blurriness in the image. However, many major microscope manufacturers also offer modulation contrast objectives such as fluorites that are designed with a higher degree of correction for optical aberrations. For example, Nikon offers 20× and 40× Plan Fluor ELWD objectives in addition to 10×, 20×, and 40× Achromat LWD objectives.

Images obtained by HMC and NAMC contain excellent specimen detail and contrast and do not suffer from annoying halo effects often encountered with other contrasting techniques such as phase contrast. In addition, unlike other contrasting techniques in which the sample is placed between two polarizers, HMC or NAMC is not affected by the presence of birefringent materials such as plastic culture dishes in or near the sample plane since the specimen is not placed between the two polarizers. The cost of modulation contrast accessories is also considerably lower than some other contrasting techniques. However, to generate the high level of detail necessary for evaluating sperm morphology based on MSOME criteria, a different type of contrast technique called differential interference contrast, or DIC, is used during IMSI as described in the following section.

Differential Interference Contrast in IMSI and Switching from MSOME to Microinjection

In order to achieve the high level of detail required for sperm selection based on MSOME criteria, a high numerical aperture, 60× or 100×, oil immersion DIC objective lens is typically used. DIC, or differential interference contrast, utilizes a beam-shearing interference system to generate a monochromatic shadow-cast image that effectively displays the gradient of optical paths as contrast. The images produced by DIC are not unlike those produced by HMC or NAMC in their pseudo shadow-cast appearance. However, the mechanisms of contrast generation are completely different. Unlike in HMC or NAMC, the optical components required for DIC microscopy do not obstruct or mask the objective and condenser diaphragms and thus enable their full numerical apertures to be utilized. This results in a significant improvement in resolution. By using high numerical aperture objective and condenser lenses, very fine gradients in optical paths can be detected and translated to contrast in the resulting image (see Fig. 9.1 for examples of sperm imaged by DIC). In extreme high-resolution versions of DIC, mainly used in cell biology and biophysics fields, even single microtubules of 25 nm width can be visualized.

The basic optical components required for achieving DIC are a strain-free objective lens, usually specified as a DIC lens, two matched birefringent prisms (specific for the objective lens) and two polarizers (the second polarizer is commonly referred to as an "analyzer"). See Fig. 9.5a for the locations of the following DIC components on a typical inverted microscope.

- *Linear Polarizer*: The first polarizer, installed between the illumination light source and the condenser turret acts to produce the necessary plane-polarized light for interference imaging.
- *Condenser Prism*: Linear polarized light leaving the first polarizer is sheared into orthogonal polarized components by the first prism housed in the condenser turret near the front focal plane of the condenser. The prisms used in DIC are birefringent compound prisms termed Nomarski (or Wollaston) prisms that act to shear incident plane polarized light into orthogonal polarized components which are spatially separated by a miniscule distance that is typically less than a micrometer. The degree of shear of the condenser prism is dictated by the numerical aperture of the objective to be used. Different numerical aperture

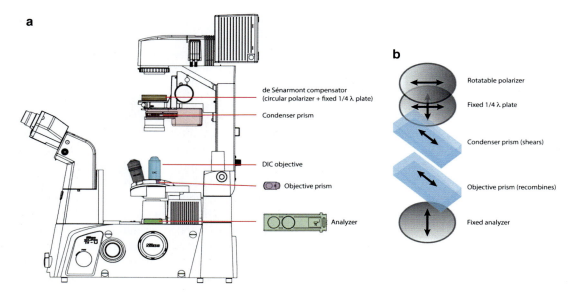

Fig. 9.5 Differential Interference Contrast setup. Panel (**a**) shows the DIC components on a typical inverted microscope. In this example, a de Sénarmont compensator (*yellow*) consisting of a rotating polarizer and fixed ¼ λ plate is positioned between the light source and the condenser turret (*pink*). The first Nomarski prism (condenser prism) is housed in the condenser turret (*pink*) while the second Nomarski prism (objective prism; *purple*) is located in the nosepiece, just underneath the DIC objective (*blue*). The analyzer is located underneath the nosepiece, usually in a manual slider (*green*) or in a filter turret (not shown). Panel (**b**) shows the vibrational axes of the polarizer and analyzer (at 90° to each other) and the shear axes of the prisms, which are oriented at a 45° angle to the polarizer and analyzer. The ¼ wavelength retardation plate is oriented such that its slow axis is parallel to the analyzer and its fast axis is parallel to the polarizer. On a Nikon system configured for both DIC and NAMC, switching from DIC imaging (for MSOME) to NAMC microscopy for microinjection is relatively simple. The user simply rotates the nosepiece to position the NAMC objective lens in the light path, rotates the condenser turret to select for the appropriate slit aperture for the NAMC lens, and pulls out the analyzer (or rotates the filter turret to move the analyzer out of the light path; not shown)

objectives have corresponding prisms often designated as "DIC L" (<0.5 N.A.), "DIC M" (>0.5 to 0.9 N.A.) and "DIC H" (>0.9 N.A.).

- *Objective Prism*: These sheared, orthogonally polarized wavefront pairs then illuminate the specimen and are recombined by a matched, inverted Nomarski prism that's housed near the back focal plane of the objective lens. In a Nikon DIC system, the second inverted prism is installed in a slot underneath the objective lens in the nosepiece turret. This configuration allows for easy removal of the prism for non-DIC applications such as fluorescence. Objective prisms are likewise dictated by the objective's numerical aperture as well as other optical properties unique to the objective. Therefore, there can be multiple prisms available for a given magnification and correct selection is required for optimal DIC imaging results.
- *Analyzer*: The second polarizer, or "analyzer", is typically positioned downstream of the objective lens with its vibrational axis at a 90° angle to the first polarizer, in a "cross polarized" fashion (Fig. 9.5b). In a Nikon DIC system, the analyzer can be housed either in a manual slider under the objective holder or in a filter turret which can be motorized to enable automatic removal of the analyzer from the optical path for non-DIC applications. If the specimen has a homogenous refractive index, the pairs of sheared wavefronts will be unchanged in their phase relationship to one another and when recombined by the second prism, will produce linearly polarized light that is blocked by the analyzer. However, if

the pairs of sheared wavefronts experience different optical path lengths in the specimen, a phase shift will occur between the pair of wavefronts and when recombined, will produce elliptically polarized light that will pass through the analyzer and interfere to form an image. In this configuration, phase gradients are superimposed on a very dark, or black background and take on the appearance of a darkfield image. In addition, only large phase gradients present in the specimen are visible. In order to produce the typical three dimensional, shadow-cast appearance of DIC images (Fig. 9.1), a method called bias retardation is introduced into the system.

- *Compensator for Bias Retardation*: There are a couple of different ways to introduce bias retardation, or phase shifts between the pairs of sheared wavefronts. In a Nikon DIC system, a quarter-wavelength retardation plate is physically coupled to the first polarizer (and contained in the same housing) to introduce bias retardation into the optical train. These two components together are also referred to as a de Sénarmont compensator. By rotating the polarizer relative to the fast axis of the retardation plate, the amount of retardation can be altered. Other manufacturers introduce bias retardation by translating one of the prisms, usually the objective prism, across the optical path of the microscope. Both methods of bias retardation produce the same net result of changing the intensity levels of phase gradients in the specimen and generating an orientation-dependent bright highlights and dark shadows superimposed on a lighter background. By altering the bias retardation users can modulate the degree of contrast as well as the shadow-cast orientation in the image.

DIC is a highly effective method for imparting contrast to very small structures and producing thin optical sections of specimens that provide sharp images at each focal plane that are devoid of out-of-focus blur. As such, DIC is the contrasting method of choice for high-resolution, high-magnification sperm morphology examination for IMSI applications. Nikon offers several choices for IMSI objectives including high numerical aperture Plan Apochromat Lambda 100×/1.45 N.A. and 60×/1.40 N.A. oil immersion lenses. The 60× lens is often preferred over the 100× lens for sperm morphology examination and selection because of its larger field of view and greater depth of focus. However, there are several caveats for using DIC to examine sperm prior to microinjection. Since DIC microscopy relies on the placement of the specimen between two polarizers (see Fig. 9.4a), birefringent material such as plastic cell culture dishes may not be used as sample holders. Sperm samples must be plated on glass-bottom dishes for IMSI. The thickness of the glass-bottom must be 0.17 mm— the thickness of a standard #1.5 coverglass. Oil immersion objective lenses have been corrected for optical aberrations arising when using a #1.5 coverglass. Therefore, using coverslips of an alternate thickness (not 0.17 mm) will result in poor image quality. Another point to consider when performing IMSI is that the higher numerical aperture (N.A.) lenses used for MSOME (e.g. Nikon's Plan Apo Lambda 100× and 60× oil immersion DIC lenses) tend to be oil immersion lenses whereas microinjection or ICSI is typically carried out using a lower magnification dry objective lens such as the NAMC lenses described in the previous section. Therefore, when switching from MSOME to microinjection, the immersion oil left on the bottom of the specimen dish after imaging with the high N.A. oil immersion lens has to be cleaned off prior to imaging with the dry objective. Cleaning the bottom of the specimen dish results in time delays in the IMSI procedure and can also introduce unwanted mechanical disturbances to the sample. To remove this MSOME-ICSI transition problem, Nikon developed a Plan LWD 100×/0.85 N.A. Dry DIC objective lens which can be used for MSOME without the need for immersion oil. To further aid in the switch from MSOME to ICSI or DIC to NAMC, Nikon's IMSI polarizer is designed for use with both DIC and NAMC objective lenses. The only components that need to be moved (aside from the objective lenses) when transitioning between MSOME and ICSI are the modules in the condenser turret (DIC prisms and NAMC slit apertures) which are easily switched by simply rotating the turret and the analyzer (used for DIC) which needs to be removed from the light path when carrying out NAMC microscopy for ICSI (see Fig. 9.5a and figure legend). For those who prefer to use the higher numerical aperture oil immersion lenses for MSOME, Nikon also provides oil immersion, lower magnification DIC lenses that can be used for ICSI instead of the dry NAMC objective lenses. When switching between Achromat- or Plan Fluor-type NAMC objectives and either Plan LWD 100× dry or Plan Apo Lambda 100× oil immersion lenses, parfocality issues may arise. To minimize the need to change focus when switching between these lenses, Nikon also provides parfocality shims that can be installed beneath each objective.

Generation of >6,000× Magnification for MSOME

In order to examine sperm morphology and the status of sub-cellular organelles using the MSOME criteria, a magnification of >6,000× is required. This level of magnification can be achieved by using a high-magnification objective lens such as a 60× or 100× combined with a magnification changer (such as a >1× tube lens), a videozoom (either in the form of a fixed magnification camera coupler or a zooming adaptor set that provides a zooming range from 0.9 to 2.25×), and a digital camera and imaging system to add digital zoom. The final magnification is calculated by the following formula:

Total magnification = (magnification of the objective lens) × (magnification of the magnification changer) × (magnification of the videozoom) × (diagonal length of the final display screen/diagonal length of the CCD).

For example, if using a 60× objective lens with a 1.5× tube lens, a 2.5× camera coupler, a digital camera with a 0.66 inch diagonal chip (such as Nikon's digital camera DS-Qi1) and a 19 in. monitor, the total magnification would be = 60 × 1.5 × 2.5 × (19/0.66) = 6,477×. It is interesting to note that much of this magnification is "empty magnification" in which there is no gain in resolution. However, vacuoles in the sperm head and morphological detail of the sperm head itself become easier to detect at this level of magnification.

Microscope Body Considerations

IMSI should be carried out on a stable microscope body or base that prevents or minimizes the transmission of vibrations. A stable base is particularly important when performing intracytoplasmic microinjections as small amounts of vibrations in the environment can be transmitted to the injection and holding needles. Microscope bodies which offer additional magnification changers are also very useful for generating the necessary >6,000× magnification. Nikon's Eclipse Ti-U inverted microscope provides two tube lenses, one for 1× magnification and a second for 1.5× magnification. Users can quickly switch between the two magnifications with an easily accessible lever positioned at the front of the microscope. The Ti-U with its large, stable base is designed and manufactured to resist thermal fluctuations and vibrations, an ideal platform for carrying out vibration-free microinjections. The Ti-U microscope is configured for either left-side port or right-side port camera placement depending on user preference or stage handle placement. An optional model provides a beam splitter (20/80) that splits 20 % of the light the binocular port and 80 % to the left port, enabling simultaneous imaging by eye and the camera mounted on the left port. This configuration is convenient for teaching purposes and for archival recording. The Ti-U can also be configured with a variety of different stages to suit the needs of the application including a basic mechanical stage that provides a large stable surface for mounting various micromanipulators and for performing sperm examination and selection. As described in a following section, integrated stage-micromanipulator systems such as the Integra 3™ by Research Instruments Ltd. can also be easily mounted on Nikon's Ti-U microscope.

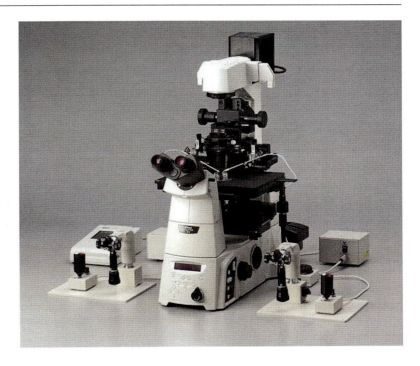

Fig. 9.6 An example of an ICSI/IMSI microscope. A Nikon Eclipse Ti-E (a fully motorized version of a Ti-U) configured with a Nikon/Narishige NT88 V3 micromanipulation and microinjection system

A high-intensity light source should be used for performing DIC and NAMC imaging. Typically, a 100 W halogen light source is used. A heat absorbing filter and either a green or NCB11 (Nikon color balancing filter #11) filter are typically inserted in between the halogen lamp housing and field diaphragm and are recommended for sample viability and to obtain the clearest NAMC and DIC images. In recent years, powerful LED light sources are also becoming a popular choice for their fast on/off cycles, minimal heat production, and longevity. For housing DIC and NAMC condenser modules, a turret-type condenser carrier that can hold multiple modules is preferred. Nikon offers non-motorized and motorized condenser turrets. For the objective lens holder or nosepiece, Nikon provides a DIC-specific nosepiece, which contains slots under each objective lens for nosepiece prisms. Nosepieces also come in non-motorized and motorized versions. The fluorescence filter turret, which can be used to house the analyzer used in DIC, can also be motorized. Using motorized components enables the acquisition software such as Nikon's NIS-Elements to program specific condenser and filter turret positions for each objective lens so that the user can simply click one button in the software to change from DIC to NAMC imaging (see Fig. 9.6 for a fully motorized inverted microscope configured for ICSI/IMSI).

Camera and Digital Imaging

The camera and digital imaging system are critical components of an IMSI setup as they provide the additional magnifications necessary to achieve the >6,000× total magnification required for MSOME, as described in a previous section. The camera is typically coupled to the microscope with a camera coupler that contains either a fixed magnifier (e.g. 2.5×) or a zooming adaptor set that provides a zooming range (e.g. from 0.9 to 2.25×), also to provide the additional magnification necessary for MSOME. The camera used for IMSI also has to have high sensitivity and fast capture rates in order to capture snapshots of extremely fast moving sperm. Consideration to pixel size must also be given in order to ensure extraction of maximum detail from the sample. For example, a camera with very large pixels would defeat the purpose of using a high numerical aperture imaging system. Nikon's DS-Qi1 cooled digital camera with its small 6.45 μm pixels, high quantum efficiency detector, wide dynamic range, fast analog-to-digital converter, and low read noise is a typical CCD camera used for IMSI applications. The new scientific CMOS cameras with their extreme frame rates, large chip sizes, small pixels, and high sensitivity, present an interesting alternative to the standard interline CCDs for IMSI applications.

Maintaining Sample Temperature

Maintaining the correct temperature is critical for sperm and oocyte viability. There are a variety of methods and commercially available products for regulating temperature during microscopic imaging. For example, there are ITO (indium tin oxide)-coated transparent glass thermal heating plates that can be inserted in the microscope stage, which impart heat to the specimen through the bottom of the petri dish or coverslip. However, the high-magnification objective lenses typically used for MSOME have short working distances. These objectives cannot focus through both the specimen dish and the thermal plate. As a solution to this problem, Tokai Hit developed a thermal plate with a hole in the center that allows short working distance objectives to focus directly through the specimen carrier (Fig. 9.7; Thermo Plate). The Thermo Plate by Tokai Hit is made of metal for improved thermal stability. Another consideration when performing MSOME is that oil immersion objective lenses act as heat syncs, drawing heat away from the specimens resulting in temperature fluctuations at the sample. Utilizing a lens heater can significantly improve temperature stability at the specimen. Lens heaters can come in the form of heating elements that wrap around the objective lens barrel such as those offered by Tokai Hit (Fig. 9.7) or

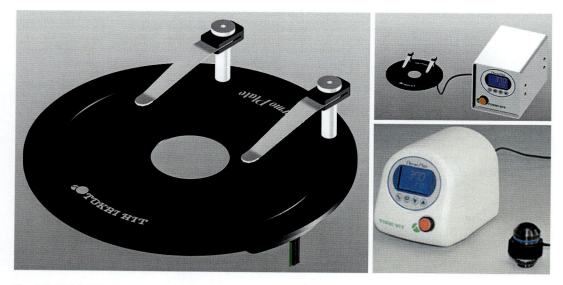

Fig. 9.7 Tokai Hit's Thermo Plate and accessories. The thermo plate is made of metal for thermal stability and features a round cutout in the middle for use with short working distance objectives such as the high-magnification, high-numerical aperture, oil immersion lenses used for MSOME. The insets show the control unit that accompanies the Thermo Plate (*top*) as well as an objective lens heater made by Tokai Hit (*bottom*)

heated air streams directed towards the objective lens under the stage (Research Instruments' Integra 3 Thermosafe™).

Options for Micromanipulators

Intracytoplasmic injection of sperm into oocytes requires precise and fine control for converting hand motion to the needle or pipette tip. Needles/pipettes and samples need to be changed frequently so a mechanism for easy exchange and the ability to quickly return the needle or pipette to the same prior position can be very helpful. In addition, many IMSI and ICSI practitioners often perform large numbers of injections and sperm selection so there is an ergonomic requirement for IMSI/ICSI setups.

Micromanipulators can be hydraulic- (using oil), mechanical or motor-based. Hydraulic systems, which use oil, provide smooth three-dimensional movements but can suffer from oil leakage, deterioration of oil caused by UV light, and entrapment of air bubbles in the lines, impeding performance. Motorized micromanipulators are useful for recording positional information but the movements can be jumpy since the motors only move in *x* and *y* directions. Mechanical systems using gear reduction systems that convert coarse mechanical movement to fine micro-movements are becoming increasingly popular due to the smooth movements they offer as well as the increased reliability provided by eliminating the risk of oil leakage, deterioration, and trapped air bubbles.

Joystick orientations can be hanging or upright. Hanging joystick type, available on Nikon/Narishige NT88-V3 or the Integra 3™ by Research Instruments are generally preferred as they offer more ergonomic hand positioning for long periods of use.

- *Nikon/Narishige NT88 V3 Micromanipulator System* utilizes electronic coarse micromanipulator positioning coupled with hydraulic fine control. The coarse electronic control has both speed control as well as "turbo" button for extra fast movement on an upright-type joystick. The hydraulic fine control utilizes a hanging joystick for ergonomic positioning. See Fig. 9.6 for an example of a NT88 V3 system on a Nikon inverted microscope.
- *Research Instruments Ltd Integra 3*™ is a completely integrated micromanipulator system consisting of a XY mechanical stage with three-stage heating, mechanical coarse, and fine micromanipulator system with hanging joystick design. There are two heated metal plates: an inner plate with a 16 mm aperture and an outer plate, as well as a mechanism called Thermosafe that gently blows warm air under the stage to warm all the objectives eliminating heat-sync scenarios when switching between objectives. Setting and controlling each heater independently ensures even heat across the stage and at the specimen plane. Audible alarms are triggered and error logs are saved if the temperature fluctuates beyond the desired mark. The mechanical design of this micromanipulator system allow for easy and precise pipette positioning as well as fast pipette exchange and one step angle adjustment. See Fig. 9.8 for an example of an Integra 3™ system on a Nikon inverted microscope.

Microinjectors are used to deliver microliter volumes of liquid into cells. They are also used to aspirate small quantities of liquid, or in the case of IMSI a single spermatozoon. Microinjectors with appropriate sized pipette types can be used for a variety of applications including oocyte holding, microinjection/ICSI, as well as polar body, blastomere, and trophectoderm biopsies. Microinjectors can be oil-filled or pneumatic (air). Both systems offer precise control for holding, aspiration, and injection. Oil-filled syringes present similar drawbacks to oil hydraulic micromanipulators namely, leakage and oil breakdown due to UV exposure. Pneumatic microinjector series SAS and SAS-SE, often referred to as "mushroom" due to their upright handle and large base design, offered by Research Instruments Ltd., are well accepted and widely used.

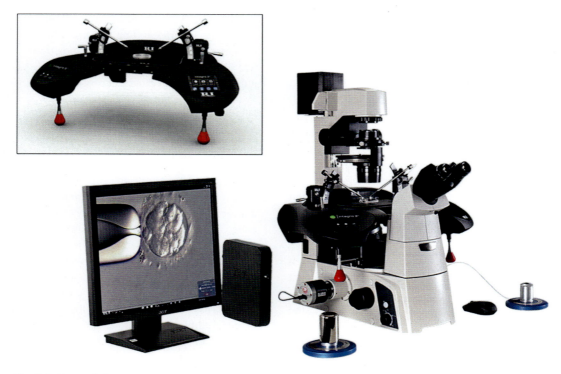

Fig. 9.8 Research Instruments Ltd Integra 3™ system configured on a Nikon Eclipse series inverted microscope. The integrated stage, heating, and micromanipulator system is shown in the *inset*

Conclusion

IMSI requires higher magnification, higher resolution imaging capability than the normal ICSI microscope. A standard ICSI microscope utilizes a 40× objective with numerical aperture ranging from 0.55 to 0.6 N.A. as the highest magnification objective. In order to visualize the most morphologically normal sperm, thereby increasing the potential for successful IVF, higher magnification, and numerical aperture objectives with DIC capability as well as a high-magnification digital imaging strategy needs to be employed. Increasing magnification without increasing numerical aperture only produces "empty magnification" as no additional information is being resolved. As magnification and corresponding numerical aperture increase, the need for thinner coverglass dishes is required. In order to achieve the highest possible magnification/numerical aperture combination possible, oil immersion becomes a necessity, thereby requiring the oil to be removed after IMSI and prior to ICSI. This can be difficult to achieve and may in fact dislodge the selected sperm from their holding droplet of PVP. Nikon has introduced a LWD 100× dry objective that offers the best compromise between high magnification (100×), high numerical aperture (0.85 N.A.), long working distance (0.95–1.3 mm) and comes with a correction collar to correct for optical aberrations that may occur at different imaging depths or when using coverglass of varying thicknesses. Differential Interference Contrast (DIC) is the desired contrasting technique as it utilizes the full apertures of the objective and the condenser to maximize the resolving power of the imaging system. DIC also produces crisp, clean, pseudo three-dimensional images that are optimal for visualizing the morphology of sperm and their intracellular detail. Because DIC is dependent upon polarized light, plastic dishes cannot be used and glass-bottom dishes need to be used.

Microscope features such as a 1.5× internal magnification factor and high-magnification video couplers are desired in order to achieve the >6,000× magnification required for successful IMSI imaging. Digital camera selection with a large chip and fast processing speed is required. Careful consideration must also be given to heating (and maintaining a stable temperature), and the types of micromanipulator and microinjectors to be used as these factors will affect both MSOME and ICSI steps which are typically performed on the same microscope with the same equipment within minutes of each other during IMSI.

References

1. Kruger TF, Acosta AA, Simmons KF, Swanson RJ, Matta JF, Veeck LL, Morshedi M, Brugo S. New method of evaluating sperm morphology with predictive value for human in vitro fertilization. Urology. 1987;30(3):248–51.
2. Kruger TF, Menkveld R, Stander FS, Lombard CJ, Van der Merwe JP, van Zyl JA, Smith K. Sperm morphologic features as a prognostic factor in in vitro fertilization. Fertil Steril. 1986;46(6):1118–23.
3. Donnelly ET, Lewis SE, McNally JA, Thompson W. In vitro fertilization and pregnancy rates: the influence of sperm motility and morphology on IVF outcome. Fertil Steril. 1998;70(2):305–14.
4. Palermo G, Joris H, Devroey P, Van Steirteghem AC. Pregnancies after intracytoplasmic injection of single spermatozoon into an oocyte. Lancet. 1992;340(8810):17–8.
5. Miller JE, Smith TT. The effect of intracytoplasmic sperm injection and semen parameters on blastocyst development in vitro. Hum Reprod. 2001;16(5):918–24.
6. De Vos A, Van De Velde H, Joris H, Verheyen G, Devroey P, Van Steirteghem A. Influence of individual sperm morphology on fertilization, embryo morphology, and pregnancy outcome of intra- cytoplasmic sperm injection. Fertil Steril. 2003;79(1):42–8.
7. Bartoov B, Berkovitz A, Eltes F, Kogosowski A, Menezo Y, Barak Y. Real-time fine morphology of motile human sperm cells is associated with IVF-ICSI outcome. J Androl. 2002;23(1):1–8.
8. Antinori M, Licata E, Dani G, Cerusico F, Versaci C, d'Angelo D. Antinori S Intracytoplasmic morphologically selected sperm injection: a prospective randomized trial. Reprod Biomed Online. 2008;16(6):835–41.
9. Bartoov B, Berkovitz A, Eltes F, Kogosovski A, Yagoda A, Lederman H, Artzi S, Gross M, Barak Y. Pregnancy rates are higher with intracytoplasmic morphologically selected sperm injection than with conventional intracytoplasmic injection. Fertil Steril. 2003;80(6):1413–9.

The Technical Background of Advanced IMSI Systems

10

Mikhail Levtonov, Klaus Rink, and Paul Gassner

IMSI (*I*ntracytoplasmic, *m*orphologically selected *s*perm *i*njection) is high magnification analysis of the sperm head ultrastructure (Fig. 10.1) prior to ICSI in order to exclude abnormal sperm from being microinjected. Besides abnormal head shape and size, the main structures to select against with IMSI are vacuoles in the sperm head. As a side effect, midpiece and tail defects will be detectable as well. Several publications addressed the application and the positive outcome of using IMSI instead of ICSI on selected patient collectives [1–8].

The main difference between conventional ICSI and IMSI is sperm selection which for IMSI is done under much higher optical resolution and magnification than for ICSI. Appropriate technical equipment as well as sufficient time and experience are required to integrate the IMSI procedure into daily routine.

In some way IMSI—on a basic level—was always done during ICSI procedures [9]. Typically, ICSI is done using a 20× lens and 10× eyepieces. Alternatively, the embryologist was using a 40× objective combined with the intermediate magnification to have a closer look at sperm morphology.

The total magnification of a microscope (Fig. 10.2) is the product of the magnifications of both the lens and the eyepieces. The resolution of a microscope basically depends on the numerical aperture (N.A.) of the condenser lens and the objective used. The typical N.A. of 20× and the 40× lenses is ranging between 0.3 and 0.5. Most long working distance condensers used for IVF have an N.A. between 0.35 and 0.6. Working distance is a limiting factor as most micromanipulators need at least 30–40 mm distance between the front lens of the condenser and the microscope stage. The working distance of the objective is determined by the thickness of the bottom of a culture dish and possibly by the use of a heated glass stage.

All this limits the resolution and the possible useful magnification factor for sperm morphology assessment during standard ICSI. For IMSI the sperm are observed and checked with much better resolution and magnification in order to select against morphological abnormalities with the best possible accuracy. Several optical and opto-electronic components combined with special software are needed for upgrading a standard ICSI workplace to an IMSI station.

An important factor with respect to image quality is the use of glass bottom dishes. Plastic dishes have many advantages for routine IVF but several disadvantages restricting their use for IMSI. The advantages are price, an easier workflow (no need to transfer sperm to other dishes for assessment) and better handling.

M. Levtonov, PhD (✉) • K. Rink, PhD
Octax Microscience GmbH, Dr.-Pauling-Str. 9,
Bruckberg 84079, Germany
e-mail: levtonov@octax.de; klaus.rink@octax.de

P. Gassner, PhD
MTG Medical Technology Vertriebs-GmbH,
Dr.-Pauling-Str. 9, Bruckberg 84079, Germany

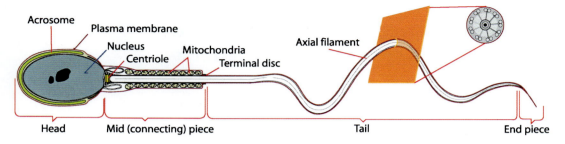

Fig. 10.1 Human spermatozoon

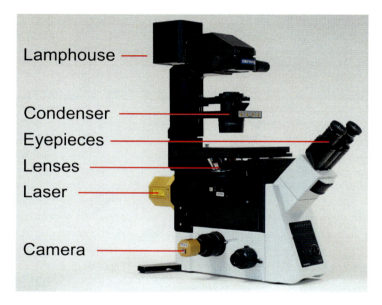

Fig. 10.2 Modern microscope intended for IMSI (micromanipulators not shown)

A major disadvantage, however, is an inferior optical quality which will limit the resolution of the whole optical system. Second, the thickness of the plastic layer (typically 1 mm) limits the number of suitable objectives with appropriate working distance.

Figure 10.3 shows the typical image quality at the end of the nineties using analog cameras. Both the resolution and image quality strongly were limiting the potential of detecting morphological details of the sperm head like vacuoles [10].

The first study on living sperm ultramorphology, done by Bartoov et al. [1] significantly improved this situation by using higher resolution optics and cameras; however, his technology was based on a combination of standard components from the microscope manufacturers. His system was based on classical Nomarski interference contrast, also called differential interference contrast (DIC) using a 100× oil immersion lens which could only work on glass bottom dishes.

In 2007, OCTAX® Microscience GmbH showed the first oil-free IMSI system called cytoScreen™. It combined a conventional relief contrast condenser of minimum 0.5 N.A. with a 60× high resolution dry objective, a custom-made high-resolution digital camera and adapted software featuring a digital zooming function. The system was able to significantly improve image quality and at the same time target the practical

Fig. 10.3 Typical image of human sperm, taken in the 1990s with an analog camera

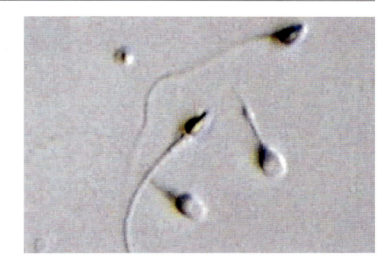

Fig. 10.4 High-magnification relief contrast image as seen with cytoScreen™ FLEX

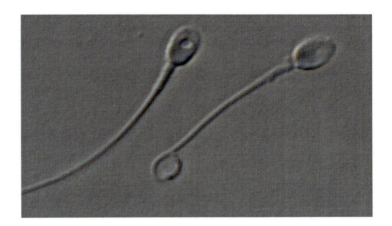

needs of the embryologist, offering a system which could work without DIC and oil immersion—a fundamental difference to the systems used by Bartoov [3]. Needless to say, this kind of system was much more universal to use and could easily combine with existing ICSI stations.

In a second step, both the versatility and image quality of cytoScreen™ were further improved in 2012, resulting in the second generation cytoScreen Flex™ (Figs. 10.4, 10.5, and 10.6). The main components of the new system are:
- A high-resolution, long working distance Adaptive Electronic Condenser (AEC)™, N.A. 0.6, offering a wide variety of contrast patterns for all IVF applications.
- A customized, long working distance optics (60× large field of view, NA 0.7, working distance up to 2 mm), specially adapted to the AEC™.
- A fast high-resolution camera (>3 Megapixels up to 40 fps) with integrated hardware zooming function.
- A special software with live image refinement features like sophisticated edge and contrast enhancement and electronic relief contrast.

As cytoScreen Flex™ is mainly based on opto-electronic and software components, expensive optical parts, e.g., a zoomable c-mount or intermediate magnification can be omitted, combining all the necessary features like high resolution and

Fig. 10.5 cytoScreen™ Flex showing edge enhancement

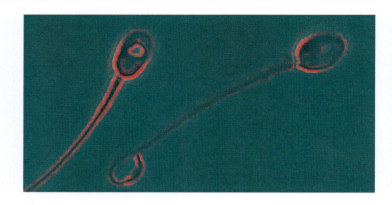

Fig. 10.6 High-magnification relief contrast image as seen with cytoScreen™ Flex

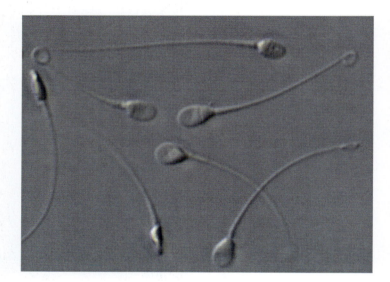

a zooming function with unprecedented flexibility and working speed. Finally, the imaging results get very close to the quality of an expensive and cumbersome DIC/Nomarski contrast system.

The name affix "Flex" is derived from the variety of conditions cytoScreen Flex™ is able to cope with: the system should be used with glass bottom dishes for the reasons indicated above but can also work with conventional plastic dishes. It can be attached to inverted microscopes equipped with either a heated glass insert or an insert plate with a central hole. Finally, it might even be combined with the use of OCTAX LaserShot™ or the movable OCTAX NaviLase™ which are working on the same software platform to immobilize sperm [11, 12] for detailed IMSI analysis.

References

1. Bartoov B, Berkovitz A, Eltes F. Selection of spermatozoa with normal nuclei to improve the pregnancy rate with intracytoplasmic sperm injection. N Engl J Med. 2001;345(14):1067–8.
2. Bartoov B, Berkovitz A, Eltes F, Kogosovsky A, Yagoda A, Lederman H, Artzi S, Gross M, Barak Y. Pregnancy rates are higher with intracytoplasmic morphologically selected sperm injection than with conventional intracytoplasmic injection. Fertil Steril. 2003;80(6):1413–9.
3. Bartoov B, Berkovitz A, Eltes F, Kogosowski A, Menezo Y, Barak Y. Real-time fine morphology of motile human sperm cells is associated with IVF-ICSI outcome. J Androl. 2002;23(1):1–8.
4. Antinori M, Licata E, Dani G, Cerusico F, Versaci C, d'Angelo D, Antinori S. Intracytoplasmic morphologically selected sperm injection: a prospective

randomized trial. Reprod Biomed Online. 2008;16(6): 835–41.
5. Cassuto NG, Bouret D, Plouchart JM, Jellad S, Vanderzwalmen P, Balet R, Larue L, Barak Y. A new real-time morphology classification for human spermatozoa: a link for fertilization and improved embryo quality. Fertil Steril. 2009;92(5): 1616–25.
6. Souza Setti A, Ferreira RC, Paes de Almeida Ferreira Braga D, de Cassia Savio Figueira R, Iaconelli A, Borges E. Intracytoplasmic sperm injection outcome versus intracytoplasmic morphologically selected sperm injection outcome: a meta-analysis. Reprod Biomed Online. 2010;21(4):450–5.
7. Vanderzwalmen P, Hiemer A, Rubner P, Bach M, Neyer A, Stecher A, Uher P, Zintz M, Lejeune B, Vanderzwalmen S, Cassuto G, Zech NH. Blastocyst development after sperm selection at high magnification is associated with size and number of nuclear vacuoles. Reprod Biomed Online. 2008;17(5): 617–27.
8. Garolla A, Fortini D, Menegazzo M, De Toni L, Nicoletti V, Moretti A, Selice R, Engl B, Foresta C. High-power microscopy for selecting spermatozoa for ICSI by physiological status. Reprod Biomed Online. 2008;17(5):610–6.
9. Berkovitz A, Eltes F, Lederman H, Peer S, Ellenbogen A, Feldberg B, Bartoov B. How to improve IVF-ICSI outcome by sperm selection. Reprod Biomed Online. 2006;12(5):634–8.
10. Franco JG, Baruffi RLR, Mauri AL, Petersen CG, Oliveira JBA, Vagnini L. Significance of large nuclear vacuoles in human spermatozoa: implications for ICSI. Reprod Biomed Online. 2008;17(1):42–5.
11. Aktan TM, Montag M, Duman S, Gorkemli H, Rink K, Yurdakul T. Use of a laser to detect viable but immotile spermatozoa. Andrologia. 2004;36(6):366–9.
12. Nordhoff V, Schuering AN, Krallmann C, Zitzmann M, Schlatt S, Kiesel L, Kliesch S. Optimizing TESE-ICSI by laser-assisted selection of immotile spermatozoa and polarization microscopy for selection of oocytes. Andrology. 2013;1(1):67–74.

Sperm Vacuoles: Origin and Implications

11

Pierre Vanderzwalmen, Nicolas Zech, Bernard Lejeune, Anton Neyer, S. Perrier d'Hauterive, Francoise Puissant, Astrid Stecher, Sabine Vanderzwalmen, Barbara Wirleitner, and Olivier Gaspard

Introduction

Since the beginning of the 1990s and the establishment of intracytoplasmic sperm injection (ICSI) [1] it is nowadays possible to help infertile couples due to male factors, e.g., severe oligoastenoteratozoospermia or azoospermia by injecting single spermatozoa from ejaculate, [2], epididymal or testicular sperm [3].

Under in vivo conditions or conventional in vitro fertilization (IVF), there is continuous natural selection against inherited factors which reduce fertility. Natural barriers occur within the male and female tract to remove faulty gametes. If we keep in mind that ICSI bypasses the natural barriers of spermatozoa selection, fertilization with abnormal spermatozoon bears the danger of potential genome enrichment with pathological alleles for the future generations [4].

With such an conceivable scenario that genetic infertility factors may be propagated via subfertile males, it might be reasonable to develop specific techniques for more accurate spermatozoa selection. As still few possibilities are available for a "positive" selection of spermatozoa, which can be later on used for injection of oocytes, particularly refined morphology assessment would be eligible.

The assessment of sperm morphology by Kruger´s strict criteria (spermocytogramme) is routinely applied and widely accepted as one of the most important predictor that correlated with a reduction of the fertilizing potential [4, 5]. This highlights the notion that sperm morphology evaluation is a very important task in the treatment of infertile couples.

P. Vanderzwalmen, Bio-Eng. (✉)
IVF Unit, IVF Centers Prof. Zech,
Römerstraße 2, Bregenz 6900, Austria

Centre de Procréation Médicalement Assistée,
Centre Hospitalier Inter Régional Cavell (CHIREC),
Rue Wayez, 35, Braine l'Alleud 1420, Belgium

Av. Du bois de chapelle, 4, B1380, Lasne, Belgium
e-mail: pierrevdz@hotmail.com

N. Zech, MD, PhD • A. Neyer, BSc
A. Stecher, BSc • B. Wirleitner, PhD
IVF Unit, IVF Centers Prof. Zech,
Römerstraße 2, Bregenz 6900, Austria
e-mail: n.zech@ivf.at; a.neyer@ivf.at;
a.stecher@ivf.at; b.wirleitener@ivf.at

B. Lejeune, MD, PhD • S. Vanderzwalmen, BSc
Centre de Procréation Médicalement Assistée,
Centre Hospitalier Inter Régional Cavell (CHIREC),
Rue Wayez, 35, Braine l'Alleud 1420, Belgium
e-mail: Blj@yucom.be; vdzsabine@hotmail.com

S.P. d'Hauterive, MD, PhD • O. Gaspard, BSc
Centre de Procréation Médicalement Assistée de
l'Université de Liège, CHR de la Citadelle, Boulevard
du Douzième de Ligne, 1, Liège 4000, Belgium
e-mail: sperrierdh@gmail.com;
olivier.gaspard@gmail.com

F. Puissant, MD, PhD
Centre de Procréation Médicalement Assistée,
Centre Hospitalier Inter Régional Cavell (CHIREC),
Edith Cavell 32, Uccle 1180, Belgium
e-mail: michel.vanrysselberge@pandora.be

Bartoov et al. [6] reported that quantitative ultramorphological sperm analysis using scanning electron microscopy (SEM) and transmission electron microscopy (TEM) is clinically informative, and is recommended when the male infertility factor cannot be clearly diagnosed by routine tests prior to first assisted reproductive technique (ART) trial. However, such as for classical spermocytogramme, morphological assessment is performed after fixation and staining processes.

In order to counteract the problem of morphological evaluation on stained spermatozoa, Bartoov et al. [7] introduced the MSOME. With the use of Nomarski differential interference contrast optics (DIC), a better three-dimensional view of the head became available. It is possible to observe in real time details, such as the so-called vacuoles, on the surface of motile sperm head.

Cephalic vacuoles are the subject of debates and controversies [8] and raised several issues regarding their origin, the reason for the occurrence of vacuoles and their pathological character with potential implications in infertility.

In Vivo Formation of Vacuole-Like Structures

When Are They Produced?

Using DIC optic, vacuoles appear as depressions at the cell surface, like lunar craters that are visible with the tangent sunlight. This observations shows that the terminology "vacuole" for these structures is misleading. With different microscopic approaches, the vacuole-like structures on the sperm head were termed craters [9] concavities [10], hollows [11] or lacunae [12]. Boitrelle et al. [10] observed that the sperm plasma membrane was intact and invaginated nearby the vacuole and that the sperm-head's thickness falls to 300 nm at the site of the large vacuole. They concluded that vacuole-like structures are nuclear depressions which correspond to a concavity in the plasma membrane rather than a hole.

The origin of vacuoles is still not fully elucidated. Literature referring to animal models [13, 14] as well as to human spermatozoa [15–18] describes the formation of nuclear vacuoles during the spermiogenesis. The same hypothesis was set up for human spermatozoa, in 1989 Baccetti et al. suggested that the nuclear and acrosomal invaginations are formed during spermiogenesis [15–18] According to these findings, the presence of vacuoles is already noticeable in elongated spermatids after testicular retrieval. The presence of vacuoles in round spermatids was demonstrated recently by Tanaka et al. [18]. Based on the classification of Clermont et al. [19], Tanaka et al. [18] and Mansour et al. [20] there are low rates (18 %) of vacuoles in spermatids entering cap phase (stage Sb1), their occurrence increases during stage Sb2 to reach a high level of 93.8 % when they are at the acrosomal phase (stage Sc; these stages of spermiogenesis).

If it is obvious that small and large vacuoles are observed in the majority of ejaculated spermatozoa and their frequency differs according to the severity of the male infertility. If it is often difficult to observe vacuole-free sperm cells in ejaculates from infertile men, in contrast to semen derived from proven fertile men. Tresholds were established for fertility, for example, Falagario et al. [21] identified a cut off of 20 % for sperm nuclear vacuolization on the total of sperm in a seminal sample. According to De Vos et al. [22] the prevalence of vacuoles in normal shaped spermatozoa seems to be low. Under high magnification, they analyzed the frequency of vacuoles in 330 male infertility semen. They reported that almost 33.3 % of the spermatozoa were morphologically normal and exhibited less than two small vacuoles. Normal shape spermatozoa with more than two small vacuoles or at least one large vacuole represent 12.3 % of the population. Finally 54.4 % showed abnormal head shapes with or without large vacuoles in conjunction with other abnormalities.

Silva et al. [23] investigated the influence of paternal age on sperm quality by MSOME. The frequency of large nuclear vacuoles was significantly higher in the older group (>41 years age) compared to the younger age groups. Such observation corroborated the study of De Almeida Ferreira Braga et al. [24].

How to Consider Vacuole-Like Structures: As a Sign of Nuclear Dysfunction or as a Normal Stage in the Acrosomial Process?

Vacuole-Like Structure and Nuclear Dysfunction

The most interesting question in connection with vacuoles is, whether these large intranuclear lacunae or structure like vacuoles are the morphological manifestation of nuclear dysfunction. Assuming that they seem to appear during the last maturation step of round spermatids, do they originate from a natural process or, more likely, from pathological (stress) situations during spermiogenesis or even early in the first stage of the spermatogenesis? In other words, what hides behind spermatozoa with large nuclear vacuoles?

The literature is controversial, while some studies report that there is no relationship between the presence of sperm head vacuoles and sperm function suggesting that sperm vacuoles should be regarded as a normal feature of the sperm head [11, 18], others mentioned that it is related to male subfertility [25]. However, Tanaka et al. [18] highlighted that the size of the vacuoles is of importance and suggested that spermatozoa with large vacuoles should not be used for injection.

A multitude of studies concluded that vacuoles reveal indirectly nuclear dysfunction in terms of lower mitochondrial potential [26], DNA integrity, aneuploidy rate and problems related with chromatin condensation.

Out of ten studies [10, 11, 26–31] determining the degree of DNA fragmentation usually with Tunnel assay, five [24, 27, 29, 31, 32] reported that vacuole-free spermatozoa yields lower rates of DNA fragmentation as compared with vacuolated spermatozoa. Perdrix et al. [27] observed for vacuolated spermatozoa a significant increase in the rates of aneuploidy and diploidy. However, for Boitrelle et al.[30] and de Almeida Ferreira Braga et al. [24], the presence of sperm aneuploidy was not correlated with the presence of nuclear vacuoles. Assuming that DNA fragmentation is mostly due to oxidative attack, and that sperm DNA condensation is a protection against ROS (reactive oxygen species), it may result that the apparent divergences between these papers could be explained by different levels of oxidative stress in patients, leading to different levels of DNA fragmentation [33].

Several DNA and chromatin staining assays including aniline blue and chromomycin A3 (CMA3) were applied in order to assess more precisely information about integrity of DNA in vacuolated spermatozoa. A negative correlation between the incidence of vacuoles and abnormally condensed chromatin was observed in all the nine conducted studies [10, 11, 26–32]. In these manuscripts, spermatozoa with large vacuoles were selected by micromanipulation before being studied by different microscopy and immunocytochemistry techniques. All the conducted studies concluded that vacuoles did not take their origin in the acrosome but that they are linked to areas of chromatin decondensation [10].

The presence of craters most likely reflect molecular defects responsible for anomalies of sperm chromatin packaging and abnormal chromatin remodeling during sperm maturation [34–36]. Boitrelle et al. [10, 30] observed chromatin condensation at the site of the vacuole and concluded that a large vacuole appears to be a nuclear "thumbprint" linked to failure of chromatin condensation. This was also confirmed in another study of Boitrelle and colleagues for small head vacuoles [10] Perdrix et al. [37] recently published their observations of the correlation between the presence of large nuclear vacuoles and chromosome architecture modifications, adding a new argument for the association between nuclear vacuole-like structure and chromatin disorganization.

According to the growing body of literature adding new arguments for the association between vacuoles and chromatin disorganization, an association between the two becomes more and more obvious. With the disorganization of the chromatin and the vacuoles in the sperm head, the spermatozoa and its DNA becomes more assailable to attacks by ROS [38–40]. Thereby, DNA fragmentation would depend on two steps, the occurrence of vacuoles in connection with insufficient chromatin condensation and on the presence of ROS. This could explain why the correlation between the presence of vacuoles on the rate of DNA fragmentation is not observed unanimously.

Chemes and Alvarez Sedo [41] studied the morphology of the sperm head by TEM. They proposed that the small lacunae observed in spermatozoa nucleus characterize the site of a normal proteolytic activity linked to histone to protamine transition. However, Haraguchi et al. [42] suggested that larger lacunae may be the result of a deregulated histone-protamine transition during spermiogenesis due to an overactive or disregulated ubiquitin proteasome system.

Could vacuoles be a selective mechanism for defective sperm to be removed in the natural selection-process? We know that in sperm "incomplete apoptosis" is a common phenomenon [43]. Spermatozoa which do not pass the "quality control" due to, e.g., DNA-defects or other aberrations during spermatogenesis undergo the normal pathway towards apoptosis but are not removed by phagocytes. Maybe the formation of vacuoles is a mechanism for abnormal spermatozoa to be attacked by ROS during storage and thereby being discarded.

In the light of these studies, we know that during spermiogenesis, spermatids undergo a complex restructuring program in which, in addition to acrosome and sperm tail formation, DNA is tightly packed leading to a drastic reduction in the size of the nucleus. These unique cellular reconstruction process requires spermatid-specific genes to execute their regulatory roles. It is estimated that 600–1.000 germ cell-specific genes participate in spermiogenesis, and specific genes such as Prm1, Prm2, Tnp1, Tnp2, and H1t2 are involved in chromosomal packaging [44].

Chromatin condensation takes place during spermiogenesis allowing protection of the paternal genome during the transit from the male to the oocyte prior to fertilization. The chromatin is radically reorganized and undergoes an extreme condensation resulting in a shift from a nucleosome-based genome organization to the sperm-specific, highly compacted nucleoprotamine structure [45]. About 85 % of human sperm histones is replaced with protamines, whereas only 15 % of the DNA remain organized by histones or is attached to the nuclear matrix [46]. Recently, Rousseaux et al. [47] demonstrated a new key stone in DNA compaction in humans and murines. They found that a testis-specific protein called bromodomain testis-specific protein (BRDT), which possesses two bromodomains capable of interactions with hyperacetylated histones, is likely to be at least partially responsible for the replacement of histones by protamines. The genome-wide incorporation of a new histone variant called testis-specific histone 2B (TH2B) might also play an important role in this histone to protamine transition as shown in murine models [48].

Prior to histone replacement by protamines, the nucleosomes are destabilized by hyperacetylation and by DNA methylation [49, 50]. Moreover the distribution of the remaining 15 % nucleosomes after the 85 % nucleosomes to nucleoprotamine replacement is not random but concerns gene regions involved in the epigenetic control and the early embryonic development [46, 50–52]. On the other side, the ratio between the two protamine subtypes protamine 1 and 2, which should normally be close to 1, can have a significant negative impact on fertility when disturbed [53]. Taken together, these data supports the idea that bad condensation of sperm DNA has a great impact on male fertility. All these potential epigenetic pattern disturbances may represent the basis of numerous human disorders.

Beside that epigenetic role of sperm chromatin condensation, particular organization of sperm DNA is also important for its protection, especially against fragmentation, during spermatozoa journey through male and female genital tracts [43].

Vacuole-Like Structure: A Receptacle of Acrosomal Enzymes?

As vacuoles are mostly localized in the anterior part of sperm head, in the region of the acrosome, one of the hypothesis on the origin of vacuoles was that they were mostly of acrosomal origin [54]. Kacem et al. stated that sperm nuclear vacuoles are mainly associated with the presence of acrosomal enzymes such as trypsin-like acrosin that may induce a harmful effect after oocyte injection. As consequence, they concluded that a large majority of normal, regularly shaped spermatozoa showing no vacuoles have already undergone their acrosome reaction and should be selected for injection.

Montjean et al. [55] tested the effect of inducers of the acrosome reaction. After incubation of sperm in either hyaluronic acid or follicular fluid for 90 min, they observed a highly significant decrease in the presence of vacuoles as a consequence of the acrosome reaction.

The study of Neyer et al. [56] did not corroborate those of Kacem and Montjean [54, 55]. In a time-lapse set-up they monitored single spermatozoa in sperm capture channel during 24 h and observed that the induction of the acrosome reaction using calcium ionophore A23587 did not lead to any modifications in pre-existing vacuole appearance, disappearance or formation [56].

In a recent paper, Gatimel et al. [57] described the MSOME performed on the semen of two men suffering from globozoospermia. In these two patients, all the spermatozoa totally lacked acrosomal structures, as confirmed by TEM and SEM, but vacuoles were present in the majority of cells (92 and 76 %), at a rate comparable to that observed in fertile controls. From those studies, we may conclude that there is a negative relation between the presence of vacuoles and the sperm capacity to undergo acrosome reaction. For Boitrelle et al. [10, 30], sperm membrane and acrosome cap are intact at the site of these depressions.

Likewise, Perdrix et al. [27] demonstrated an exclusive nuclear origin of these large head surface depressions using TEM supporting their severe impact on sperm quality.

In Vitro Formation of Vacuole-Like Structures: A Reality?

Peer et al. [58] compared the impact of incubating prepared sperm at 37 °C or at 21 °C. They concluded that after 2 h of incubation at 37 °C in culture media, the incidence of spermatozoa with vacuolated nuclei was significantly higher, so that prolonged sperm manipulations for assisted reproduction therapy should be performed at 21 °C rather than 37 °C. Schwarz et al. [59] reported a significant increase in sperm nuclear vacuolization in washed sperm but not in swim-up sperm. They concluded that the method used for sperm preparation influences sperm nuclear vacuolization and that vacuolization is unaffected by temperature in motile sperm isolated by swim-up.

Neyer et al. [56] developed a system called sperm-microcapture channels that permits an accurate observation of the same population of living spermatozoa over a period of 24 h. They analyzed whether incubation temperature (20 or 37 °C) or oxidative stress stimulates the formation of nuclear vacuoles. They observed that neither incubation at 37 °C nor induction of oxidative stress induce de-novo formation of nuclear vacuoles. According to these observations, they concluded that nuclear vacuoles on the sperm head are already produced at earlier stages of sperm maturation and are not induced or modulated by routine laboratory procedures.

However, Boitrelle et al. [60] observed that cryopreservation of human spermatozoa induces nuclear vacuolization and increases the proportion of spermatozoa with noncondensed chromatin, while Gatimel et al. [61] did not corroborate this conclusion.

Vacuole-Like Structure and Embryo Development

If vacuoles are associated with impaired chromatin packaging and with DNA fragmentation, one crucial question to investigate concerns the significance of vacuoles on the outcome in terms of fertilization, embryo development, pregnancy, miscarriage and health babies born.

This question was studied and reported by a few recent papers. It has been demonstrated that sperm nuclear vacuole size and number, as seen with DIC Nomarski optics, negatively affects blastocyst development. In four successive papers [62–65] it was shown that the occurrence of large nuclear vacuoles and/or abnormal shape reduces the percentage of good-quality embryos reaching the blastocyst stage after culture until day 5. Following the outcome of each embryo after injection of spermatozoa, they clearly demonstrated that the use of spermatozoa with no vacuoles or less than two small vacuoles can be associated with significantly higher blastocyst rates than injection with spermatozoa showing more than two small vacuoles or one large vacuole with or without abnormal shape. These studies support the previously issued hypothesis that the impact of male infertility may be at an early stage (early paternal effect), when spermatozoa is not able to attain, penetrate and/or activate the oocyte, or at a late stage (late paternal effect) when it could not support embryo development, implantation and pregnancy to term. Late paternal effects are observed after paternal genome activation and blastocyst development failure is one of their first manifestations [66–68].

The link between sperm head vacuoles and impaired chromatin condensation, and the occurrence of DNA fragmentation in the presence of ROS may explain why vacuoles can be related with impaired human embryo development [39, 65, 69] and pregnancy outcomes [67, 70–72].

Vacuole-Like Structures, Pregnancies, and Miscarriages

A more specific analysis of the impact of sperm cells with normal nuclear shape but with large vacuoles was first carried out by Berkovitz et al. [73] on two matched IMSI groups of 28 patients each. Spermatozoa with strictly defined normal nuclear shape but large vacuoles were selected for injection and compared to a control group that included normal nuclear shape spermatozoa lacking vacuoles.

No difference in the fertilization and early embryo development up to day 3 were reported. However, injection of spermatozoa with strictly normal nuclear shape but large vacuoles appeared to significantly reduce pregnancy outcomes (18 % versus 50 %) and seemed to be associated with early abortions (80 % versus 7 %).

Other studies showed also that selection of normal shape spermatozoa with a vacuole-free head was positively associated with pregnancy and lower abortion rates after day 3 or day 5 embryo transfers in couples with previous and repeated implantation failures [62, 74–82], in patients with an elevated degree of DNA fragmented spermatozoa [36] and in patients with a high degree of teratozoospermia [83]. In a recent prospective randomized study, Setti et al. [84] show the beneficial effect of performing IMSI in cases of advanced maternal age (women age ≥ 37 years old).

However, some other studies failed to show any effect of selecting vacuole-free sperm on ART outcome [82, 85, 86]. One possible explanation therefore is the patient selection. Probably IMSI indications are not precise enough, and doing IMSI in an unselected or a bad-selected population will not be advantageous. Another point is that IMSI seems to promote blastocyst development when selecting vacuole-free spermatozoa (see precious point on vacuoles and embryo development). So in addition to implantation and pregnancy rates, we have to take in account pregnancies obtained with frozen-thawed supernumerary embryos, and to calculate cumulative pregnancy rate (fresh + frozen/thawed embryo transfers) per follicle puncture. Knez et al. [65] showed that there was no significant difference in the pregnancy rates between IMSI and ICSI procedures after blastocyst transfer. However, after ICSI more pregnancies terminated by spontaneous abortion, whereas after IMSI there was no spontaneous abortion. One explanation could be that IMSI procedure permits to select spermatozoa without defect and as consequence provide more "healthy" blastocysts, possibly, in spite of very comparable development and morphology in ICSI-derived blastocysts.

Vacuole-Like Structures and Postnatal Data

Still concerns remain about the long-term safety of injecting spermatozoa carrying vacuoles. We have to be cautious, especially in the light of Aitken's work [33] on the putative negative effects of sperm DNA fragmentation for the next generation. Depending on the level of sperm nuclear DNA fragmentation, oocytes may partially repair fragmented DNA, producing blastocysts able to implant and develop up to live offspring. However the incomplete repair may lead to long-term pathologies. The work of Fernandez-Gonzalez et al. [87] on the mouse model indicates that the use of DNA-fragmented spermatozoa in ICSI can generate effects that only emerge in later life, such as, aberrant growth, premature aging, abnormal behavior and tumors derived from the mesenchymal lineage. Moreover the association of vacuoles with defects in chromatin packaging, which has an important role in epigenetic control of paternal genome as discussed earlier, is an argument in favor of the selection of vacuole-free sperm for oocyte injection.

Up to now, there are in sufficient numbers published studies concerning the health of children born after ICSI to draw any firm conclusions about the long-term safety of this procedure. However, it is important to emphasize that animal data are absolutely unequivocal on this point and clearly indicate that DNA damage in the male germ line is potentially hazardous for the embryo and therefore for the resulting offspring. According to two recently published papers, paper, sperm nucleus morphological normalcy, assessed at high magnification, could decrease the prevalence of de novo major fetal malformations in ICSI children [88, 89].

Conclusions

The introduction of MSOME and IMSI points to embryologists that more attention has to be paid during sperm selection, even when it is done with a conventional optic.

It is now confirmed in the literature that the occurrence of vacuole-like structures on the sperm head is related with sperm chromatin immaturity. However, the background and the relation between the two are still unclear. Do we face a chicken-and-egg problem? Do both, vacuoles and abnormal chromatin condensation occur at the same time or is one the consequence of the other? At this point the most probable explanation is that the vacuoles, which are in fact concavities in the sperm head membrane, first appear during the spermiogenesis rendering the nucleosome and DNA and connected molecules more vulnerable to intrinsic or extrinsic attacks by ROS. According to the level of ROS, DNA fragmentation may appear. More research on this area will bring light in these processes.

So the application of IMSI leads to more blastocysts of higher quality, increasing the chance to transfer an embryo with a high implantation potential and to obtain the birth of a healthy baby.

Seeing that this simple, noninvasive technique still arises debates and scepticism exists about its efficiency, mainly due to a low number of controlled randomized studies published yet, one fundamental question is whether we should—with the knowledge that sperm vacuoles are related with abnormal chromatin packaging and possibly with DNA fragmentation—select spermatozoa with these defects for injection if we have only to change the optics? As far as we know, there is no reason for not selecting the morphologically best spermatozoa.

References

1. Palermo G, Joris H, Devroey P, Van Steirteghem AC. Pregnancies after intracytoplasmic injection of single spermatozoon into an oocyte. Lancet. 1992;340: 17–8.
2. Van Steirteghem AC, Nagy Z, Joris H, Liu J, Staessen C, Smitz J, Wisanto A, Devroey P. High fertilization and implantation rates after intracytoplasmic sperm injection. Hum Reprod. 1993;8:1061–6.
3. Schoysman R, Vanderzwalmen P, Nijs M, Segal L, Segal-Bertin G, Geerts L, van Roosendaal E, Schoysman D. Pregnancy after fertilisation with human testicular spermatozoa. Lancet. 1993;342:1237.
4. Moretti E, Collodel G. Electron microscopy in the study of human sperm pathologies. In: Méndez-Vilas A, editor. Current microscopy contributions to advances in science and technology. Badajoz: Formatex; 2012. p. 343–51.
5. Vawda A, Gunby J, Younglai E. Semen parameters as predictors of in-vitro fertilization: the importance of strict criteria morphology. Hum Reprod. 1996;11: 1445–50.
6. Bartoov B, Eltes F, Pansky M, Langzam J, Reichart M, Soffer Y. Improved diagnosis of male fertility potential via a combination of quantitative ultramorphology and routine semen analysis. Hum Reprod. 1994;9:2069–75.

7. Bartoov B, Berkovitz A, Eltes F. Selection of spermatozoa with normal nuclei to improve the pregnancy rate with intracytoplasmic sperm injection. N Engl J Med. 2001;345:1067–8.
8. Perdrix A, Rives N. Motile sperm organelle morphology examination (MSOME) and sperm head vacuoles: state of the art in 2013. Hum Reprod Update. 2013;19:527–41.
9. Westbrook VA, Diekman AB, Klotz KL, Khole VV, von Kap-Herr C, Golden WL, Eddy RL, Shows TB, Stoler MH, Lee CY, Flickinger CJ, Herr JC. Spermatid-specific expression of the novel X-linked gene product SPAN-X localized to the nucleus of human spermatozoa. Biol Reprod. 2000;63:469–81.
10. Boitrelle F, Ferfouri F, Petit JM, Segretain D, Tourain C, Bergere M, Bailly M, Vialard F, Albert M, Selva J. Large human sperm vacuoles observed in motile spermatozoa under high magnification: nuclear thumbprints linked to failure of chromatin condensation. Hum Reprod. 2011;26:1650–8.
11. Watanabe S, Tanaka A, Fujii S, Mizunuma H. No relationship between chromosome aberrations and vacuole-like structures on human sperm head. Hum Reprod. 2009;24:i96.
12. Chemes HE, Alvarez Sedo C. Tales of the tail and sperm head aches: changing concepts on the prognostic significance of sperm pathologies affecting the head, neck and tail. Asian J Androl. 2012;141:14–23.
13. Johnson LA, Hurtgen JP. The morphological and ultrastructural appearance of the crater defect in stallion spermatozoa. Mol Reprod. 1985;12:41–6.
14. Czaker R. On the origin of nuclear vacuoles in spermatozoa: a fine structural and cytochemical study in mice. Andrologia. 1985;17:547–57.
15. Baccetti B, Burrini AG, Collodel G, Magnano AR, Piomboni P, Renieri T, Sensini C. Crater defect in human spermatozoa. Mol Reprod Develop. 1989;22:249–55.
16. Francavilla S, Bianco MA, Cordeschi G, D'Abrizio P, De Stefano C, Properzi G, Francavilla F. Ultrastructural analysis of chromatin defects in testicular spermatids in azoospermic men submitted to TESE-ICSI. Hum Reprod. 2001;16:1440–8.
17. Sardi-Segovia LM, Rocher AE, Pugliese MN, Chenlo P, Curi S, Ariagno J, Repetto H, Cohen M, Mendeluk GR, Palaoro LA. Prognostic value of germ cells in the ejaculate: a case study. Biotech Histochem. 2010;86:232–41.
18. Tanaka A, Nagayoshi M, Tanaka I, Kuzunoki H. Human sperm head vacuoles are physiological structures formed during the sperm development and maturation process. Fertil Stertil. 2012;98:315–20.
19. Clermont Y. The cycle of the seminiferous epithelium in man. Am J Anat. 1963;112:35–51.
20. Mansour RT, Fahmy IM, Taha AK, Tawab NA, Serour GL, Aboulghar MA. Intracytoplasmic spermatid injection can result in the delivery of normal offspring. J Androl. 2003;24:757–64.
21. Falagario D, Brucculeri A, Depalo R, Trerotoli P, Cittadini E, Ruvolo G. Sperm head vacuolization affects clinical outcome in ICSI cycle. A proposal of a cut-off value. J Assist Reprod Genet. 2012;29:1281–7.
22. De Vos A, Van de Velde H, Bocken G, Eylenbosch G, Franceus N, Meersdom G, Tistaert S, Vankelecom A, Tournaye H, Verheyen G. Does intracytoplasmic morphologically selected sperm injection improve embryo development? A randomized sibling-oocyte study. Hum Reprod. 2013;28:617–26.
23. Silva L, Oliveira J, Petersen C, Mauri A, Massaro F, Cavagna M, Baruffi RL, Franco Jr JG. The effects of male age on sperm analysis by motile sperm organelle morphology examination (MSOME). Reprod Biol Endocrinol. 2012;10:19.
24. De Almeida Ferreira Braga DP, Setti AS, Figueira RC, Nichi M, Martinhago CD, Iaconelli Jr A, Borges Jr E. Sperm organelle morphologic abnormalities: contributing factors and effects on intracytoplasmic sperm injection cycles outcomes. Urology. 2011;78:786–91.
25. Mundy AJ, Ryder TA, Edmonds DK. A quantitative study of sperm head ultrastructure in subfertile males with excess sperm precursors. Fertil Steril. 1994;61:751–4.
26. Garolla A, Fortini D, Menegazzo M, De Toni L, Nicoletti V, Moretti A, Selice R, Engl B, Foresta C. High power magnification microscopy and functional status analysis of sperm in the evaluation and selection before ICSI. Reprod Biomed Online. 2008;17:610–6.
27. Perdrix A, Travers A, Chelli MH, Escalier D, Do Rego JL, Milazzo JP, Mousset-Siméon N, Macé B, Rives N. Assessment of acrosome and nuclear abnormalities in human spermatozoa with large vacuoles. Hum Reprod. 2011;26:47–58.
28. Cassuto NG, Hazout A, Hammoud I, Balet R, Bouret D, Barak Y, Jellad S, Plouchart JM, Selva J, Yazbeck C. Correlation between DNA defect and sperm-head morphology. Reprod Biomed Online. 2012;24:211–8.
29. Franco Jr JG, Mauri AL, Petersen CG, Massaro FC, Silva LF, Felipe V, Cavagna M, Pontes A, Baruffi RL, Oliveira JB, Vagnini LD. Large nuclear vacuoles are indicative of abnormal chromatin packaging in human spermatozoa. Int J Androl. 2012;35:46–51.
30. Boitrelle F, Albert M, Petit J-M, Ferfouri F, Wainer R, Bergere M, Bailly M, Vialard F, Selva J. Small human sperm vacuoles observed under high magnification are pocket-like nuclear concavities linked to chromatin condensation failure. Reprod Biomed Online. 2013;27:201–11.
31. Wilding M, Coppola G, di Matteo L, Palagiano A, Fusco E, Dale B. Intracytoplasmic injection of morphologically selected spermatozoa (IMSI) improves outcome after assisted reproduction by deselecting physiologically poor quality spermatozoa. J Assist Reprod Genet. 2011;28:253–62.
32. Hammoud I, Boitrelle F, Ferfouri F, Vialard F, Bergere M, Wainer B, Bailly M, Albert M, Selva J. Selection of normal spermatozoa with a vacuole-free head (×6300) improves selection of spermatozoa with

intact DNA in patients with high sperm DNA fragmentation rates. Andrologia. 2013;45:163–70.
33. Aitken RJ, De Iuliis GN. Origins and consequences of DNA damage in male germ cells. Reprod Biomed Online. 2007;14:727–33.
34. Cayli S, Jakab A, Ovari L, Delpiano E, Celik-Ozenci C, Sakkas D, Ward D, Huszar G. Biochemical markers of sperm function: male fertility and sperm selection for ICSI. Reprod Biomed Online. 2003;7:462–8.
35. Berkovitz A, Eltes F, Yaari S, Katz N, Barr I, Fishman A, Bartoov B. The morphological normalcy of the sperm nucleus and pregnancy rate of intracytoplasmic injection with morphologically selected sperm. Hum Reprod. 2005;20:185–90.
36. Hazout A, Dumont-Hassan M, Junca AM, Cohen Bacrie P, Tesarik J. High-magnification ICSI overcomes paternal effect resistant to conventional ICSI. Reprod Biomed Online. 2006;12:19–25.
37. Perdrix A, Travers A, Clatot F, Sibert L, Mitchell V, Jumeau F, Macé B, Rives N. Modification of chromosomal architecture in human spermatozoa with large vacuoles. Andrology. 2013;1:57–66.
38. Gopalkrishnan K, Padwal V, Meherji PK, Gokral JS, Shah R, Juneja HS. Poor quality of sperm as it affects repeated early pregnancy loss. Arch Androl. 2000;45:111–7.
39. Hammadeh ME, Nkemayim DC, Georg T, Rosenbaum P, Schmidt W. Sperm morphology and chromatin condensation before and after semen processing. Arch Androl. 2000;44:221–6.
40. Mahfouz R, Sharma R, Thiyagarajan A, Kale V, Gupta S, Sabanegh E, Agarwal A. Semen characteristics and sperm DNA fragmentation in infertile men with low and high levels of seminal reactive oxygen species. Fertil Steril. 2010;94:2141–6.
41. Chemes HE, Alvarez Sedo C. Tales of the tail and sperm head aches: changing concepts on the prognostic significance of sperm pathologies affecting the head, neck and tail. Asian J Androl. 2012;14(1): 14–23.
42. Haraguchi CM, Mabuchi T, Hirata S, Shoda T, Tokumoto T, Hoshi K, Yokota S. Possible function of caudal nuclear pocket: degradation of nucleoproteins by ubiquitin-proteasome system in rat spermatids and human sperm. J Histochem Cytochem. 2007;55:585–95.
43. Aitken RJ, Koppers AJ. Apoptosis and DNA damage in human spermatozoa. Asian J Androl. 2011;13:36–42.
44. Zheng H, Stratton C, Morozumi K, Jin J, Yanagimachi R, Yan W. Lack of Spem1 causes aberrant cytoplasm removal, sperm deformation, and male infertility. Proc Natl Acad Sci U S A. 2007;104:6852–7.
45. Auger J, Dadoune JP. Nuclear status of human sperm cells by transmission electron microscopy and image cytometry: changes in nuclear shape and chromatin texture during spermiogenesis and epididymal transit. Biol Reprod. 1993;49:166–75.
46. Ward WS. Function of sperm chromatin structural elements in fertilization and development. Mol Hum Reprod. 2010;16:30–6.
47. Rousseaux S, Boussouar F, Gaucher J, Reynoird N, Montellier E, Curtet S, Vitte AL, Khochbin S. Molecular models for post-meiotic male genome reprogramming. Syst Biol Reprod Med. 2011;57:50–3.
48. Montellier E, Boussouar F, Rousseaux S, Zhang K, Buchou T, Fenaille F, Shiota H, Debernardi A, Héry P, Curtet S, Jamshidikia M, Barral S, Holota H, Bergon A, Lopez F, Guardiola P, Pernet K, Imbert J, Petosa C, Tan M, Zhao Y, Gérard M, Khochbin S. Chromatin-to-nucleoprotamine transition is controlled by the histone H2B variant TH2B. Genes Dev. 2013;27:1680–92.
49. Palermo GD, Neri QV, Takeuchi T, Squires J, Moy F, Rosenwaks Z. Genetic and epigenetic characteristics of ICSI children. Reprod Biomed Online. 2008;17:820–33.
50. Miller D, Brinkworth M, Iles D. Paternal DNA packaging in spermatozoa: more than the sum of its parts? DNA, histones, protamines and epigenetics. Reproduction. 2010;139:287–301.
51. Tavalaee M, Razavi S, Nasr-Esfahani MH. Influence of sperm chromatin anomalies on assisted reproductive technology outcome. Fertil Steril. 2009;91:1119–26.
52. Oliva R, Ballesca JL. Altered histone retention and epigenetic modifications in the sperm of infertile men. Asian J Androl. 2012;14:239–40.
53. Hammoud SS, Nix DA, Hammoud AO, Gibson M, Cairns BR, Carrell DT. Genome-wide analysis identifies changes in histone retention and epigenetic modifications at developmental and imprinted gene loci in the sperm of infertile men. Hum Reprod. 2011;26:2558–69.
54. Kacem O, Sifer C, Barraud-Lange V, Ducot B, De Ziegler D, Poirot C, Wolf J. Sperm nuclear vacuoles, as assessed by motile sperm organellar morphological examination, are mostly of acrosomal origin. Reprod Biomed Online. 2010;20:132–7.
55. Montjean D, Belloc S, Benkhalifa M, Dalleac A, Ménézo Y. Sperm vacuoles are linked to capacitation and acrosomal status. Hum Reprod. 2012;27:2927–32.
56. Neyer A, Vanderzwalmen P, Bach M, Stecher A, Spitzer D, Zech N. Sperm head vacuoles are not affected by in-vitro conditions, as analysed by a system of sperm-microcapture channels. Reprod Biomed Online. 2013;26:368–77.
57. Gatimel N, Léandri RD, Foliguet B, Bujan L, Parinaud J. Sperm cephalic vacuoles: new arguments for their non acrosomal origin in two cases of total globozoospermia. Andrology. 2013;1:52–6.
58. Peer S, Eltes F, Berkovitz A, Yehuda R, Itsykson P, Bartoov B. Is fine morphology of the human sperm nuclei affected by in vitro incubation at 37 degrees C°? Fertil Steril. 2007;88:1589–94.
59. Schwarz C, Köster M, van der Ven K, Montag M. Temperature-induced sperm nuclear vacuolization is dependent on sperm preparation. Andrologia. 2012;44 Suppl 1:126–9.

60. Boitrelle F, Albert M, Theillac C, Ferfouri F, Bergere M, Vialard F, Wainer R, Bailly M, Selva J. Cryopreservation of human spermatozoa decreases the number of motile normal spermatozoa, induces nuclear vacuolization and chromatin decondensation. J Androl. 2012;33:1371–8.
61. Gatimel N, Leandri R, Parinaud J. Sperm vacuoles are not modified by freezing-thawing procedures. Reprod Biomed Online. 2012;26:240–6.
62. Vanderzwalmen P, Hiemer A, Rubner P, Bach M, Neyer A, Stecher A, Uher P, Zintz M, Lejeune B, Vanderzwalmen S, Cassuto G, Zech NH. Blastocyst development after sperm selection at high magnification is associated with size and number of nuclear vacuoles. Reprod Biomed Online. 2008;17:617–27.
63. Cassuto NG, Bouret D, Plouchart JM, Jellad S, Vanderzwalmen P, Balet R, Larue L, Barak Y. A new real-time morphology classification for human spermatozoa: a link for fertilization and improved embryo quality. Fertil Steril. 2009;92:1616–25.
64. Knez K, Tomazevic T, Vrtacnik-Bokal E, Virant-Klun I. Developmental dynamics of IMSI-derived embryos: a time-lapse prospective study. Reprod Biomed Online. 2013;27(2):161–71.
65. Knez K, Zorn B, Tomazevic T, Vrtacnik-Bokal E, Virant-Klun I. The IMSI procedure improves poor embryo development in the same infertile couples with poor semen quality: a comparative prospective randomized study. Reprod Biol Endocrinol. 2011;9:123.
66. Shoukir Y, Chardonnens D, Campana A, Sakkas D. Blastocyst development from supernumerary embryos after intracytoplasmic sperm injection: a paternal influence? Hum Reprod. 1998;13:1632–7.
67. Tesarik J, Greco E, Mendoza C. Late, but not early, paternal effect on human embryo development is related to sperm DNA fragmentation. Hum Reprod. 2004;19:611–5.
68. Tesarik J, Mendoza C, Greco E. Paternal effects acting during the first cell cycle of human preimplantation development after ICSI. Hum Reprod. 2002;17:184–9.
69. Virro MR, Larson-Cook KL, Evenson DP. Sperm chromatin structure assay (SCSA) parameters are related to fertilization, blastocyst development, and ongoing pregnancy in in vitro fertilization and intracytoplasmic sperm injection cycles. Fertil Steril. 2004;81:1289–95.
70. Larson KL, DeJonge CJ, Barnes AM, Jost LK, Evenson DP. Sperm chromatin structure assay parameters as predictors of failed pregnancy following assisted reproductive techniques. Hum Reprod. 2000;15:1717–22.
71. Nasr-Esfahani MH, Salehi M, Razavi S, Anjomshoa M, Rozbahani S, Moulavi F, Mardani M. Effect of sperm DNA damage and sperm protamine deficiency on fertilization and embryo development post-ICSI. Reprod Biomed Online. 2005;11:198–205.
72. Talebi AR, Vahidi S, Aflatoonian A, Ghasemi N, Ghasemzadeh J, Firoozabadi RD, Moein MR. Cytochemical evaluation of sperm chromatin and DNA integrity in couples with unexplained recurrent spontaneous abortions. Andrologia. 2012;44 Suppl 1:462–70.
73. Berkovitz A, Eltes F, Ellenbogen A, Peer S, Feldberg D, Bartoov B. Does the presence of nuclear vacuoles in human sperm selected for ICSI affect pregnancy outcome? Hum Reprod. 2006;21:1787–90.
74. Bartoov B, Berkovitz A, Eltes F, Kogosovsky A, Yagoda A, Lederman H, Artzi S, Gross M, Barak Y. Pregnancy rates are higher with intracytoplasmic morphologically selected sperm injection than with conventional intracytoplasmic injection. Fertil Steril. 2003;80:1413–9.
75. Bartoov B, Berkovitz A, Eltes F, Kogosowski A, Menezo Y, Barak Y. Real-time fine morphology of motile human sperm cells is associated with IVF-ICSI outcome. J Androl. 2002;23:1–8.
76. Delaroche L, Yazbeck C, Gout C, Kahn V, Oger P, Rougier N. Intracytoplasmic morphologically selected sperm injection (IMSI) after repeated IVF or ICSI failures: a prospective comparative study. Eur J Obstet Gynecol Reprod Biol. 2013;167:76–80.
77. Greco E, Scarselli F, Fabozzi G, Colasante A, Zavaglia D, Alviggi E, Litwicka K, Varricchio MT, Minasi MG, Tesarik J. Sperm vacuoles negatively affect outcomes in intracytoplasmic morphologically selected sperm injection in terms of pregnancy, implantation, and live-birth rates. Fertil Steril. 2013;100:379–85.
78. Klement AH, Koren-Morag N, Itsykson P, Berkovitz A. Intracytoplasmic morphologically selected sperm injection versus intracytoplasmic sperm injection: a step toward a clinical algorithm. Fertil Steril. 2013;99:1290–3.
79. Antinori M, Licata E, Dani G, Cerusico F, Versaci C, D'Angelo D, Antinori S. Intracytoplasmic morphologically selected sperm injection: a prospective randomized trial. Reprod Biomed Online. 2008;16:835–41.
80. Nadalini M, Tarozzi N, Distratis V, Scaravelli G, Borini A. Impact of intracytoplasmic morphologically selected sperm injection on assisted reproduction outcome: a review. Reprod Biomed Online. 2009;19:45–55.
81. Balaban B, Yakin K, Alatas C, Oktem O, Isiklar A, Urman B. Clinical outcome of intracytoplasmic injection of spermatozoa morphologically selected under high magnification: a prospective randomized study. Reprod Biomed Online. 2011;22:472–6.
82. Setti SA, Ferreira RC, Paes de Almeida Ferreira Braga D, de Cassia Savio Figueira R, Iaconelli Jr A, Borges Jr E. Intracytoplasmic sperm injection outcome versus intracytoplasmic morphologically selected sperm injection outcome: a meta-analysis. Reprod Biomed Online. 2010;21:450–5.
83. El Khattabi L, Dupont C, Sermondade N, Hugues JN, Poncelet C, Porcher R, Cedrin-Durnerin I, Lévy R, Sifer C. Is intracytoplasmic morphologically selected sperm injection effective in patients with infertility related to teratozoospermia or repeated implantation failure? Fertil Steril. 2013;100:62–8.
84. Setti A, Figueira R, Braga D, Aoki T, Iaconelli Jr T, Borges Jr E. Intracytoplasmic morphologically selected sperm injection is beneficial in cases of

advanced maternal age: a prospective randomized study. Eur J Obstet Gynecol. 2013;171(2):286–90.
85. Leandri RD, Gachet A, Pfeffer J, Celebi C, Rives N, Carre-Pigeon F, Kulski O, Mitchell V, Parinaud J. Is intracytoplasmic morphologically selected sperm injection (IMSI) beneficial in the first ART cycle? A multicentric randomized controlled trial. Andrology. 2013;1(5):692–7.
86. Marci R, Murisier F, Lo Monte G, Soave I, Chanson A, Urner F, Germond M. Clinical outcome after IMSI procedure in an unselected infertile population: a pilot study. Reprod Health. 2013;10:16.
87. Fernández-Gonzalez R, Moreira PN, Pérez-Crespo M, Sánchez-Martín M, Ramirez MA, Pericuesta E, Bilbao A, Bermejo-Alvarez P, de Dios Hourcade J, de Fonseca FR, Gutiérrez-Adán A. Long-term effects of mouse intracytoplasmic sperm injection with DNA-fragmented sperm on health and behavior of adult offspring. Biol Reprod. 2008;78:761–72.
88. Cassuto NG, Hazout A, Bouret D, Balet R, Larue L, Benifla JL, Viot G. Low birth defects by deselecting abnormal spermatozoa before ICSI. Reprod Biomed Online. 2013;28(1):47–53. doi:10.1016/j.rbmo.2013.08.013.
89. Berkovitz A, Eltes F, Paul M, Adrian E, Benjamin B. The chance of having a healthy normal child following intracytoplasmic Morphologically-selected sperm injection (IMSI) treatment is higher compared to conventional IVF-ICSI treatment. Fertil Steril. 2007;88 Suppl 1:S20.

MSOME: Conventional Semen Analysis, Sperm Manipulation, and Cryopreservation

12

Amanda S. Setti and Edson Borges Jr.

MSOME and Conventional Semen Analysis

Evaluation of sperm morphology plays a crucial role in the diagnosis of male fertility potential and has demonstrated a predictive value for IVF-ICSI treatments [1–3]. MSOME provides an accurate description of spermatozoa abnormalities, particularly the presence of head vacuoles [4]. However, no consensus has been established concerning normal or abnormal MSOME criteria, despite being essential to transposing MSOME analysis into routine evaluation of male infertility [5]. Therefore, some studies have analyzed the relationship between sperm normalcy according to the World Health Organization (WHO) or Tygerberg criteria and MSOME.

Bartoov et al. [4] investigated the relationship between normal spermatozoa according to the WHO reference values [6] and MSOME in 20 patients and found no significant correlations between the percentage of morphologically normal spermatozoa as defined by the WHO and the percentage of morphologically normal spermatozoa as defined by MSOME. Conversely, a strong positive correlation between the percentage of normal sperm forms according to the Tygerberg criteria and MSOME was observed by Oliveira et al. [7]. Nevertheless, both studies found that MSOME was shown to be much more restrictive, presenting significantly lower normality percentages for the semen samples in comparison to those observed after analysis according to the Tygerberg or WHO criteria.

Later, Cassuto et al. [8] found significant correlations between the incidence of score-0 spermatozoa (presenting an abnormal head, one or several vacuoles, and an abnormal base) and sperm concentration, motility, and morphology.

Conventional semen analysis and MSOME evaluation were performed simultaneously in sperm samples from 440 patients [5]. The results showed that sperm head vacuoles were significantly larger in abnormal semen samples. Relative vacuolar area (RVA), defined as vacuole area (μm^2)/head area (μm^2) × 100, was the most discriminative MSOME criterion between normal and abnormal semen samples, and was negatively correlated with poor sperm morphology.

It is noteworthy that routine morphological examination is performed on the entire semen sample, whereas the most remarkable feature of MSOME is the focus on motile sperm fractions,

A.S. Setti, BSc
Instituto Sapientiae - Centro de Estudos e Pesquisa em Reprodução Assistida,
Av. Brigadeiro Luis Antonio, 4545, Sao Paulo, SP 01401-002, Brazil
e-mail: amanda@sapientiae.org.br

E. Borges Jr, MD, PhD (✉)
Fertility - Centro de Fertilização Assistida,
Av. Brigadeiro Luis Antonio, 4545, Sao Paulo, SP 01401-002, Brazil
e-mail: edson@fertility.com.br

providing information about the sperm fraction referred for ICSI. Moreover, MSOME is a reliable technique for analyzing semen and has been suggested as a routine technique for semen analysis [9].

MSOME and Sperm Preparation and Manipulation

During semen sample liquefaction, the spermatozoa are exposed to round cells and leukocytes, both potential sources of reactive oxygen species (ROS) that are positively correlated with sperm head morphological abnormalities [10]. Moreover, the concentration of ROS may produce crater defects in the form of deep vacuoles in mammals [11].

Despite the origin of sperm vacuoles remains disappointingly unknown, the use of MSOME may be a helpful tool for the selection of spermatozoa. However, whether or not specific in vitro conditions during sperm preparation and manipulation results in the formation of sperm vacuoles is still under debate.

It has previously been demonstrated that extended in vitro culture at 37 °C may reduce sperm viability [12]. Since the morphological evaluation of sperm under high magnification is a time-consuming technique [13], there has been some investigation regarding the impact of semen sample incubation at 37 °C on the sperm nucleus morphology. It has been demonstrated that after 2 h of incubation at 37 °C there was a significant increase in the frequency of vacuolated nuclei [14]. No significant morphological changes in sperm nuclei were observed upon prolonged incubation at 21 °C. Additionally, after 2 h of incubation, the incidence of spermatozoa with vacuolated nuclei was significantly higher at 37 °C compared with 21 °C [14]. Similarly, Schwarz et al. [15] reported a negative impact of temperature on the morphological integrity of sperm nuclei. Conversely, using the sperm-microcapture channels in a 24-h period, Neyer et al. [16] demonstrated that sperm vacuoles are not generated by incubation at 37 °C.

Several semen preparation techniques have been established to separate the sperm fraction for use in assisted reproductive techniques. The most commonly used protocols are density-gradient centrifugation and swim-up [17]. Several studies addressed whether there was any differences between these two methods regarding sperm motility and concentration after semen preparation and the outcomes of intrauterine insemination [18–22]. It is of great importance to select a processing technique that improves the sample with spermatozoids that show a low amount of nuclear vacuolization after preparation.

Monqaut et al. [23] evaluated sperm morphology under high magnification before and after swim-up and density gradient centrifugation and classified recovered spermatozoa according to the degree of vacuolization. Despite both methods showed a positive effect on sperm quality, the swim-up method produced significantly higher incidence of morphologically normal spermatozoa than gradient centrifugation.

Borges et al. [24] compared the results of intracytoplasmic morphologically selected sperm injection between cycles in which the swim-up or the density gradient centrifugation techniques were used for sperm preparation. Implantation, pregnancy, and miscarriage rates were not statistically different between the groups. Both techniques recovered improved sperm fractions and resulted in similar IMSI outcomes.

MSOME and Sperm Cryopreservation

Human sperm cryopreservation has been routinely practiced for several years. Despite the success of sperm cryopreservation technique, the freezing–thawing process has proven to be associated with modifications in seminal quality, particularly the decrease in sperm motility and increase in morphological abnormalities [25].

During the cryopreservation of spermatozoa, both the formation of intracellular ice crystals [26] and the crystallization of the extracellular medium [27] are associated with mechanical damage and may result in rupture of the plasma membrane and disturbance of cellular organelles [28]. Moreover, sperm cryopreservation has been correlated with an increase in the levels of some apoptosis markers [29]. Lastly, cryopreservation was found to induce chromatin decondensation [30], DNA denaturation [31] and increased sperm DNA fragmentation [32]. However, it is still under debate whether or not cryopreservation can induce sperm nuclear damage. Most of the techniques used to evaluate sperm damage are invasive. It would be advantageous to recognize negative effects of cryopreservation that might appear in post-thaw spermatozoa. Hence, a few studies evaluated the sperm morphology by MSOME in frozen-thawed sperm.

Boitrelle et al. [33] evaluated whether or not cryopreservation modifies motile sperm morphology under high magnification and/or is associated with chromatin decondensation. Cryopreservation induced sperm nuclear vacuolization, decreased the incidence of grade I+II spermatozoa and the sperm viability rate and increased the incidence of sperm with noncondensed chromatin.

Conversely, Gatimel et al. [28] demonstrated that the cryopreservation has no effect on human sperm vacuoles. The main difference between the two studies is that Boitrelle et al. studied men from infertile couples, while only samples from recently fertile men were included in the study by Gatimel et al. Moreover, the dilution ratio with the cryoprotectant was different; and Boitrelle et al. used a morphological classification that included not only vacuoles but also other sperm abnormalities.

and the density-gradient centrifugation techniques recover improved sperm fractions and result in similar IMSI outcomes. Sperm cryopreservation may result in the appearance of vacuoles due to mechanical stress during the procedure. As long as the precise reasons for vacuole formation are still unknown, it is important to avoid prolonged sperm manipulation.

References

1. Kruger TF, Acosta AA, Simmons KF, Swanson RJ, Matta JF, Oehninger S. Predictive value of abnormal sperm morphology in in vitro fertilization. Fertil Steril. 1988;49(1):112–7.
2. Kruger TF, Acosta AA, Simmons KF, Swanson RJ, Matta JF, Veeck LL, et al. New method of evaluating sperm morphology with predictive value for human in vitro fertilization. Urology. 1987;30(3):248–51.
3. Kruger TF, Menkveld R, Stander FS, Lombard CJ, Van der Merwe JP, van Zyl JA, et al. Sperm morphologic features as a prognostic factor in in vitro fertilization. Fertil Steril. 1986;46(6):1118–23.
4. Bartoov B, Berkovitz A, Eltes F, Kogosowski A, Menezo Y, Barak Y. Real-time fine morphology of motile human sperm cells is associated with IVF-ICSI outcome. J Androl. 2002;23(1):1–8.
5. Perdrix A, Saidi R, Menard JF, Gruel E, Milazzo JP, Mace B, et al. Relationship between conventional sperm parameters and motile sperm organelle morphology examination (MSOME). Int J Androl. 2012;35(4):491–8.
6. WHO. WHO laboratory manual for the examination of human semen and sperm-cervical mucus interaction. 4th ed. Cambridge: Published on behalf of the World Health Organization by Cambridge University Press; 1999.
7. Oliveira JB, Massaro FC, Mauri AL, Petersen CG, Nicoletti AP, Baruffi RL, et al. Motile sperm organelle morphology examination is stricter than Tygerberg criteria. Reprod Biomed Online. 2009;18(3):320–6.
8. Cassuto NG, Hazout A, Hammoud I, Balet R, Bouret D, Barak Y, et al. Correlation between DNA defect and sperm-head morphology. Reprod Biomed Online. 2012;24(2):211–8.
9. Oliveira JB, Petersen CG, Massaro FC, Baruffi RL, Mauri AL, Silva LF, et al. Motile sperm organelle morphology examination (MSOME): intervariation study of normal sperm and sperm with large nuclear vacuoles. Reprod Biol Endocrinol. 2010;8:56.
10. Agarwal A, Said TM. Role of sperm chromatin abnormalities and DNA damage in male infertility. Hum Reprod Update. 2003;9(4):331–45.
11. Tremellen K, Tunc O. Macrophage activity in semen is significantly correlated with sperm quality in infertile men. Int J Androl. 2010;33(6):823–31.

Conclusion

The available literature seems to support that MSOME is a much stricter criterion of sperm morphology evaluation, since it identifies vacuoles that are not identified by the conventional semen analysis. Any technique that increases the quality of recovered spermatozoa and/or decreases the extent of vacuolated sperm could present an advantage in treatment's outcomes. Nevertheless, it appears that both the swim-up

12. Calamera JC, Fernandez PJ, Buffone MG, Acosta AA, Doncel GF. Effects of long-term in vitro incubation of human spermatozoa: functional parameters and catalase effect. Andrologia. 2001;33(2):79–86.
13. Berkovitz A, Eltes F, Yaari S, Katz N, Barr I, Fishman A, et al. The morphological normalcy of the sperm nucleus and pregnancy rate of intracytoplasmic injection with morphologically selected sperm. Hum Reprod. 2005;20(1):185–90.
14. Peer S, Eltes F, Berkovitz A, Yehuda R, Itsykson P, Bartoov B. Is fine morphology of the human sperm nuclei affected by in vitro incubation at 37 degrees C? Fertil Steril. 2007;88(6):1589–94.
15. Schwarz C, Koster M, van der Ven K, Montag M. Temperature-induced sperm nuclear vacuolisation is dependent on sperm preparation. Andrologia. 2012; 44 Suppl 1:126–9.
16. Neyer A, Vanderzwalmen P, Bach M, Stecher A, Spitzer D, Zech N. Sperm head vacuoles are not affected by in-vitro conditions, as analysed by a system of sperm-microcapture channels. Reprod Biomed Online. 2013;26(4):368–77.
17. Enciso M, Iglesias M, Galan I, Sarasa J, Gosalvez A, Gosalvez J. The ability of sperm selection techniques to remove single- or double-strand DNA damage. Asian J Androl. 2011;13(5):764–8.
18. Dodson WC, Moessner J, Miller J, Legro RS, Gnatuk CL. A randomized comparison of the methods of sperm preparation for intrauterine insemination. Fertil Steril. 1998;70(3):574–5.
19. Boomsma CM, Heineman MJ, Cohlen BJ, Farquhar C. Semen preparation techniques for intrauterine insemination. Cochrane Database Syst Rev. 2004;3, CD004507.
20. Xu L, Lu RK, Chen L, Zheng YL. Comparative study on efficacy of three sperm-separation techniques. Asian J Androl. 2000;2(2):131–4.
21. Allamaneni SS, Agarwal A, Rama S, Ranganathan P, Sharma RK. Comparative study on density gradients and swim-up preparation techniques utilizing neat and cryopreserved spermatozoa. Asian J Androl. 2005;7(1):86–92.
22. Sakkas D, Manicardi GC, Tomlinson M, Mandrioli M, Bizzaro D, Bianchi PG, et al. The use of two density gradient centrifugation techniques and the swim-up method to separate spermatozoa with chromatin and nuclear DNA anomalies. Hum Reprod. 2000; 15(5): 1112–6.
23. Monqaut AL, Zavaleta C, Lopez G, Lafuente R, Brassesco M. Use of high-magnification microscopy for the assessment of sperm recovered after two different sperm processing methods. Fertil Steril. 2011; 95(1):277–80.
24. Borges Jr E, Setti AS, Vingris L, Figueira Rde C, Braga DP, Iaconelli Jr A. Intracytoplasmic morphologically selected sperm injection outcomes: the role of sperm preparation techniques. J Assist Reprod Genet. 2013;30(6):849–54.
25. O'Connell M, McClure N, Lewis SE. The effects of cryopreservation on sperm morphology, motility and mitochondrial function. Hum Reprod. 2002;17(3):704–9.
26. Muldrew K, McGann LE. Mechanisms of intracellular ice formation. Biophys J. 1990;57(3):525–32.
27. Donnelly ET, McClure N, Lewis SE. Cryopreservation of human semen and prepared sperm: effects on motility parameters and DNA integrity. Fertil Steril. 2001;76(5):892–900.
28. Gatimel N, Leandri R, Parinaud J. Sperm vacuoles are not modified by freezing–thawing procedures. Reprod Biomed Online. 2013;26(3):240–6.
29. Said TM, Gaglani A, Agarwal A. Implication of apoptosis in sperm cryoinjury. Reprod Biomed Online. 2010;21(4):456–62.
30. Fortunato A, Leo R, Liguori F. Effects of cryostorage on human sperm chromatin integrity. Zygote. 2012; 21(4):330–6.
31. Dejarkom S, Kunathikom S. Evaluation of cryo-injury of sperm chromatin according to computer controlled rate freezing method part 2. J Med Assoc Thai. 2007; 90(5):852–6.
32. Gosalvez J, Nunez R, Fernandez JL, Lopez-Fernandez C, Caballero P. Dynamics of sperm DNA damage in fresh versus frozen-thawed and gradient processed ejaculates in human donors. Andrologia. 2011;43(6): 373–7.
33. Boitrelle F, Albert M, Theillac C, Ferfouri F, Bergere M, Vialard F, et al. Cryopreservation of human spermatozoa decreases the number of motile normal spermatozoa, induces nuclear vacuolization and chromatin decondensation. J Androl. 2012;33(6):1371–8.

MSOME and Sperm Chromatin Status

Florence Boitrelle and Martine Albert

Since the first use of intracytoplasmic sperm injection (ICSI) in the early 1990s [1], this technique has become a powerful tool for infertile couples—particularly in cases of severe male infertility and low sperm counts [1]. However, although the "best-looking" or the "morphologically most normal" live spermatozoon is chosen in ICSI, it is well known that this selection does not guarantee nuclear quality or enable nuclear defects to be detected [2, 3]. Over the last decade, several methods for better evaluation of the nuclear quality of live spermatozoa have been developed. For example, motile sperm organelle morphology examination (MSOME, using Nomarski differential interferential contrast microscopy and high magnification, >6,300×) was first performed in the early 2000s [4]. This sperm observation technique reportedly enables better assessment of a spermatozoon's morphology and better visualization of sperm head vacuoles—structures that are not visible at a conventional ICSI-like magnification (particularly if the vacuole is small, i.e., if it occupies <4 % of the sperm head's area) [4]. Sperm head vacuoles can be classified in terms of their size (large or small), position (anterior or posterior), depth (deep or superficial), number (single or multiple), and frequency. They are found in semen with normal characteristics as well as in semen with abnormal characteristics. In a recent systematic review of the literature [5], we discussed the links between the presence of vacuoles and embryo development following intracytoplasmic morphologically selected sperm injection (IMSI). In fact, individual spermatozoa differ in their ability to produce an embryo capable of implanting. Several studies have concluded that IMSI with morphometrically normal spermatozoa with no vacuoles or only one small vacuole is associated with significantly higher blastocyst and/or pregnancy rates [6, 7] (relative to IMSI with morphometrically abnormal spermatozoa or morphometrically normal spermatozoa with two or more small vacuoles or one large vacuole). Hence, we sought to answer the following questions. What underlies the putative relationships between blastocyst and/or pregnancy rates, sperm chromatin status and the spermatozoon's vacuolar status? Are vacuoles markers of sperm quality? Are they nuclear in nature and related to sperm chromatin status? And if vacuoles do reflect sperm chromatin status, is there any value in selecting vacuole-free spermatozoa for oocyte injection? Before studying the relationships between vacuoles and chromatin status, we first summarize links between vacuoles and chromatin structural abnormalities.

F. Boitrelle, MD (✉) • M. Albert, MD
Department of Reproductive Biology and Cytogenetics, Poissy General Hospital, 10, Champ Gaillard Street, 78303 Poissy, France

EA 2493, Versailles University of Medicine and Science, 78000 Versailles, France
e-mail: florenceboitrelle@yahoo.fr

Structural Aspects of Vacuoles: Links Between Vacuoles and Chromatin Structural Morphology

A normal sperm nucleus has been described as being convex, smooth, homogeneous and regular [8]. Human sperm vacuoles were first described as "nuclear holes" when examined by electron microscopy and two-dimensional imaging [9]. Using the same techniques, Chemes et al. reported that vacuoles were chromatin lacunae that could function as proteolytic centers to eliminate protein residues in sperm nuclei [10]. Thanks to the availability of higher-resolution techniques and technical progress in microscopy, it was shown that vacuoles were nuclear concavities rather than nuclear holes [11–13].

Atomic force microscopy is a nanometer-resolution type of scanning microscopy. Using this technique, large vacuoles (i.e., occupying more than 25 % of the sperm head area) have been described as thin nuclear areas where the plasma membrane was intact but sunken [11] or where the sperm plasma membrane subsided [12]. The vacuoles were then referred to as "hollows" or "concavities" (for more details, see Fig. 13.1 (reproduced from [11])). Use of three-dimensional (3D) deconvolution microscopy (a technique with a resolution of about 100 nm) confirmed that large and small vacuoles were respectively thumbprint-like and pocket-like nuclear concavities [11, 13]. Three-dimensional deconvolution microscopy with 4′,6-diamino-2-phenylindole (DAPI) staining of the DNA provided a description of the surroundings of the nucleus (for more details, see Fig. 13.2 (reproduced from [11]) and Fig. 13.3

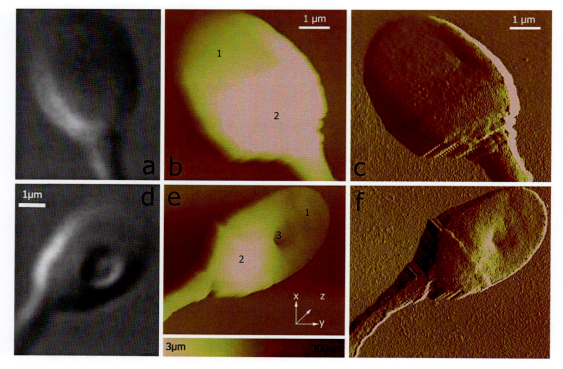

Fig. 13.1 Atomic force microscopy images. (**a**) a "top" spermatozoon observed under high magnification (10,000×) light microscopy with Nomarski contrast; (**b**) the same "top" spermatozoon observed using atomic force microscopy (AFM), with a z color scale indicating the thickness profiles of the head region; (**c**) the same "top" spermatozoon viewed with AFM, with a scale bar to measure the length and width. (**d**) a spermatozoon with a large vacuole observed under high magnification (10,000×) light microscopy with Nomarski contrast; (**e**) the same "vacuolated" spermatozoon observed using AFM, with a z color scale indicating the height profiles of the head region; (**f**) the same "vacuolated" spermatozoon using AFM with a scale bar to measure the length and width. Figure from [11]

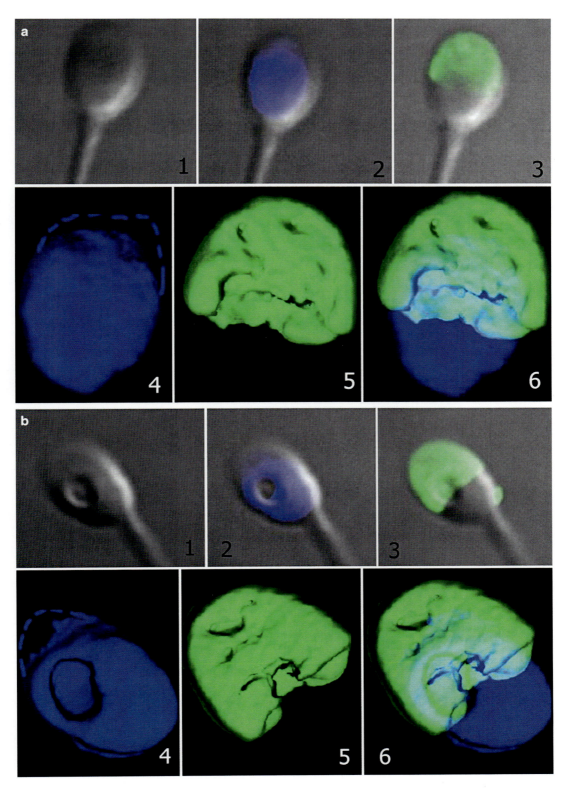

Fig. 13.2 Three-dimensional (3D) deconvolution microscopy images. (**a**) a "top" spermatozoon observed under high magnification with Nomarski contrast (differential interference contrast, DIC) (a1), a DIC/DAPI merge (a2) and a DIC/PSA (*Pisum sativum* agglutinin) *lectin* merge (a3). (a4–a6) 3D-reconstructed images of the same "top" spermatozoon. DAPI fluoresces blue (a4) and PSA lectin fluoresces green (a5). Colocalization of fluorescent probes (a6).

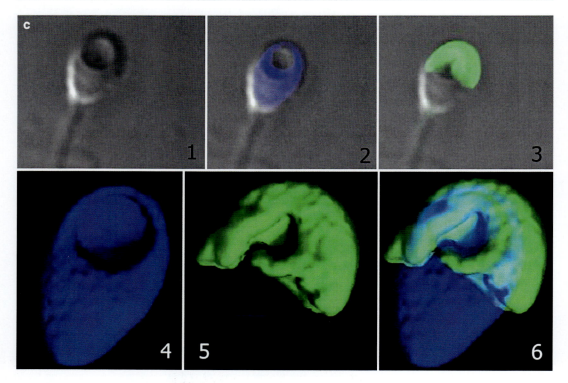

Fig. 13.2 (continued) (**b** and **c**) two spermatozoa with a large vacuole observed under high magnification with DIC (b1, c1), a DIC/DAPI merge (b2, c2) and a DIC/PSA lectin merge (b3, c3). (b4 and c4, b5 and c5, b6 and c6) 3D reconstructed images of the same "vacuolated" spermatozoa. DAPI fluoresces blue (b4, c4) and PSA lectin fluoresces green (b5, c5). Colocalization of fluorescent probes (b6, c6). Figure from [11]

(reproduced from [13])). Interestingly, use of a 3D reconstruction software package revealed that small vacuoles were deep, pocket-like, DAPI-negative concavities (for more details, see Fig. 13.4 (reproduced from [13])). These concavities were larger and deeper than expected from surface imaging alone (e.g., the vacuole indicated by a white arrow in the Figure). In summary, structural studies have described vacuoles as nuclear concavities of various sizes and at various depths. Hence, one could hypothesize that the presence of chromatin concavities in the sperm nucleus might have a negative impact on chromatin organization and status. In order to test this hypothesis, we and others have compared the chromatin status of various types of spermatozoa (vacuole-free spermatozoa and spermatozoa with small or large vacuoles).

The Relationship Between Sperm Head Vacuoles and Sperm Chromatin Condensation Status

Physiologically, a sum of complex events causes the sperm chromatin to condense very tightly (by up to six times more than in a somatic cell). Chromatin condensation takes place during the late stage of spermatogenesis (i.e., spermiogenesis), when most of the histones are replaced first by transition proteins and then by protamines. This replacement process leads to the generation of a mature spermatozoon with correctly condensed chromatin, i.e., chromatin in which 85 % of the DNA is bound to protamines and only 15 % remains bound to histones (for a review, see [14]). This histone–protamine

13 MSOME and Sperm Chromatin Status

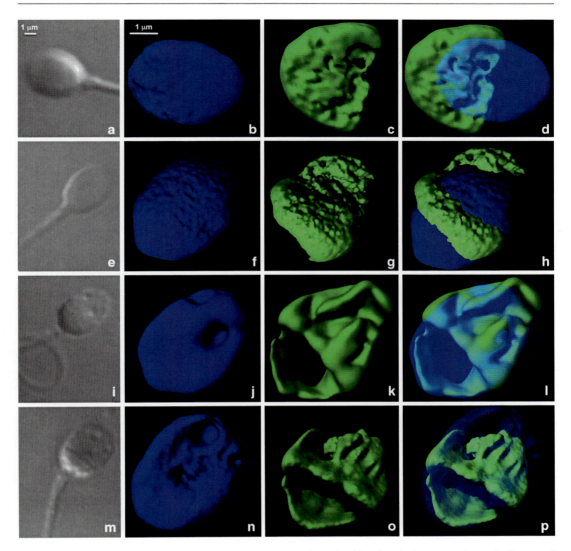

Fig. 13.3 3D deconvolution microscopy images. (**a** and **e**) two morphometrically normal spermatozoa with a vacuole-free head, observed at high magnification with DIC. (**b–d** and **f–h**) 3D-reconstructed images of the same, normal spermatozoon. DAPI fluoresces blue (**b** and **f**) and PSA fluoresces green (**c** and **g**). Colocalization of the fluorescent probes (**d** and **h**). (**i** and **m**) two morphometrically normal spermatozoa with multiple, small vacuoles observed at high magnification with DIC. (**j–l** and **n–p**) 3D reconstructed images of the same spermatozoa. DAPI fluoresces blue (**j** and **n**) and PSA fluoresces green (**k** and **o**). Colocalization of fluorescent probes (**l** and **p**). Figure from [13]

replacement is the end result of many complex epigenetic events, including the incorporation of histone variants and posttranslational histone modifications (e.g., methylation and acetylation). These events appear to influence embryo development after fertilization [15, 16]. Furthermore, it has recently been reported that sperm samples containing a high number of spermatozoa with non-condensed chromatin were involved in recurrent implantation failures [17, 18].

Several assays are available for quantifying protamines and evaluating chromatin condensation in spermatozoa, including direct methods (such as protamine extraction, electrophoretic separation and staining with Coomassie Blue) and indirect methods (such as chromomycin A3

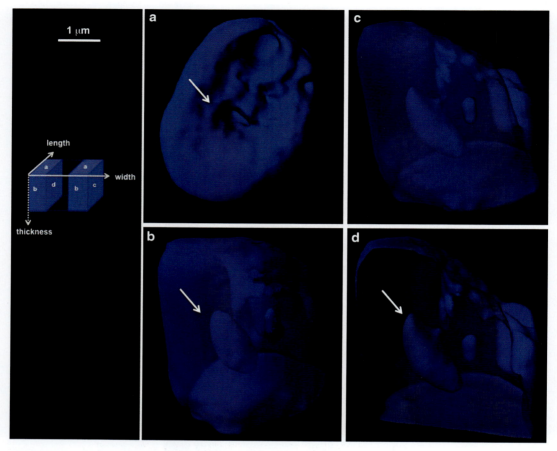

Fig. 13.4 Three-dimensional microscopy images (viewed in several planes) of the nucleus of the spermatozoon labelled as "**m**" in Fig. 13.3. (**a**) The nucleus surface (face *a* of the schematic cube) of spermatozoon **m**. (**b**) Posterior view (face *b*) of the nuclear contents. The *white arrow* shows a nuclear pocket (concavity) linked to a surface vacuole. (**c**) Right-side view (face *c*) of the nuclear contents. (**d**) Sagittal section of the nucleus (face *d* of the schematic cube), showing internal features. The *white arrow* shows a nuclear pocket linked to a surface vacuole. Figure from [13]

staining and aniline blue staining). For vacuoles, the two most frequently used chromatin condensation assays are chromomycin A3 (CMA3) staining (based on in situ competition with protamines) and aniline blue (AB) staining (based on the detection of residual histones in the sperm head).

As we recently reported in a review article [19], the relationship between the presence of vacuoles and the degree of sperm chromatin condensation has been extensively studied (for an overview, see Table 13.1 (reproduced from [19])). Some researchers have focused on chromatin condensation in spermatozoa with large vacuoles.

Below, we deliberately mention whether the studies in question assessed the chromatin condensation of spermatozoa with large vacuoles (regardless of the potential presence of other sperm abnormalities) or with a single, large vacuole as the only abnormality (i.e., in otherwise morphologically normal sperm). Indeed, we have found that spermatozoa's morphology (and particularly the size and shape of the head) is related to chromatin status (unpublished data). Hence, when seeking to establish robust links between vacuoles and chromatin status, we consider that it is essential to study vacuolated spermatozoa with no other morphological abnormalities.

Table 13.1 Relationships between sperm head vacuoles and sperm chromatin condensation status

	Number of patients	Chromatin condensation assessment	Vacuolated spermatozoa — Number and size of vacuoles	Presence of other potential abnormalities	Proportion of vacuolated spermatozoa with non-condensed chromatin (%)	Spermatozoa used as "controls" — Type of spermatozoa used as "controls"	Proportion of "control" spermatozoa with non-condensed chromatin (%)	P
Cassuto 2012 [20]	26	AB	At least one vacuole (size not specified)	Yes	19.5	Unselected spermatozoa (obtained after two-layer density centrifugation)	10.1	**p < 0.0001**
Perdrix 2011 [21]	20	AB	A single vacuole occupying >13 % of the sperm head area	Yes	50.4	Whole sperm	26.5	**p < 0.0001**
Franco 2012 [22]	66	CMA3	At least one vacuole occupying >50 % of the sperm head area	Yes	53.2	Morphologically normal and vacuole-free	40.3	**p < 0.0001**
Boitrelle 2011 [11]	15	AB	A single vacuole occupying >25 % of the sperm head area	No	36.2	Morphologically normal and vacuole-free	7.6	**p < 0.0001**
Boitrelle 2013 [13]	15	AB	At least three vacuoles occupying each <4 % of the sperm head area	No	39.8	Morphologically normal and vacuole-free	9.3	**p < 0.0001**

Studies (with sample sizes and methodological details) evaluating the relationship between the presence or absence of vacuoles and sperm chromatin condensation status. *AB* aniline blue staining, *CMA3* chromomycin A3 staining. *P* values in bold type are statistically significant. Table from [19], an Open Access article distributed under the terms of the Creative Commons Attribution License (http://creativecommons.org/licenses/by/2.0), which permits unrestricted use, distribution, and reproduction in any medium, provided the original work is properly cited

Firstly, in Cassuto et al.'s study of 26 patients, spermatozoa with an abnormally shaped head (i.e., an abnormal base and/or an asymmetric nuclear extrusion) and at least one large vacuole (although the size was not specified) were selected under high magnification [20]. This type of spermatozoa was referred to as "score-0." The researchers compared the degree of chromatin condensation (according to AB staining) of score-0 spermatozoa with that seen in unselected spermatozoa (i.e., those present in the sperm after two-layer density centrifugation). The proportion of spermatozoa with chromatin condensation failure was higher for the score-0 sample than for unselected spermatozoa (19.5 % vs. 10.1 %, respectively; $p<0.0001$). Perdrix et al. studied 20 patients and selected spermatozoa with one large vacuole (occupying >13 % of the sperm head area), regardless of whether or not the spermatozoa presented other morphological abnormalities [21]. The proportion of spermatozoa with chromatin condensation failure (according to AB staining) was higher for spermatozoa with large vacuoles than for spermatozoa from whole sperm (50.4 % vs. 26.5 %, respectively; $p<0.0001$). Franco et al. [22] studied 66 patients and selected spermatozoa with one or more large vacuole (occupying ≥ 50 % of the sperm head area)—again, regardless of whether or not these spermatozoa presented other morphological abnormalities. The researchers found that the spermatozoa with large vacuoles were more likely to present abnormal chromatin packaging (as assessed by the CMA3 assay) than morphologically normal, vacuole-free spermatozoa were (53.2 % vs. 40.3 %, respectively; $p<0.0001$). Once again, we consider that it is essential to study vacuolated spermatozoa with no other morphological abnormalities when seeking to establish robust links between vacuoles and chromatin status. We have thus adopted this approach. In a study of 15 patients, morphologically normal spermatozoa with one large vacuole (>25 % of the head area) were more likely to present chromatin condensation failure (as assessed by AB staining) than vacuole-free, morphologically normal spermatozoa (36.2 % vs. 7.6 %, respectively; $p<0.0001$) [11]. In summary, the above-mentioned studies all reported an association between the presence of one or more large vacuoles on one hand and chromatin condensation failure on the other. However, only one group has studied the nature of small vacuoles [13]. Spermatozoa with more than two small vacuoles (each occupying less than 4 % of the sperm head area) but that were otherwise normal (i.e., free of morphological abnormalities) were more likely to have non-condensed chromatin (as assessed by AB staining) than morphologically normal spermatozoa without vacuoles (39.8 % vs. 9.3 %, respectively; $p<0.0001$). Hence, several concordant studies have established links between the presence of vacuoles and chromatin condensation failure. One can thus legitimately hypothesize that human sperm-head vacuoles reflect nuclear quality. This notion is important for understanding how IMSI could benefit patients with recurrent implantation failures following ICSI or recurrent miscarriages; by giving us a "clearer view" of spermatozoa, IMSI enables better selection of spermatozoa with correctly condensed chromatin and helps avoid "at-risk" spermatozoa with vacuoles and chromatin condensation failure.

In addition to these links between vacuoles and chromatin condensation status, it is important to bear in mind that chromatin condensation is necessary for protecting the spermatozoon's nucleus during its long journey though the male and female genital tracts. Indeed, chromatin condensation failure confers susceptibility to external damage and then nuclear DNA damage (DNA denaturation or fragmentation, for example). Again, one can hypothesize that the presence of sperm vacuoles is associated with the degree of sperm DNA damage. Several research groups have studied these putative links (for a review, see [19]), which are discussed in another chapter.

In conclusion, most of the data gathered to date indicate that vacuoles are nuclear in nature and are associated with chromatin condensation failure and a potential increase in susceptibility to DNA damage. Hence, a decade after the first description of MSOME in the 2000s, this noninvasive technique enables (1) the visualization of nuclear structures that are associated with nuclear chromatin condensation failure and (2) the selection of spermatozoa with the highest quality nuclear chromatin.

References

1. Palermo G, Joris H, Devroey P, Van Steirteghem AC. Pregnancies after intracytoplasmic injection of single spermatozoon into an oocyte. Lancet. 1992; 340(8810):17–8.
2. Avendano C, Franchi A, Duran H, Oehninger S. DNA fragmentation of normal spermatozoa negatively impacts embryo quality and intracytoplasmic sperm injection outcome. Fertil Steril. 2010;94(2):549–57.
3. Abu DA, Franken DR, Hoffman B, Henkel R. Sequential analysis of sperm functional aspects involved in fertilisation: a pilot study. Andrologia. 2012;44 Suppl 1:175–81.
4. Bartoov B, Berkovitz A, Eltes F. Selection of spermatozoa with normal nuclei to improve the pregnancy rate with intracytoplasmic sperm injection. N Engl J Med. 2001;345(14):1067–8.
5. Boitrelle F, Guthauser B, Alter L, Bailly M, Bergere M, Wainer R, Vialard F, Albert M, Selva J. High-magnification selection of spermatozoa prior to oocyte injection: confirmed and potential indications. Reprod Biomed Online. 2014;28(1):6–13.
6. Vanderzwalmen P, Hiemer A, Rubner P, Bach M, Neyer A, Stecher A, Uher P, Zintz M, Lejeune B, Vanderzwalmen S, Cassuto G, Zech NH. Blastocyst development after sperm selection at high magnification is associated with size and number of nuclear vacuoles. Reprod Biomed Online. 2008;17(5):617–27.
7. Knez K, Tomazevic T, Zorn B, Vrtacnik-Bokal E, Virant-Klun I. Intracytoplasmic morphologically selected sperm injection improves development and quality of preimplantation embryos in teratozoospermia patients. Reprod Biomed Online. 2012;25(2): 168–79.
8. Auger J, Eustache F, Andersen AG, Irvine DS, Jorgensen N, Skakkebaek NE, Suominen J, Toppari J, Vierula M, Jouannet P. Sperm morphological defects related to environment, lifestyle and medical history of 1001 male partners of pregnant women from four European cities. Hum Reprod. 2001;16(12):2710–7.
9. Zamboni L. The ultrastructural pathology of the spermatozoon as a cause of infertility: the role of electron microscopy in the evaluation of semen quality. Fertil Steril. 1987;48(5):711–34.
10. Chemes HE, Alvarez SC. Tales of the tail and sperm head aches: changing concepts on the prognostic significance of sperm pathologies affecting the head, neck and tail. Asian J Androl. 2012;14(1):14–23.
11. Boitrelle F, Ferfouri F, Petit JM, Segretain D, Tourain C, Bergere M, Bailly M, Vialard F, Albert M, Selva J. Large human sperm vacuoles observed in motile spermatozoa under high magnification: nuclear thumbprints linked to failure of chromatin condensation. Hum Reprod. 2011;26(7):1650–8.
12. Watanabe S, Tanaka A, Fujii S, Mizunuma H, Fukui A, Fukuhara R, Nakamura R, Yamada K, Tanaka I, Awata S, Nagayoshi M. An investigation of the potential effect of vacuoles in human sperm on DNA damage using a chromosome assay and the TUNEL assay. Hum Reprod. 2011;26(5):978–86.
13. Boitrelle F, Albert M, Petit JM, Ferfouri F, Wainer R, Bergere M, Bailly M, Vialard F, Selva J. Small human sperm vacuoles observed under high magnification are pocket-like nuclear concavities linked to chromatin condensation failure. Reprod Biomed Online. 2013;27(2):201–11.
14. Oliva R, de Mateo S. Medical implications of sperm nuclear quality. In: Rousseaux S, Khochbin S, editors. Epigenetics and human reproduction. 1st ed. New York, NY: Springer; 2011.
15. Carrell DT, Hammoud SS. The human sperm epigenome and its potential role in embryonic development. Mol Hum Reprod. 2010;16(1):37–47.
16. Carrell DT. Epigenetics of the male gamete. Fertil Steril. 2012;97(2):267–74.
17. Kazerooni T, Asadi N, Jadid L, Kazerooni M, Ghanadi A, Ghaffarpasand F, Kazerooni Y, Zolghadr J. Evaluation of sperm's chromatin quality with acridine orange test, chromomycin A3 and aniline blue staining in couples with unexplained recurrent abortion. J Assist Reprod Genet. 2009;26(11–12):591–6.
18. Talebi AR, Vahidi S, Aflatoonian A, Ghasemi N, Ghasemzadeh J, Firoozabadi RD, Moein MR. Cytochemical evaluation of sperm chromatin and DNA integrity in couples with unexplained recurrent spontaneous abortions. Andrologia. 2012;44 Suppl 1:462–70.
19. Boitrelle F, Guthauser B, Alter L, Bailly M, Wainer R, Vialard F, Albert M, Selva J. The nature of human sperm head vacuoles: a systematic literature review. Basic Clin Androl. 2013;23:3.
20. Cassuto NG, Hazout A, Hammoud I, Balet R, Bouret D, Barak Y, Jellad S, Plouchart JM, Selva J, Yazbeck C. Correlation between DNA defect and sperm-head morphology. Reprod Biomed Online. 2012;24(2):211–8.
21. Perdrix A, Travers A, Chelli MH, Escalier D, Do Rego JL, Milazzo JP, Mousset-Simeon N, Mace B, Rives N. Assessment of acrosome and nuclear abnormalities in human spermatozoa with large vacuoles. Hum Reprod. 2011;26(1):47–58.
22. Franco Jr JG, Mauri AL, Petersen CG, Massaro FC, Silva LF, Felipe V, Cavagna M, Pontes A, Baruffi RL, Oliveira JB, Vagnini LD. Large nuclear vacuoles are indicative of abnormal chromatin packaging in human spermatozoa. Int J Androl. 2012;35(1):46–51.

MSOME and Sperm DNA Integrity: Biological and Clinical Considerations

14

Jan Tesarik

Introduction

Motile sperm organellar morphology examination (MSOME) has been introduced to human reproductive medicine as a tool for detecting subtle sperm morphological abnormalities, not detectable at the magnification used in standard intracytoplasmic sperm injection (ICSI) [1]. Intracytoplasmic morphologically selected sperm injection (IMSI), which uses MSOME for sperm selection, has been shown to improve assisted reproduction outcomes in some, though not all, andrological indications (reviewed in [2]).

The rationale of the use of MSOME-ICSI was to overcome the negative paternal effects on the early embryo development after conventional ICSI [3, 4]. Among these paternal effects, two patterns have been distinguished. The one, called the early paternal effect, impairs morphology and cleavage speed of the early embryonic cleavage divisions, whereas the other, called the late paternal effect, impairs implantation and the early post-implantation development without producing perceptible perturbations of embryo cleavage and blastocyst development [4]. The late paternal effect, but not the early one, has been shown to be associated with sperm DNA fragmentation [5, 6].

It has been suggested that MSOME can serve to select spermatozoa with intact DNA to be injected to oocytes [7], but conflicting observations have been reported in the literature. In this chapter the place of MSOME/IMSI in assisted reproduction in cases with pathologically increased sperm DNA damage is critically reviewed with regard to the current knowledge of etiology and diagnosis of sperm DNA damage, and alternative treatment methods to overcome its consequences.

Sperm DNA Fragmentation

The phenomenon of human sperm DNA fragmentation, and its relationship with sperm fertilizing ability and the developmental potential of the embryo, has been studied extensively over the past 10 years [7–9]. Abundant information is now available as to the etiology of sperm DNA fragmentation, methods of its evaluation, and its impact on sperm reproductive potential in vivo and in vitro.

Etiology of Sperm DNA Fragmentation

Sperm DNA fragmentation can be caused by different etiological factors. These include abnormalities of sperm chromatin remodeling during spermiogenesis [10, 11], an incomplete process

J. Tesarik, MD, PhD (✉)
Molecular Assisted Reproduction and Genetics,
MAR&Gen Clinic, Camino De Ronda 2,
Granada 18004, Spain
e-mail: jan_tesarik@yahoo.es; clinicamargen@gmail.com

of programmed cell death [12], and oxidative stress [13, 14].

Sperm chromatin remodeling during mammalian spermiogenesis involves the formation of DNA strand breaks in elongating spermatids [15]. In mice, these DNA strand breaks are normally marked by a histone phosphorylation event and later repaired by topoisomerase [16]. Failure of this repair process can be expected to lead to the persistence of the DNA strand breaks, created during spermiogenesis, in mature spermatozoa [17].

Programmed cell death is a physiological process in the testis, which is responsible for the regulation of the cell number ratio between germ cells and Sertoli cells [18] but also for the removal of damaged germ cells in different pathological conditions (reviewed in [7]). Germ cells undergoing programmed cell death in the human testis are removed through phagocytosis by Sertoli cells, and they are not released to the lumen of the seminiferous tubules [19]. Thus, DNA damage detected in ejaculated spermatozoa is unlikely to be caused by the classical programmed cell death pathway, as also supported by the lack of association between DNA fragmentation in human ejaculated spermatozoa and the presence of the typical markers of programmed cell death, such as caspase activity [19] or expression of *Bcl-x* and *p53* [12].

Oxidative stress appears to be the main factor responsible for DNA fragmentation in human spermatozoa. In spite of its protection by the highly condensed protamines, sperm nuclear DNA is still exposed to the action of reactive oxygen species (ROS) [17]. The risk of sperm DNA damage by ROS is especially high when the concentration of ROS in the proximity of spermatozoa is pathologically elevated or when the concentration of physiological antioxidant protective factors in the epididymis or seminal plasma is pathologically low.

Excessively high ROS concentrations can be generated by spermatozoa themselves [20], but they can also derive from leukocytic infiltration into the ejaculate caused by infection [21, 22]. Loss of antioxidant production, in its turn, can be related to smoking [23], or a decrease in the levels of antioxidant factors, such as vitamin C [24], carnitin [25] and co-enzyme Q_{10} [26], in the seminal plasma.

Evaluation of Sperm DNA Fragmentation

A number of diagnostic tests for the evaluation of sperm DNA fragmentation have been proposed. These include TUNEL [27], comet [28], chromomycin A3 assay [29], in-situ nick translation [30], DNA breakage detection fluorescence in situ hybridization [31], sperm chromatin dispersion test (SCD) [32], and the sperm chromatin structure assay (SCSA) [33]. Of these, TUNEL, SCSA, SCD, and Comet are the most currently used ones nowadays [7]. These tests evaluate the percentage of spermatozoa with fragmented DNA in a sperm sample. However, their results have to be interpreted in the context of available clinical comparisons between the percentage of DNA-fragmented spermatozoa and the outcome of an assisted reproduction attempt. This evaluation is not easy because it may be influenced by a number of factors not related to sperm DNA fragmentation, such as the age of the female partner, the technique of assisted reproduction used, and the characteristics of different evaluation methods. As a matter of example, Table 14.1 shows the supposed published thresholds of DNA integrity normalcy with TUNEL and SCSA in the clinical context of intrauterine insemination, in vitro fertilization, and ICSI [7].

The clinical context in which sperm DNA integrity is evaluated is of utmost importance. The number of previous failed assisted reproduction attempts, the female age, and the ovarian reserve are very important factors to predict the chance of assisted reproduction success with a given value of sperm fragmentation test [7].

Sperm DNA Fragmentation and Fertility

Excessive sperm DNA fragmentation has been reported to be associated with infertility, miscarriage, and birth defects in the offspring (reviewed in [9]). This condition is also known to impair results of assisted reproduction, including ICSI (reviewed in [7]). More specifically, sperm DNA fragmentation has been shown to be related to the

Table 14.1 Discriminating threshold values of SCSA and TUNEL suggested for prediction of assisted reproduction treatment outcome (presented in chronological order of publication)

Technique	Threshold (%)	Clinical context	Reference
TUNEL (M)	12; TUNEL+[a]	IUI	Duran et al. [71]
TUNEL (M)	18; TUNEL+[a]	ICSI	Benchaib et al. [72]
TUNEL (M)	24.3; TUNEL+[a]	ICSI	Henkel et al. [73]
TUNEL (M)	36.5; TUNEL+[a]	IVF	Henkel et al. [73, 74]
SCSA (FC)	27; DFI[b]	IVF, ICSI	Larson-Cook et al. [75]
SCSA (FC)	30; DFI[b]	IVF, ICSI	Virro et al. [61]
SCSA (FC)	27-30; DFI[b]	IUI, IVF	Evenson and Wixon [76]
TUNEL (M)	15; TUNEL+[a]	ICSI	Greco et al. [64]
TUNEL (FC)	30; TUNEL+[a]	ICSI	Hazout et al. [43]

Reprinted from Tesarik (2006) [7]
FC flow cytometry, *ICSI* intracytoplasmic sperm injection, *IUI* intrauterine insemination, *M* microscopy, *SCSA* sperm chromatin structure assay, *TUNEL* terminal deoxyribonucleotidyl transferase-mediated dUTP fluorescein–dUTP nick-end labeling
[a]TUNEL+ stands for the percentage of TUNEL-positive spermatozoa determined in a sample
[b]DFI is DNA fragmentation index, calculated as a product of the number of red-stained spermatozoa (single-stranded DNA) divided by the sum of red-stained and green-stained (double-stranded DNA) spermatozoa

so called "late paternal effect" on embryo development [5, 6]. This means that, rather than impairing fertilization and the development of early cleaving embryos, sperm DNA fragmentation has an impact on blastocyst formation [34], implantation and post-implantation development [35].

The Concept of MSOME

The concept of Motile Sperm Organellar Morphology Examination (MSOME) has been introduced by Bartoov et al. [1, 36, 37]. This method is based on a morphological analysis of isolated motile spermatozoa in real time at high magnification (up to ×6,600). MSOME has been applied to the selection of spermatozoa for ICSI—this combination has been given the name of Intracytoplasmic Morphologically selected Sperm Injection (IMSI) [1, 36–38].

The first publications demonstrated an increase in the pregnancy rate using IMSI compared with ICSI [1, 37]. However, subsequent studies comparing the success rates of IMSI and ICSI gave contradictory results. Some studies have shown that IMSI improves reproductive outcomes in case of male infertility factor and/or previous failed ICSI attempts in terms of implantation and clinical pregnancy rate as compared to conventional ICSI [39, 40]. On the other hand, IMSI and conventional ICSI seem to provide comparable laboratory and clinical results when an unselected infertile population is evaluated [41, 42]. Hence, the advantage of using IMSI instead of ICSI appears to be associated with some particular sperm pathologies. Indirect evidence has suggested that sperm DNA fragmentation may be one of them [7, 43].

How Can Spermatozoa with Damaged DNA Be Detected by MSOME?

It is well known that, in addition to its ability to identify common sperm organellar alterations, such as abnormalities of acrosome, postacrosomal lamina, neck, mitochondria, and tail, MSOME is also able to identify anomalies of sperm chromatin packaging reflected by the presence of sperm head vacuoles [1]. It was suggested that spermatozoa suffering this chromatin abnormality are particularly prone to DNA damage, and their use for assisted reproduction should thus be avoided [7]. However, this view has been contested by several other studies, and it is only

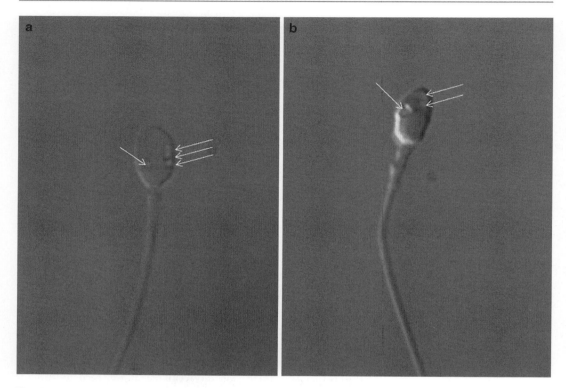

Fig. 14.1 Images of human spermatozoa by MSOME. (**a**) A spermatozoon with normal head shape and a few small vacuoles (<4 % of the head volume). (**b**) A spermatozoon with abnormal head shape and one large and several small vacuoles. *Arrows* indicate vacuoles. Reprinted from Greco et al. (2013) [60]

recently that the relationship between the presence of intranuclear vacuoles and sperm DNA damage has been demonstrated unequivocally.

Biological Considerations

Sperm intranuclear vacuoles were first observed by transmission electron microscopy [44]. These vacuoles were later observed by atomic force microscopy (a very-high-resolution type of scanning electron microscopy) and shown to correspond to pocket-like nuclear concavities linked to failure of chromatin condensation [45]. As compared with these high-resolution observational techniques that cannot be applied to living cells, MSOME, which works with living spermatozoa, cannot locate the vacuoles unequivocally with respect to other sperm-head structural components such as the plasma membrane and the acrosome (Fig. 14.1). Even though some vacuoles observed in the sperm head by MSOME may be of acrosomal origin, there are strong arguments supporting the nuclear location of these structures. For instance, MSOME has revealed vacuoles also in the heads of spermatozoa from patients with globozoospermia which lack an acrosome [46], and the induction of the acrosome reaction, leading to acrosomal vesiculation, did not modify the percentage of spermatozoa with sperm head vacuoles observed by MSOME [45, 47]. It is thus evident that most of the sperm head vacuoles observed by MSOME correspond to nuclear regions with defective chromatin condensation.

Sperm chromatin condensation occurs during spermiogenesis, and the replacement of the nuclear basic proteins histones by protamines is a key-event in this process. Evidently, testicular pathologies impairing this final phase of spermatogenesis can disturb this process. In fact, several concordant studies have established links between the presence of vacuoles and chromatin condensation failure [45, 48, 49].

The replacement of histones with protamines, required for sperm chromatin condensation during spermiogenesis, is known to protect sperm nuclear DNA against damage after the release of spermatozoa from the testis and their passage through epididymis [50, 51]. Oxidative stress, leading to sperm DNA fragmentation, is a major adverse factor to which spermatozoa are exposed after their release from the protective environment created by Sertoli cells with the testicular seminiferous tubules [7]. It is thus reasonable to suspect that sperm nuclear DNA is particularly prone to oxidative DNA damage in regions with defects of chromatin condensation, visualized as intranuclear vacuoles by MSOME. In fact, individually selected spermatozoa with large vacuoles [52, 53] or several large or small vacuoles [54, 55] have been found to present high levels of DNA damage.

Moreover, a recent study evaluating simultaneously sperm head morphology and the presence of nuclear vacuoles, on the one hand, and sperm DNA fragmentation, on the other hand, in the same single spermatozoa confirmed these observations [56]. In the latter study individual spermatozoa were first selected by MSOME and then subjected to Sperm Chromatin Dispersion (SCD) test to assess DNA integrity status (Fig. 14.2). The results show that all spermatozoa presenting a normal morphology and no traces of vacuolization by MSOME are free of DNA damage. As to spermatozoa with abnormal head morphology and/or intranuclear vacuoles, they are at risk of bearing fragmented DNA, but many of them are free of DNA damage [56]. These observations match perfectly with the idea that defects of sperm chromatin condensation expose spermatozoa to an increased risk of DNA damage when exposed to risk factors [7]. On the other hand, it seems that spermatozoa with defects of nuclear chromatin condensation can be entirely free of DNA damage if not exposed to potential DNA damaging factors. In agreement with this hypothesis, unpublished results obtained at our clinic show that the probability of DNA damage in a population of MSOME-selected spermatozoa with intranuclear vacuoles is higher as compared to vacuole-free spermatozoa only in cases in which the proportion of DNA-fragmented spermatozoa is pathologically increased, but not in cases with normal degrees of sperm DNA fragmentation.

Clinical Considerations

Several studies have shown that the chance of ongoing pregnancy after ICSI performed with spermatozoa with abnormal sperm head morphology and/or sperm head vacuoles, as evidenced by MSOME (IMSI), is lower as compared to cases with normal sperm head morphology [37, 39, 40, 57]. Accordingly, blastocyst development after sperm selection at high magnification is associated with the size and the number of nuclear vacuoles [58].

On the other hand, IMSI and conventional ICSI seem to provide comparable laboratory and clinical results when an unselected infertile population is evaluated [41, 59]. These findings are not surprising in the light of the observation that the presence of sperm nuclear vacuoles is not associated with an increased risk of DNA fragmentation in patients in whom the percentage of DNA-fragmented spermatozoa in the ejaculate is not pathologically elevated.

In some cases no morphologically normal and vacuole-free spermatozoa can be found by MSOME in the sperm sample to be used for IMSI. A recent study shows that this condition entails a significant impairment of pregnancy, implantation, and live birth rates as compared to cases in which morphologically normal and vacuole-free spermatozoa can be selected [60]. It has been suggested that sperm DNA fragmentation produces a so-called late paternal effect on early embryonic development, which means that the paternal effect can influence negatively late

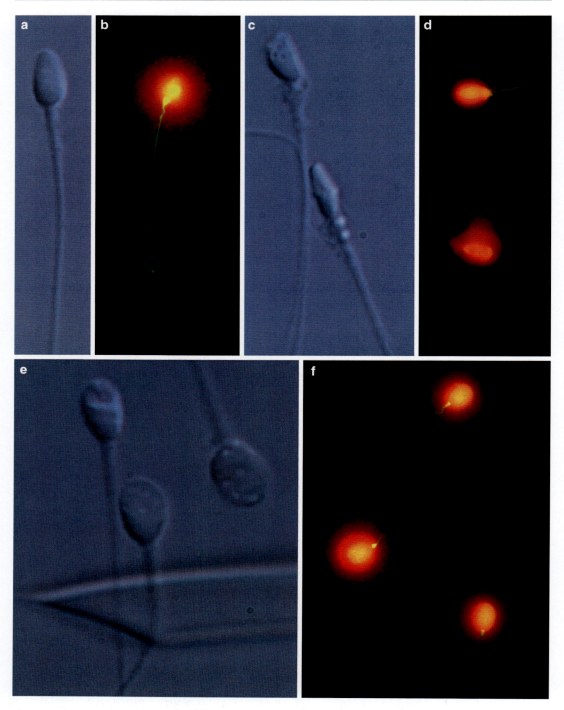

Fig. 14.2 Visualization of sperm morphology using MSOME and DNA fragmentation assessment using SCD test in selected spermatozoa. Normal spermatozoa showing absence of vacuoles (**a**) and absence of DNA damage in the same spermatozoa (**b**). Two highly abnormal spermatozoa (**c**) and presence of DNA fragmentation in both cases (**d**). Three spermatozoa showing presence of vacuolization (**e**) and lack of DNA fragmentation (**f**). Reprinted from Gosálves et al. (2013) [56]

pre-implantation and post-implantation embryo development as well as the clinical outcomes in the absence of any detectable impairment of zygote development, cleaving speed, and early pre-implantation embryo quality [5, 6]. In agreement with this idea, other studies have shown that blastocyst development [34, 61] and pregnancy outcome [6, 62] are impaired in cases of pathologically increased rates of sperm DNA fragmentation.

The Place for MSOME as Part of Diagnostic and Therapeutic Methods to Be Used in Cases of Pathologically Increased Sperm DNA Fragmentation

MSOME and Diagnosis of Sperm DNA Fragmentation

As outlined in the previous sections, MSOME is not a direct measure of sperm DNA damage extent. It provides information about sperm chromatin condensation status which is related to the vulnerability of sperm DNA to different kinds of potentially damaging factors. Hence, MSOME is probably not an examination to begin with if sperm DNA damage is suspected. In fact, MSOME outcomes can be properly interpreted only on the basis of previous knowledge about sperm DNA fragmentation, provided by direct tests detecting sperm DNA integrity.

In cases in which no excessive sperm DNA damage is detected the recourse to MSOME as a diagnostic tool may not be required. On the other hand, MSOME is important to evaluate the chance of avoiding the injection of DNA-damaged spermatozoa by IMSI if the rate of DNA fragmentation, determined by direct tests, is pathologically elevated. The chance of pregnancy by IMSI is higher when at least a few morphologically normal and nonvacuolated spermatozoa can be found, and this information is important for the choice of the optimal therapy in patients with pathologically elevated sperm DNA fragmentation (see below).

MSOME and Treatment of Sperm DNA Fragmentation

Several in vivo and in vitro treatments have been proposed to increase the chance of success of assisted reproduction in cases of pathologically elevated sperm DNA fragmentation. Oral treatment with high-dose anti-oxidants during 2 months prior to an ICSI attempt can be considered as an approach of the first choice [7], since it has been shown to decrease significantly the percentage of DNA-fragmented spermatozoa in 76 % of the patients treated [63] and to improve the ICSI outcome [64]. MSOME and IMSI can be used after previous antioxidant treatment to further improve the chance of success. This combination is even more interesting in the light of the finding that antioxidant treatment can produce defects in sperm chromatin condensation [65]. Because the presence of sperm head vacuoles, detectable by MSOME, has been shown to reflect defects in chromatin condensation (see above), the combination of in vivo antioxidant treatment and subsequent MSOME/IMSI can be expected to enable the selection of DNA- and chromatin-intact spermatozoa for fertilization.

If oral antioxidant treatment fails to lower the percentage of DNA-fragmented spermatozoa, MSOME is one of the available in-vitro sperm selection methods to be applied. These include the use of Annexin-V columns [66, 67] and a sperm selection method based on sperm–hyaluronic acid binding [68, 69], both of which have been shown to significantly reduce the percentage of spermatozoa with DNA fragmentation. Additional selection by MSOME of spermatozoa previously selected by these techniques may further improve the efficacy of these techniques, which might be especially important in cases in which only few oocytes are available for the assisted reproduction attempt.

Finally, if all in vivo and in vitro treatments fail, ICSI with testicular spermatozoa has been reported to significantly improve pregnancy rates in cases with pathologically elevated sperm DNA fragmentation [70]. MSOME, in combination with the other in vivo and vitro treatment technique may avoid the necessity of having recourse to this invasive technique of the last chance.

Conclusions

(a) MSOME can detect spermatozoa with chromatin packaging defects whose DNA is particularly sensitive to damage when exposed to destabilizing factors.
(b) If the degree of sperm DNA fragmentation, as determined by direct tests, is normal, abnormal spermatozoa, detected by MSOME, are unlikely to have their DNA fragmented.
(c) If the degree of sperm DNA fragmentation, as determined by direct tests, is pathologically elevated, abnormal spermatozoa, detected by MSOME, are likely to bear fragmented DNA.
(d) ICSI with MSOME-selected spermatozoa (IMSI) is not indicated in cases with normal sperm DNA, as detected by direct tests, unless other indications for IMSI are present.
(e) MSOME-IMSI can be used in cases of pathologically elevated sperm DNA fragmentation which do not improve after in vivo treatment with antioxidants.
(f) MSOME-IMSI can be used in cases of pathologically elevated sperm DNA fragmentation with a good response to oral antioxidant treatment to further decrease the risk of injection of a DNA-fragmented spermatozoa, especially if only few oocytes are available.
(g) MSOME-ICSI can be combined with other in vitro selection techniques to increase sperm selection efficiency.
(h) In cases of repeated failure of MSOME-IMSI, eventually combined with other treatment strategies, the recourse to ICSI with testicular spermatozoa may be needed as a treatment of the last chance.

References

1. Bartoov B, Berkovitz A, Eltes F. Selection of spermatozoa with normal nuclei to improve the pregnancy rate with intracytoplasmic sperm injection. N Engl J Med. 2001;345:1067–8.
2. Perdrix A, Rives N. Motile sperm organelle morphology examination (MSOME) and sperm head vacuoles: state of the art in 2013. Hum. Reprod. 2013. Update, Advanced Access, doi:10.1093/humupd/dmt021.
3. Janny L, Menezo YJ. Evidence for a strong paternal effect on human preimplantation embryo development and blastocyst formation. Mol Reprod Dev. 1994;38:36–42.
4. Tesarik J, Mendoza C, Greco E. Paternal effects acting during the first cell cycle of human preimplantation development after ICSI. Hum Reprod. 2002;17:184–9.
5. Tesarik J, Greco E, Mendoza C. Late, but not early, paternal effect on human embryo development is related to sperm DNA fragmentation. Hum Reprod. 2004;19:611–5.
6. Tesarik J. The paternal effects on cell division in the human preimplantation embryo. Reprod Biomed Online. 2005;10:370–5.
7. Tesarik J, Mendoza-Tesarik R, Mendoza C. Sperm nuclear DNA damage: update on the mechanism, diagnosis and treatment. Reprod Biomed Online. 2006;12:715–21.
8. Sakkas D, Alvarez JG. Sperm DNA fragmentation: mechanisms of origin, impact on reproductive outcome, and analysis. Fertil Steril. 2010;93:1027–36.
9. Aitken RJ, De Iuliis GN, McLachlan RI. Biological and clinical significance of DNA damage in the male germ line. Int J Androl. 2009;32:46–56.
10. Sakkas D, Mariethoz E, Manicardi G, Bizzaro D, Bianchi PG, Bianchi U. Origin of DNA damage in ejaculated human spermatozoa. Rev Reprod. 1999;4:31–7.
11. Marcon L, Boissonneault G. Transient DNA strand breaks during mouse and human spermiogenesis new insights in stage specificity and link to chromatin remodelling. Biol Reprod. 2004;70:910–8.
12. Sakkas D, Moffatt O, Manicardi GC, Mariethoz E, Tarozzi N, Bizzaro D. Nature of DNA damage in ejaculated human spermatozoa and the possible involvement of apoptosis. Biol Reprod. 2002;66:1061–7.
13. Kodama H, Yamaguchi R, Fukuda J, Kasi H, Tanak T. Increased deoxyribonucleic acid damage in the spermatozoa of infertile male patients. Fertil Steril. 1997;65:519–24.
14. De Iuliis GN, Wingate JK, Koppers AJ, McLaughlin EA, Aitken RJ. Definitive evidence for the nonmitochondrial production of superoxide anion by human spermatozoa. J Clin Endocrinol Metab. 2006;91:1968–75.
15. McPherson S, Longo FJ. Chromatin structure–function alterations during mammalian spermatogenesis: DNA nicking and repair in elongating spermatids. Eur J Histochem. 1993;37:109–28.
16. Leduc F, Maquennehan V, Nkoma GB, Boissonneault G. DNA damage response during chromatin remodeling in elongating spermatids of mice. Biol Reprod. 2008;78:324–32.
17. Aitken RJ, De Iuliis GN. On the possible origins of DNA damage in human spermatozoa. On the possible

origins of DNA damage in human spermatozoa. Mol Hum Reprod. 2010;16:3–13.
18. Rodriguez I, Ody C, Araki K, Garcia I, Vassalli P. An early and massive wave of germinal cell apoptosis is required for the development of functional spermatogenesis. EMBO J. 1997;16:2262–70.
19. Tesarik J, Ubaldi F, Rienzi L, Martinez F, Iacobelli M, Mendoza C, Greco E. Caspase-dependent and-independent DNA fragmentation in sertoli and germ cells from men with primary testicular failure: relationship with histological diagnosis. Hum Reprod. 2004;19:254–61.
20. Aitken RJ, Clarkson JS. Cellular basis of defective sperm function and its association with the genesis of ROS by human spermatozoa. J Reprod Fertil. 1987;81:459–69.
21. Aitken RJ, West KM. Analysis of the relationship between reactive oxygen species production and leucocyte infiltration in fractions of human semen separated on percoll gradients. Int J Androl. 1990;13:433–51.
22. Henkel R, Maass G, Hajimohammad M, Menkveld R, Stalf T, Villegas J, Sánchez R, Kruger TF, Schill WB. Urogenital inflammation: changes of leucocytes and ROS. Andrologia. 2003;35:309–13.
23. Fraga CG, Motchnik PA, Wyrobek AJ, Rempel DM, Ames BN. Smoking and low antioxidant levels increase oxidative damage to DNA. Mutat Res. 1996;351:199–203.
24. Song GJ, Norkus EP, Lewis V. Relationship between seminal ascorbic acid and sperm DNA integrity in infertile men. Int J Androl. 2006;29:569–75.
25. De Rosa M, Boggia B, Amalfi B, Zarrilli S, Vita A, Colao A, Lombardi G. Correlation between seminal carnitine and functional spermatozoal characteristics in men with semen dysfunction of various origins. Drugs R D. 2005;6:1–9.
26. Mancini A, De Marinis L, Littarru GP, Balercia G. An update of coenzyme Q10 implications in male infertility: biochemical and therapeutic aspects. Biofactors. 2005;25:165–74.
27. Gorczyca W, Traganos F, Jesionowska H, Darzynkiewicz Z. Presence of DNA strand breaks and increased sensitivity of DNA in situ to denaturation in abnormal human sperm cells: analogy to apoptosis of somatic cells. Exp Cell Res. 1993;207:202–5.
28. Hughes C, Lewis S, McKelvey-Martin V, Thompson W. A comparison of baseline and induced DNA damage in human spermatozoa from fertile and infertile men, using a modified comet assay. Mol Hum Reprod. 1996;2:613–9.
29. Manicardi GC, Bianchi PG, Pantano S, Azzoni P, Bizzaro D, Bianchi U, Sakkas D. Presence of endogenous nicks in DNA of ejaculated human spermatozoa and its relationship to chromomycin A3 accessibility. Biol Reprod. 1995;52:864–7.
30. Bianchi PG, Manicardi GC, Bizzaro D, Bianchi U, Sakkas D. Effect of deoxyribonucleic acid protamination on fluorochrome staining and in situ nick-translation of murine and human mature spermatozoa. Biol Reprod. 1993;49:1083–8.
31. Fernandez JL, Vazquez-Gundin F, Delgado A, Goyanes VJ, Ramiro-Diaz J, de la Torre J, Gosálvez J. DNA breakage detection-FISH (DBD-FISH) in human spermatozoa: technical variants evidence different structural features. Mutat Res. 2000;453:77–82.
32. Fernandez JL, Muriel L, Rivero MT, Goyanes V, Vazquez R, Alvarez JG. The sperm chromatin dispersion test: a simple method for the determination of sperm DNA fragmentation. J Androl. 2003;24:59–66.
33. Evenson DP, Larson KL, Jost LK. Sperm chromatin structure assay: its clinical use for detecting sperm DNA fragmentation in male infertility and comparisons with other techniques. J Androl. 2002;23:25–43.
34. Seli E, Gardner DK, Schoolcraft WB, Moffatt O, Sakkas D. Extent of nuclear DNA damage in ejaculated spermatozoa impacts on blastocyst development after in vitro fertilization. Fertil Steril. 2004;82:378–83.
35. Borini A, Tarozzi N, Bizzaro D, Bonu MA, Fava L, Flamigni C, Coticchio G. Sperm DNA fragmentation: paternal effect on early post-implantation embryo development in ART. Hum Reprod. 2006;21:2876–81.
36. Bartoov B, Berkovitz A, Eltes F, Kogosowski A, Menezo YJ, Barak Y. Real-time fine morphology of motile human sperm cells is associated with IVF-ICSI outcome. J Androl. 2002;23:1–8.
37. Bartoov B, Berkovitz A, Eltes F, Kogosovsky A, Yagoda A, Lederman H, Artzi S, Gross M, Barak Y. Pregnancy rates are higher with intracytoplasmic morphologically selected sperm injection than with conventional intracytoplasmic injection. Fertil Steril. 2003;80:1413–9.
38. Berkovitz A, Eltes F, Yaari S, Katz N, Barr I, Fishman A, Bartoov B. The morphological normalcy of the sperm nucleus and pregnancy rate of intracytoplasmic injection with morphologically selected sperm. Hum Reprod. 2005;20:185–90.
39. Berkovitz A, Eltes F, Lederman H, Peer S, Ellenbogen A, Feldberg B, Bartoov B. How to improve IVF-ICSI outcome by sperm selection. Reprod Biomed Online. 2006;12:634–8.
40. Antinori M, Licata E, Dani G, Cerusico F, Versaci C, D'Angelo D, Antinori S. Intracytoplasmic morphologically selected sperm injection: a prospective randomized trial. Reprod Biomed Online. 2008;16:835–41.
41. Balaban B, Yakin K, Alatas C, Oktem O, Isiklar A, Urman B. Clinical outcome of intracytoplasmic injection of spermatozoa morphologically selected under high magnification: a prospective randomized study. Reprod Biomed Online. 2011;22:472–6.
42. Souza Setti A, Paes de Almeida Ferreira Braga D, Iaconelli Jr A, Aoki T, Borges Jr E. Twelve years of MSOME and IMSI: a review. Reprod Biomed. 2013;27(4):338–52.
43. Hazout A, Dumont-Hassan M, Junca A-M, Cohen Bacrie P, Tesarik J. High-magnification ICSI overcomes paternal effect resistant to conventional ICSI. Reprod Biomed Online. 2006;12:19–25.

44. Zamboni L. The ultrastructural pathology of the spermatozoon as a cause of infertility: the role of electron microscopy in the evaluation of semen quality. Fertil Steril. 1987;48:711–34.
45. Boitrelle F, Ferfouri F, Petit JM, Segretain D, Tourain C, Bergere M, Bailly M, Vialard F, Albert M, Selva J. Large human sperm vacuoles observed in motile spermatozoa under high magnification: nuclear thumbprints linked to failure of chromatin condensation. Hum Reprod. 2011;26:1650–8.
46. Gatimel N, Leandri RD, Foliguet B, Bujan L, Parinaud J. Sperm cephalic vacuoles: new arguments for their non acrosomal origin in two cases of total globozoospermia. Andrology. 2013;1:52–6.
47. Neyer A, Vanderzwalmen P, Bach M, Stecher A, Spitzer D, Zech N. Sperm head vacuoles are not affected by in-vitro conditions, as analysed by a system of sperm-microcapture channels. Reprod Biomed Online. 2013;26:38–377.
48. Perdrix A, Travers A, Chelli MH, Escalier D, Do Rego JL, Milazzo JP, Mousset-Simeon N, Mace B, Rives N. Assessment of acrosome and nuclear abnormalities in human spermatozoa with large vacuoles. Hum Reprod. 2011;26:47–58.
49. Franco Jr JG, Mauri AL, Petersen CG, Massaro FC, Silva LF, Felipe V, Cavagna M, Pontes A, Baruffi RL, Oliveira JB, Vagnini LD. Large nuclear vacuoles are indicative of abnormal chromatin packaging in human spermatozoa. Int J Androl. 2012;35:46–51.
50. Muratori M, Marchiani S, Maggi M, Forti G, Baldi E. Origin and biological significance of DNA fragmentation in human spermatozoa. Front Biosci. 2006;11:1491–9.
51. Tarozzi N, Nadalini M, Stronati A, Bizzaro D, Dal Prato L, Coticchio G, Borini A. Anomalies in sperm chromatin packaging: implications for assisted reproduction techniques. Reprod Biomed Online. 2009; 18:486–95.
52. Garolla A, Fortini D, Menegazzo M, De Toni L, Nicoletti V, Moretti A, Selice R, Engl B, Foresta C. High-power microscopy for selecting spermatozoa for ICSI by physiological status. Reprod Biomed Online. 2008;17:610–6.
53. Franco Jr JG, Baruffi RL, Mauri AL, Petersen CG, Oliveira JB, Vagnini L. Significance of large nuclear vacuoles in human spermatozoa: implications for ICSI. Reprod Biomed Online. 2008;17:42–5.
54. Wilding M, Coppola G, di Matteo L, Palagiano A, Fusco E, Dale B. Intracytoplasmic injection of morphologically selected spermatozoa (IMSI) improves outcome after assisted reproduction by deselecting physiologically poor quality spermatozoa. J Assist Reprod Genet. 2011;28:253–62.
55. Hammoud I, Boitrelle F, Ferfouri F, Vialard F, Bergere M, Wainer B, Bailly M, Albert M, Selva J. Selection of normal spermatozoa with a vacuole-free head (x6300) improves selection of spermatozoa with intact DNA in patients with high sperm DNA fragmentation rates. Andrologia. 2013;45:163–70.
56. Gosálves J, Migueles B, López-Fernández C, Sanchéz-Martín F, Sáchez-Martín P. Single sperm selection and DNA fragmentation analysis: the case of MSOME/IMSI. Nat Sci. 2013;5:7–14.
57. de Almeida Ferreira Braga DP, Setti AS, Figueira RC, Nichi M, Martinhago CD, Iaconelli Jr A, Borges Jr E. Sperm organelle morphologic abnormalities: contributing factors and effects on intracytoplasmic sperm injection cycles outcomes. Urology. 2011;78:786–91.
58. Vanderzwalmen S, Cassuto G, Zech NH. Blastocyst development after sperm selection at high magnification is associated with size and number of nuclear vacuoles. Reprod Biomed Online. 2008;17:617–27.
59. Marci R, Murisier F, Lo Monte G, Soave I, Chanson A, Urner F, Germond M. Clinical outcome after IMSI procedure in an unselected infertile population: a pilot study. Reprod Health. 2013;22(10):16.
60. Greco E, Scarselli FG, Colasante A, Zavaglia D, Alviggi E, Litwicka K, Varricchio MT, Minasi MG, Tesarik J. Sperm vacuoles negatively affect outcomes in intracytoplasmic morphologically selected sperm injection in terms of pregnancy, implantation, and live-birth rates. Fertil Steril. 2013;100:379–85.
61. Virro MR, Larson-Cook KL, Evenson DP. Sperm chromatin structure assay (SCSA) parameters are related to fertilization, blastocyst development, and ongoing pregnancy in in vitro fertilization and intracytoplasmic sperm injection cycles. Fertil Steril. 2004;81:1289–95.
62. Larson KL, DeJonge CJ, Barnes AM, Jost LK, Evenson DP. Sperm chromatin structure assay parameters as predictors of failed pregnancy following assisted reproductive techniques. Hum Reprod. 2000; 15:1717–22.
63. Greco E, Iacobelli M, Rienzi L, Ubaldi F, Ferrero S, Tesarik J. Reduction of the incidence of sperm DNA fragmentation by oral antioxidant treatment. J Androl. 2005;26:349–53.
64. Greco E, Romano S, Iacobelli M, Ferrero S, Baroni E, Minasi MG, Ubaldi F, Rienzi L, Tesarik J. ICSI in cases of sperm DNA damage: beneficial effect of oral antioxidant treatment. Hum Reprod. 2005;20:2590–4.
65. Ménézo Y, Hazout A, Panteix G, Robert F, Rollet J, Cohen-Bacrie P, Chapuis F, Clément P, Benkhalifa M. Antioxidants to reduce sperm DNA fragmentation: an unexpected adverse effect. Reprod Biomed Online. 2007;14:418–21.
66. Said TM, Grunewald S, Paasch U, Glander HJ, Baumann T, Kriegel C, Li L, Agarwal A. Advantage of combining magnetic cell separation with sperm preparation techniques. Reprod Biomed Online. 2005;10:740–6.
67. Said T, Agarwal A, Grunewald S, Rasch M, Baumann T, Kriegel C, Li L, Glander HJ, Thomas Jr AJ, Paasch U. Selection of nonapoptotic spermatozoa as a new tool for enhancing assisted reproduction outcomes: an in vitro model. Biol Reprod. 2006;74:530–7.
68. Jakab A, Sakkas D, Delpiano E, Cayli S, Kovanci E, Ward D, Revelli A, Huszar G. Intracytoplasmic sperm injection: a novel selection method for sperm with

normal frequency of chromosomal aneuploidies. Fertil Steril. 2005;84:1665–73.
69. Parmegiani L, Graciela Estela Cognigni GE, Bernardi S, Troilo E, Ciampaglia W, Filicori M. "Physiologic ICSI": hyaluronic acid (HA) favors selection of spermatozoa without DNA fragmentation and with normal nucleus, resulting in improvement of embryo quality. Fertil Steril. 2010;93:598–604.
70. Greco E, Scarselli F, Iacobelli M, Rienzi L, Ubaldi F, Ferrero S, Franco G, Anniballo N, Mendoza C, Tesarik J. Efficient treatment of infertility due to sperm DNA damage by ICSI with testicular spermatozoa. Hum Reprod. 2005;20:226–30.
71. Duran EH, Morshedi M, Taylor S, Oehninger S. Sperm DNA quality predicts intrauterine insemination outcome: a prospective cohort study. Hum Reprod. 2002;17:3122–8.
72. Benchaib M, Braun V, Lornage J, Hadj S, Salle B, Lejeune H, Guérin JF. Sperm DNA fragmentation decreases the pregnancy rate in an assisted reproductive technique. Hum Reprod. 2003;18:1023–8.
73. Henkel R, Kierspel E, Hajimohammad M, Stalf T, Hoogendijk C, Mehnert C, Menkveld R, Schill WB, Kruger TF. DNA fragmentation of spermatozoa and assisted reproduction technology. Reprod Biomed Online. 2003;7:477–84.
74. Henkel R, Hajimohammad M, Stalf T, et al. Influence od deoxyribonuclei acid damage on fertilization and pregnancy. Fertil Steril. 2004;81:965–72.
75. Larson-Cook KL, Brannian JD, Hansen KA, Kasperson KM, Aamold ET, Evenson DP. Relationship between the outcomes of assisted reproductive techniques and sperm DNA fragmentation as measured by the sperm chromatin structure assay. Fertil Steril. 2003;80:895–902.
76. Evenson DP, Wixon R. Clinical aspects of sperm DNA fragmentation detection and male fertility. Theriogenology. 2006;65:979–91.

MSOME and Sperm Chromosomal Constitution

15

Amanda S. Setti and Edson Borges Jr.

Introduction

It is estimated that one in seven couples will experience fertility issues throughout their reproductive lives. The male factor, which is the single most common cause of infertility, is solely responsible in 30 % and contributory in an additional 30 % of cases [1, 2]. Assisted reproductive technologies (ART) are often considered as the first-line treatment to achieve pregnancy in infertile couples.

ART bypasses seminal abnormalities, such as a reduced sperm count, motility and percentage of morphologically normal cells. Traditionally, the evaluation of male fertility potential has relied upon microscopic assessment to determine semen quality [3]. Evaluation of sperm morphology has been known as the best prognostic indicator of spontaneous pregnancies [4], intra-uterine insemination [5], and conventional IVF [6] success.

However, the standard morphology evaluation on random stained cells from the ejaculate is of limited value during intracytoplasmic sperm injection (ICSI). Because the ICSI procedure involves the direct injection of the spermatozoon into the oocyte, embryologists considered that the morphological evaluation of male gametes was of secondary importance [7].

It is now well established that the spermatozoon is not only a genetic material carrier to the oocyte. The human spermatozoon is crucial for contributing three components: (1) the paternal genome, (2) the signal to initiate oocyte activation, and (3) the centriole, which participates in the initial zygote development [8]. Therefore, ICSI has created concerns over the possibility of a paternal influence because the fertilizing spermatozoon have highly dynamic and essential participation in embryogenesis that and may be determinant of compromised embryo development [8–12].

A spermatozoon considered as morphologically normal under a magnification of 400× (Fig. 15.1) may carry minor morphological defects that impair the fertilization process and embryonic development. In the past decade a new approach involving real-time, high-magnification (up to 6,600×) observation of unstained spermatozoa, named "motile sperm organelle morphology examination" (MSOME), has been introduced [13] (Fig. 15.2). MSOME is able to identify mainly sperm head vacuoles, considered as nuclear defects (Fig. 15.3) [13] that may be associated with DNA and chromosomal abnormalities.

A.S. Setti, BSc
Instituto Sapientiae - Centro de Estudos e Pesquisa em Reprodução Assistida,
Av. Brigadeiro Luis Antonio, 4545, Sao Paulo,
SP 01401-002, Brazil
e-mail: amanda@sapientiae.org.br

E. Borges Jr, MD, PhD (✉)
Fertility - Centro de Fertilização Assistida,
Av. Brigadeiro Luis Antonio, 4545, Sao Paulo,
SP 01401-002, Brazil
e-mail: edson@fertility.com.br

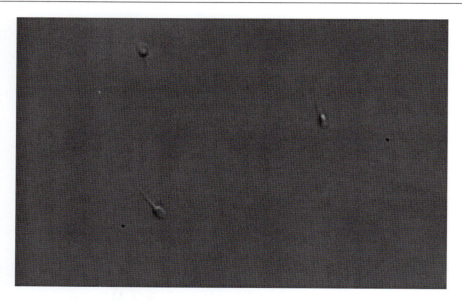

Fig. 15.1 Spermatozoa visualized under a magnification of 400×

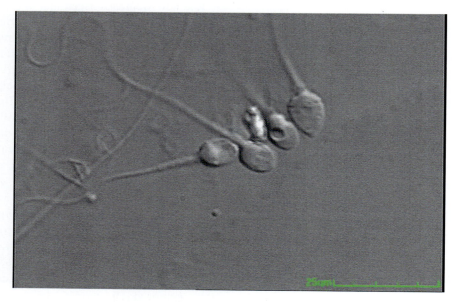

Fig. 15.2 Spermatozoa visualized by MSOME (6,600×)

Because all the available tests for functional and genetic sperm assessment are extremely cytotoxic, sperm DNA integrity, and chromosomal constitution cannot be assessed in the sperm cell used for ICSI.

Sperm Chromosomal Constitution

In males, meiosis begins with puberty and occurs continuously throughout adulthood. Through meiosis I (MI), primary spermatocytes divide into

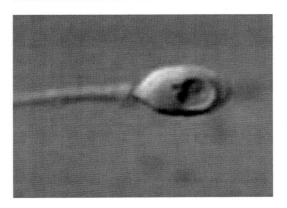

Fig. 15.3 Sperm with a large nuclear vacuole under MSOME (6,600×)

The human spermatozoon is an haploid cell ($n=23$) that contains 22 autosomes and one sex chromosome, either the X or Y. Anomalies in the sperm genetic information are known as numerical and structural chromosomal abnormalities. Numerical abnormalities comprise aneuploidies and polyploidies and structural abnormalities include chromosome breaks, gaps, inversions, insertions, deletions, translocations, and acentric fragments [14].

Techniques for Sperm Chromosomal Analysis

two secondary spermatocytes, and through meiosis II (MII) each secondary spermatocyte divides into two spermatids, which will differentiate and mature into a spermatozoon (Fig. 15.4).

Tremendous progress has been made studying the cytogenetics of male gamete. In 1970, the first chromosomal studies of spermatozoa were developed, using the differential staining of

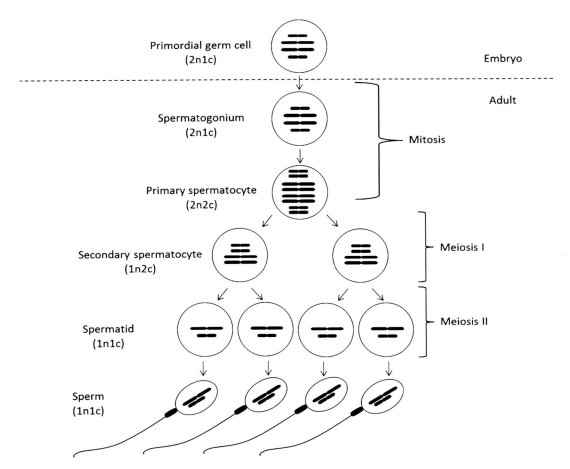

Fig. 15.4 Gamete formation in males (spermatogenesis)

specific regions of chromosomes [15]. An average aneuploidy rate of ~2 % per chromosome was reported, giving a total aneuploidy rate of 38 % if all chromosomes were considered together [16]. However, due to nonspecific staining of chromosomes, these estimates were considered excessive and untrustworthy. Thus, a more reliable technique was necessary.

In 1978, Rudak et al. [17] settled a system in which human sperm were introduced to hamster eggs which then proceeded through the initial stages of development. After that, cells were fixed and stained using karyotyping methods to observe metaphase nuclei, creating the first extended cytogenetic observation of human chromosomes, in which numerical as well as structural abnormalities could be analyzed.

In the 1990s, the first fluorescent in situ hybridization (FISH) assay was developed, offering a rapid, accurate and reliable technique for the identification of aneuploidy and polyploidy in human sperm [18]. However, due to the small size of the sperm head, FISH cannot be performed for all chromosomes because signals would overlap. Therefore, FISH is habitually performed for chromosomes related to aneuploidies that can result in live birth (chromosomes 13, 18, 21, X, and Y) [19].

Male Infertility and Chromosome Abnormalities

Human male infertility and chromosome abnormalities are frequently closely related. It has been reported that, in sperm of fertile men, the frequency of numerical and structural chromosome abnormalities varies from 1 to 2 % and 7 to 14 %, respectively [14]. Infertile patients have an increased incidence of chromosomal abnormalities [20], being the most common the aneuploidies, Y chromosome structural abnormalities, Robertsonian and reciprocal translocations, and chromosome inversions [21].

Alterations of semen parameters, including oligozoospermia, asthenozoospermia, and teratozoospermia, appear to be associated with increased sperm aneuploidy. Oligozoospermia was proven to be related to sperm chromosomal alterations [22, 23], but the highest levels are reported in men affected by severe oligoasthenoteratozoospermia and in men suffering from non-obstructive azoospermia [24, 25].

Despite aneuploid spermatozoa are still able of fertilizing eggs, their use for ICSI is associated with reduced pregnancy rates, recurrent abortion, and chromosomal aberrations in the offspring [26, 27].

MSOME and Chromosomal Abnormalities

Sperm chromosomal constitution cannot be assessed in the sperm cell used for ICSI, therefore, several studies have investigated the relationship between sperm morphology by MSOME and sperm chromosomal status.

Garolla et al. [28] evaluated the mitochondrial status, DNA integrity, DNA fragmentation, and sperm aneuploidies in normozoospermic subjects and in two groups of patients with primary testicular damage or partial obstruction of the seminal tract. Moreover, in patients with severe testicular impairment, mitochondria, DNA, and chromosomes were reanalyzed on a single spermatozoon, selected at a magnification of 13,000× on the basis of normal morphology. Patients with testicular damage showed increased sperm aneuploidies as compared to the controls. In contrast, in the PO group the mean percentage of sperm aneuploidies was not different from controls. From semen samples of the ten patients with testicular damage, a total of 20 single immotile sperm cells per patient were retrieved and classified on the basis of normal morphology and absence or presence of vacuoles. FISH analysis in these cells showed that no chromosomal alteration was present in morphologically normal sperm cells. It is important to highlight that in this study a different equipment setting, able to multiply the sperm image up to 13,000×, was adopted. The authors showed that no matter the initial status of the whole sperm sample, spermatozoa selected by this method have lower incidence of DNA and chromosome alterations and concluded that, especially in patients with severe testicular damage, the amplified use of MSOME could increase the efficacy and safety of the ICSI procedure, thus improving the outcome of male factor infertility treatment, above all in patients with severe testicular damage.

de Almeida Ferreira Braga et al. [29] investigated whether there was a connection between morphologic sperm normalcy evaluated through high magnification and sperm DNA integrity and sperm aneuploidy. The authors performed MSOME and FISH techniques in 200 sperm cells from 50 patients undergoing ICSI as a result of male infertility. The results showed that despite the presence of vacuoles and abnormal nuclear cell size was positively correlated with sperm DNA fragmentation, there was no correlation between these morphological features and aneuploidy. This result is in disagreement with the findings of Garolla et al. [28] and the authors justified that the studies' designs were very different, since de Almeida Ferreira Braga et al. analyzed the incidence of sperm aneuploidy in 200 cells, and Garolla et al. evaluated a single cell under high magnification and analyzed for sperm aneuploidies, which could explain the differences found between the studies.

Perdrix et al. [30] evaluated evaluate acrosome morphology, chromatin condensation, DNA fragmentation and sperm aneuploidy in spermatozoa with vacuoles occupying >13.0 % of sperm head area. For each of the 15 patients included in the analysis, results were compared with those obtained in spermatozoa from native semen sample. Results showed that aneuploidy and diploidy rates were significantly increased in sperm with large vacuoles. Nevertheless, due the low number of analyzed subjects, these results, as the authors themselves noted, should be interpreted with caution.

Watanabe et al. [31] utilized a human sperm chromosome assay to investigate whether the sperm vacuoles are related to DNA damage. Morphologically normal sperm (selected under 400× magnification) obtained from 17 patients and 3 fertile donors were analyzed for the presence of vacuoles under a magnification of 1,000×. In three patients and two donor samples, structural chromosomal damage was evaluated in normal sperm containing large vacuoles. The frequency of chromosomal abnormalities in sperm selected under high-magnification was not significantly different from that obtained for sperm examined under 400× magnification. Nevertheless, it is important to note that the incidence of normal-shaped sperm with large vacuoles was sporadic and therefore chromosome analysis dealt with low numbers. Since the incidence of chromosomal abnormalities was twofold higher in vacuolated sperm than the value in normal-shaped sperm without vacuoles obtained from the same patients, one might argue that that difference could reach statistical significance in the analysis of a larger number of patients. In addition, it is worth mentioning that in this study sperm morphology was examined under a magnification of 1,000× while in the majority of studies a magnification of at least 6,000× was applied.

Boitrelle et al. [32] performed high-magnification morphological evaluation (10,000×), in 15 infertile patients, to select 450 morphologically normal spermatozoa and 450 spermatozoa with a large vacuole (occupying ≥25 % of the head area). Subsequently, chromatin condensation, DNA fragmentation and the status of chromosomes X, Y, and 18 in these spermatozoa were analyzed. The results showed that despite the presence of a vacuole was associated with impaired chromatin condensation, normal and vacuolated spermatozoa did not differ significantly in terms of aneuploidy.

It has been proven that in patients with macrocephalic sperm head syndrome normal-head spermatozoa can be retrieved but these spermatozoa are often aneuploid [33]. Chelli et al. [34] investigated two infertile males with macrocephalic sperm head syndrome originated from North Africa. Norma-headed spermatozoa were selected under 400× and 1,000× magnification and the FISH analysis was performed on those selected spermatozoa. A total of 39 spermatozoa were selected under 400× and 6 were selected under 1,000×. A statistically significant decrease in diploidy and an increase in haploidy were observed in MSOME-selected spermatozoa as compared to sperm selected under 1,000×.

Despite the selection by MSOME resulted in significant elimination of sperm polyploidy and diploidy it did not eliminate the select of aneuploid spermatozoa. The authors highlighted that their results should be viewed with caution because only six spermatozoa were retrieved. Nevertheless, the absence of vacuoles after MSOME analysis was not a guarantee of normal chromosome content in these patients.

Another study evaluated whether high-magnification observation of spermatozoa in translocation carriers is related to sperm morphology and chromosomal content. Nine men carrying either a balanced reciprocal or a Robertsonian translocation were included in the study. The results showed that the absence of sperm vacuoles by MSOME was not sufficient to avoid spermatozoa with an unbalanced chromosomal content in patients carrying a reciprocal or a Robertsonian translocation [35].

Individual chromosomes reside in distinct territories [36, 37] and the preferential longitudinal positioning has been recognized for 11 chromosomes in human sperm [38]. Chromosomes X, Y, and 18 positioning has also been compared between spermatozoa with large vacuoles and normal spermatozoa analyzed and the results showed that chromosome architecture was modified in spermatozoa with large vacuoles compared with normal spermatozoa [39].

Conclusion

Recently, the MSOME, a noninvasive technique of sperm selection has been proposed to best predict ICSI outcome. The MSOME allows the selection of sperm cells with better physiological status and has been reported to result in improved implantation and pregnancy rates and reduced miscarriage rates. Few studies have investigated the chromosomal contents of morphologically normal and abnormal sperm cells selected by MSOME; however, to date, the results are still controversial. These discrepancies may be explained by (1) the lack of definition regarding the size of a large nuclear vacuole, (2) the difference in the total calculated magnification applied in sperm analysis, and (3) the characteristics of the patients analyzed in each study. Therefore, further studies are necessary to determine whether or not the presence of sperm vacuoles correlates with sperm chromosomal status.

References

1. Smit M, Romijn JC, Wildhagen MF, Weber RF, Dohle GR. Sperm chromatin structure is associated with the quality of spermatogenesis in infertile patients. Fertil Steril. 2010;94(5):1748–52.
2. Trost LW, Nehra A. Guideline-based management of male infertility: why do we need it? Ind J Urol. 2011;27(1):49–57.
3. Merchant R, Gandhi G, Allahbadia GN. In vitro fertilization/intracytoplasmic sperm injection for male infertility. Ind J Urol. 2011;27(1):121–32.
4. Bonde JP, Ernst E, Jensen TK, Hjollund NH, Kolstad H, Henriksen TB, et al. Relation between semen quality and fertility: a population-based study of 430 first-pregnancy planners. Lancet. 1998;352(9135):1172–7.
5. Van Waart J, Kruger TF, Lombard CJ, Ombelet W. Predictive value of normal sperm morphology in intrauterine insemination (IUI): a structured literature review. Hum Reprod Update. 2001;7(5):495–500.
6. Kruger TF, Menkveld R, Stander FS, Lombard CJ, Van der Merwe JP, van Zyl JA, et al. Sperm morphologic features as a prognostic factor in in vitro fertilization. Fertil Steril. 1986;46(6):1118–23.
7. Lundin K, Soderlund B, Hamberger L. The relationship between sperm morphology and rates of fertilization, pregnancy and spontaneous abortion in an in-vitro fertilization/intracytoplasmic sperm injection programme. Hum Reprod. 1997;12(12):2676–81.
8. Barroso G, Valdespin C, Vega E, Kershenovich R, Avila R, Avendano C, et al. Developmental sperm contributions: fertilization and beyond. Fertil Steril. 2009;92(3):835–48.
9. Host E, Ernst E, Lindenberg S, Smidt-Jensen S. Morphology of spermatozoa used in IVF and ICSI from oligozoospermic men. Reprod Biomed Online. 2001;3(3):212–5.
10. Lopes S, Sun JG, Jurisicova A, Meriano J, Casper RF. Sperm deoxyribonucleic acid fragmentation is increased in poor-quality semen samples and correlates with failed fertilization in intracytoplasmic sperm injection. Fertil Steril. 1998;69(3):528–32.
11. Munne S, Magli C, Bahce M, Fung J, Legator M, Morrison L, et al. Preimplantation diagnosis of the aneuploidies most commonly found in spontaneous abortions and live births: XY, 13, 14, 15, 16, 18, 21, 22. Prenat Diagn. 1998;18(13):1459–66.
12. Sakkas D, Urner F, Bianchi PG, Bizzaro D, Wagner I, Jaquenoud N, et al. Sperm chromatin anomalies can influence decondensation after intracytoplasmic sperm injection. Hum Reprod. 1996;11(4):837–43.

13. Bartoov B, Berkovitz A, Eltes F. Selection of spermatozoa with normal nuclei to improve the pregnancy rate with intracytoplasmic sperm injection. N Engl J Med. 2001;345(14):1067–8.
14. Verma RS, Babu A. Human chromosomes: manual of basic techniques. New York, NY: Pergamon Press; 1989.
15. Barlow P, Vosa CG. The Y chromosome in human spermatozoa. Nature. 1970;226(5249):961–2.
16. Pawlowitzki IH, Pearson PL. Chromosomal aneuploidy in human spermatozoa. Humangenetik. 1972;16(1):119–22.
17. Rudak E, Jacobs PA, Yanagimachi R. Direct analysis of the chromosome constitution of human spermatozoa. Nature. 1978;274(5674):911–3.
18. Ko E, Rademaker A, Martin R. Microwave decondensation and codenaturation: a new methodology to maximize FISH data from donors with very low concentrations of sperm. Cytogenet Cell Genet. 2001;95(3–4):143–5.
19. Templado C, Vidal F, Estop A. Aneuploidy in human spermatozoa. Cytogenet Genome Res. 2011;133(2–4):91–9.
20. Bourrouillou G, Dastugue N, Colombies P. Chromosome studies in 952 infertile males with a sperm count below 10 million/ml. Hum Genet. 1985;71(4):366–7.
21. Van Assche E, Bonduelle M, Tournaye H, Joris H, Verheyen G, Devroey P, et al. Cytogenetics of infertile men. Hum Reprod. 1996;11 Suppl 4:1–24. discussion 25–26.
22. Irvine DS, Twigg JP, Gordon EL, Fulton N, Milne PA, Aitken RJ. DNA integrity in human spermatozoa: relationships with semen quality. J Androl. 2000;21(1):33–44.
23. Zini A, Libman J. Sperm DNA damage: clinical significance in the era of assisted reproduction. CMAJ. 2006;175(5):495–500.
24. Shi Q, Martin RH. Aneuploidy in human spermatozoa: FISH analysis in men with constitutional chromosomal abnormalities, and in infertile men. Reproduction. 2001;121(5):655–66.
25. Shi Q, Martin RH. Aneuploidy in human sperm: a review of the frequency and distribution of aneuploidy, effects of donor age and lifestyle factors. Cytogenet Cell Genet. 2000;90(3–4):219–26.
26. Loutradi KE, Tarlatzis BC, Goulis DG, Zepiridis L, Pagou T, Chatziioannou E, et al. The effects of sperm quality on embryo development after intracytoplasmic sperm injection. J Assist Reprod Genet. 2006;23(2):69–74.
27. Egozcue S, Blanco J, Vendrell JM, Garcia F, Veiga A, Aran B, et al. Human male infertility: chromosome anomalies, meiotic disorders, abnormal spermatozoa and recurrent abortion. Hum Reprod Update. 2000;6(1):93–105.
28. Garolla A, Fortini D, Menegazzo M, De Toni L, Nicoletti V, Moretti A, et al. High-power microscopy for selecting spermatozoa for ICSI by physiological status. Reprod Biomed Online. 2008;17(5):610–6.
29. de Almeida Ferreira Braga DP, Setti AS, Figueira RC, Nichi M, Martinhago CD, Iaconelli Jr A, et al. Sperm organelle morphologic abnormalities: contributing factors and effects on intracytoplasmic sperm injection cycles outcomes. Urology. 2011;78(4):786–91.
30. Perdrix A, Travers A, Chelli MH, Escalier D, Do Rego JL, Milazzo JP, et al. Assessment of acrosome and nuclear abnormalities in human spermatozoa with large vacuoles. Hum Reprod. 2011;26(1):47–58.
31. Watanabe S, Tanaka A, Fujii S, Mizunuma H, Fukui A, Fukuhara R, et al. An investigation of the potential effect of vacuoles in human sperm on DNA damage using a chromosome assay and the TUNEL assay. Hum Reprod. 2011;26(5):978–86.
32. Boitrelle F, Ferfouri F, Petit JM, Segretain D, Tourain C, Bergere M, et al. Large human sperm vacuoles observed in motile spermatozoa under high magnification: nuclear thumbprints linked to failure of chromatin condensation. Hum Reprod. 2011;26(7):1650–8.
33. Guthauser B, Vialard F, Dakouane M, Izard V, Albert M, Selva J. Chromosomal analysis of spermatozoa with normal-sized heads in two infertile patients with macrocephalic sperm head syndrome. Fertil Steril. 2006;85(3):750.e755–7.
34. Chelli MH, Albert M, Ray PF, Guthauser B, Izard V, Hammoud I, et al. Can intracytoplasmic morphologically selected sperm injection be used to select normal-sized sperm heads in infertile patients with macrocephalic sperm head syndrome? Fertil Steril. 2010;93(4):1347.e1341–1345.
35. Cassuto NG, Le Foll N, Chantot-Bastaraud S, Balet R, Bouret D, Rouen A, et al. Sperm fluorescence in situ hybridization study in nine men carrying a Robertsonian or a reciprocal translocation: relationship between segregation modes and high-magnification sperm morphology examination. Fertil Steril. 2011;96(4):826–32.
36. Haaf T, Ward DC. Higher order nuclear structure in mammalian sperm revealed by in situ hybridization and extended chromatin fibers. Exp Cell Res. 1995;219(2):604–11.
37. Zalensky AO, Allen MJ, Kobayashi A, Zalenskaya IA, Balhorn R, Bradbury EM. Well-defined genome architecture in the human sperm nucleus. Chromosoma. 1995;103(9):577–90.
38. Zalensky A, Zalenskaya I. Organization of chromosomes in spermatozoa: an additional layer of epigenetic information? Biochem Soc Trans. 2007;35(Pt 3):609–11.
39. Perdrix A, Travers A, Clatot F, Sibert L, Mitchell V, Jumeau F, et al. Modification of chromosomal architecture in human spermatozoa with large vacuoles. Andrology. 2013;1(1):57–66.

Intracytoplasmic Morphologically Selected Sperm Injection (IMSI): Indications and Clinical Results

16

Nino Guy Cassuto and André Hazout

Introduction

The Intracytoplasmic Sperm Injection (ICSI) story started in 1992, with the first attempt offering a new and large opportunity in the field of male factor infertility treatment [1]. The success obtained in cases of oligoasthenoteratozoospermia (OAT) was, at this time, revolutionary.

Ten years later, technical progress permitted a high magnification of the spermatozoon with a new vision of Motile Sperm Organelle Morphology Examination (MSOME) [2] prior to Intracytoplasmic Morphologically Selected Sperm Injection (IMSI) improving the pregnancy rate [3, 4]. This can achieve magnification ranging from 6,100× to more. Several approaches were used to classify morphological abnormalities of human spermatozoa at high magnification, invisible with the standard optical of 400×, which is commonly used for selecting spermatozoon in ICSI routine. Recently, it has been reported that ICSI of sperm with vacuoles tends to result in decreased blastocysts and pregnancy rates [5, 6] and causes early miscarriages, [7] and it has been proposed that vacuoles are not just a polymorphism but pose a risk for an abnormality that is associated with DNA injury [8].

N.G. Cassuto, MD (✉) • A. Hazout, MD
Art Unit, Drouot Laboratory,
Drouot Street 21, Paris 75009, France
e-mail: guycassuto@labodrouot.com

On the other hand, examining the incidence of vacuoles in spermatozoa at various developmental and maturation stages, other authors performed an IMSI using motile normal-shaped sperm with or without vacuoles; surprisingly they found that human sperm vacuoles did not affect ICSI outcomes [9]. However, a consensual definition of a "so-called" normal spermatozoon is still unknown and this is the reason why the results are still conflicting.

In this chapter we try to clarify the main indications of IMSI according to our proper classification and experience and discuss unsolved matters.

Materials and Methods

Sperm Preparation and Technical Considerations

The intracytoplasmic morphologically selected sperm injection (IMSI) uses a Nomarski system which enables to choose and select spermatozoon at high magnification (6,100×) as opposed to ICSI, performed at low magnification (400×).

These techniques are completely similar but differ in the observation time that is longer for IMSI. The examination of the sperm head and nucleus by MSOME allows one to see what remain invisible with standard ICSI. According to the description given by Bartoov [2] the morphological normalcy of the spermatozoon is evaluated with the nucleus in terms of shape (smooth, symmetric, and oval) and chromatin content (homogeneous chromatin containing no more than one vacuole that occupies <4 % of the nuclear area). But for neck, cytoplasmic droplet, and tail, low magnification is enough. The problem is that today, even in light of the work of Tanaka [9] nobody is able to define normal sperm or assess the real impact of nuclear vacuoles.

This new approach is still a matter of debate because some authors find that the completion time is long and that the price of the material is high in relation to the results.

Spermatozoon Selection

After preparation in a centrifuged bilayer gradient (low density and high density), the motile spermatozoa were observed in three dimensions (3D) at high-magnification under an inverted microscope equipped with Differential Inferential Contrast (DIC) optics called Nomarski, producing 3D vision thanks to a polarization light. This provided high magnification of 1,500× with a zoom of up to 6,100× and higher.

In a glass-bottom culture dish the fresh washed pellet was placed and the motile spermatozoon examined. Assessment of morphology was carried out as previously described by Cassuto–Barak [10]. Briefly, we established a detailed classification scoring scale ranging from 0 to 6. The morphology of spermatozoon defined the head and base shape, the presence or absence of vacuole in the nucleus. The formula for the scoring scale counts two points for a normal head, three for a head without vacuole, and one for a normal base. A range of spermatozoa with different scores and grading sketches are shown in Fig. 16.1.

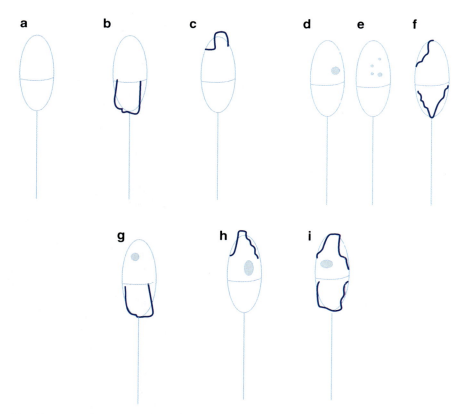

Fig. 16.1 Sperm-scoring sketches according to the Cassuto–Barak Classification: 2HN+3VN+1BN (HN= normal head; VN=no vacuole; BN=normal base). Maximum score is 6. (**a**) Score 6: HN+VN+BN. (**b**) Score 5: HN+VN. (**c**) Score 4: VN+BN. (**d**, **e**) Score 3: HN+BN or VN (**f**). (**g**) Score 2: HN. (**h**) Score 1: BN. (**i**) Score 0

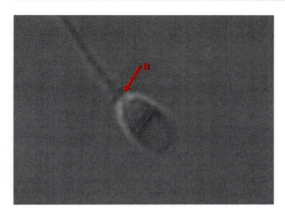

Fig. 16.2 Score-6 Top Spermatozoon with a normal base

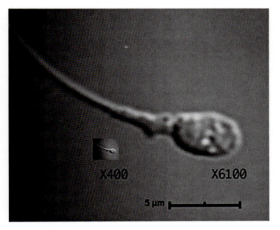

Fig. 16.3 Score-0 Spermatozoon at high and low magnification. Bar = 5 μm

A "top" spermatozoon with a score of 6 points is shown in Fig. 16.2.

A score of 0 was defined by a nuclear-shape disorder with an abnormal base and/or a nuclear asymmetrical extrusion and/or invagination of the nuclear membrane and at least one large or several vacuoles (Fig. 16.3).

Impact of Sperm Morphology

According to our sperm classification, there was a clear positive correlation between the head morphology of the spermatozoon, fertilization, and expanded blastocyst rate. Cassuto et al. have shown that ultramorphological criteria previously established with a scoring scale according to sperm head, vacuole, and base appear to be unrelated to chromosomal abnormalities [11] but related to DNA damage, particularly with chromatin decondensation which may affect embryo development [8].

Spermatozoa chosen for ICSI may have morphological abnormalities which could decrease the implantation and pregnancy rates [12]. However, when using high magnification, several studies have shown an increased blastocyst and pregnancy rates by selecting physiologically normal spermatozoa [4, 5, 13, 14]. The contribution of maternal age in correlation to sperm score revealed a distinction between oocytes originating from women younger than 30 years and oocytes from women aged 30 and older [10].

Moreover, in a recent study, it has been shown that in couples with advanced maternal age, IMSI performance results in higher blastocyst formation, implantation, and clinical pregnancy rates as compared with conventional ICSI [15]. More recently it has been shown that the use of IMSI minimizes the risk of major malformations in offspring [16].

Impact of Sperm DNA Structure

The clinical significance of DNA damage in the male germ line has been the subject of much discussion and the source of some confusion.

There is an extensive literature addressing the relationship between DNA damage in spermatozoa and fertility, defined in a variety of ways and under diverse circumstances including natural conception [17]. These data mainly showed a weak relationship between DNA damage and fertility. The most powerful associations appear to be with natural conceptions, IUI, and IVF, but weak with ICSI. This has led some societies not to recommend sperm DNA testing under the pretext that they are not really helpful. In reality, it would appear clear that there is no direct relationship between the status of DNA in a sperm nucleus and the fertilizing potential of the cell. The sperm nucleus is tightly compacted, inert to the point of transcriptional silence and plays no active role in the processes of capacitating and fertilization [18].

DNA in the sperm nucleus is more sensitive to oxidative damage than to the mechanisms regulating sperm fertilization. That may be due to collateral damage to the sperm plasma membrane as a result of extensive lipid peroxidation.

Moreover, perfectly normal spermatozoa, in terms of both their appearance and function, may still carry DNA damage, creating a problem when it comes to selecting spermatozoa for ICSI [19]. The significance of DNA damage in spermatozoa is not about predicting fertility but rather about its potential to modify the genetic constitution of the embryo. It is today indisputable that DNA damage in the father's sperm can influence embryonic development. The assessment of such damage is underestimated because of the repair capacity of oocytes, particularly in young women, explaining the conflicting results of several studies.

High magnification is a tool permitting to identify and to discard abnormal sperm with a chromatin decondensation, in real time.

Review of the Literature and Results

IMSI has a theoretical potential to improve reproductive outcomes among couples undergoing assisted reproduction techniques (ART).

In a recent Cochrane database [20] study comparing ICSI and IMSI, the authors retrieved 294 records; from those, nine parallel design studies were included, comprising 2,014 couples (IMSI = 1,002; ICSI = 1,012). Live birth was evaluated by only one trial and there was no significant evidence of a difference between IMSI and ICSI (risk ratio (RR) 1.14, 95 % confidence interval (CI) 0.79–1.64), but these results concerning only 168 women, the evidence was of low quality. IMSI was associated with a significant improvement in clinical pregnancy rate (RR 1.29, 95 % CI 1.07–1.56, 9 RCTs, 2,014 women, $I(2) = 57$ %, with very-low-quality evidence also). In their study the authors did not find a significant difference in miscarriage rate between IMSI and ICSI (RR 0.82, 95 % CI 0.59–1.14, 6 RCTs, 552 clinical pregnancies, $I(2) = 17$ %, very-low-quality evidence). None of the included studies reported congenital abnormalities. Thereby results from RCTs do not support the clinical use of IMSI. There is no evidence of effect on live birth or miscarriage and the fact that IMSI improves clinical pregnancy is of very low quality.

Recently, Klement et al. [21] studied 1,891 IVF-ICSI cycles and 577 IVF-IMSI cycles. In the first IVF treatment, pregnancy rates (PRs) were 46 % and 47 %, respectively, and delivery rates were 23 % versus 30 %, respectively. In the second cycle to follow a failed ICSI, PRs and delivery rates were significantly higher for patients who chose to shift to the IMSI technique compared with patients who chose to go through a second IVF-ICSI cycle (56 % vs. 38 % PRs and 28 % vs. 18 % delivery rates, respectively). In the following cycles a significant difference was demonstrated in both PR and delivery rates in favor of patients shifting between treatments. In a multivariate analysis an approximate threefold increased chance existed for both pregnancy and delivery only in case of couples failing an ICSI attempt who shifted to IMSI. The authors recommend IMSI only after ICSI failures.

Marci et al. [22] studying the outcome after 51 IMSI and 281 ICSI in an unselected patients group found no statistically significant differences between implantation rate (ICSI: 16.83 %; IMSI: 16.67 %), fertilization rate (ICSI: 77.27 %; IMSI: 80.00 %), and pregnancy rate (ICSI: 25.30 %; IMSI: 23.50 %). Both groups were comparable when considering live birth rate (ICSI: 11.39 %; IMSI: 13.72 %), ongoing pregnancy rate (ICSI: 7.47 %; IMSI: 5.88 %), and miscarriage rate (ICSI: 17.78 %; IMSI: 5.26 %). The subgroup analyzed did not show a statistical difference between ICSI and IMSI neither in male factor infertility subgroup nor in patients with more than one previous ICSI attempt. A trend towards better laboratory and clinical outcomes was detected in the male factor infertility subgroup when IMSI was applied. They concluded that IMSI technique does not significantly improve IVF outcome in an unselected infertile population.

De Vos et al. [23] in a randomized sibling oocyte study, focusing on the presence of nuclear vacuoles in 350 ICSI cycles, graded the semen samples (five grades) and microinjected 3,105 oocytes showing the same fertilization rate between IMSI and ICSI as well as the same pregnancy rate. They concluded that the clinical outcome was similar for IMSI and conventional ICSI. No firm conclusions could be drawn on cycle rank as a possible indication for IMSI. However, according to semen sample quality (either real-time IMSI morphology or total number of progressive motile spermatozoa in the semen sample), IMSI and ICSI showed similar clinical efficiency.

In a clinical randomized study Balaban et al. [24] compared the clinical outcome of 87 IMSI cycles with 81 conventional (ICSI) cycles in an unselected infertile population. IMSI did not provide a significant improvement in the clinical outcome compared with ICSI although there were trends for higher implantation (28.9 % versus 19.5 %), clinical pregnancy (54.0 % versus 44.4 %), and live birth rates (43.7 % versus 38.3 %) in the IMSI group. However, severe male factor patients benefited from the IMSI procedure as shown by significantly higher implantation rates compared with their counterparts in the ICSI group (29.6 % versus 15.2 %, $P=0.01$). These results suggest that IMSI may improve IVF success rates in a selected group of patients with male factor infertility.

Several previous studies demonstrated, on the contrary, a real beneficial effect of IMSI in selected infertile populations.

Antinori et al. [13] in a prospective randomized study compared ICSI and IMSI in cases of 446 male severe OATS using ICSI in 219 couples and IMSI in 227 couples. The data showed that IMSI resulted in a higher clinical pregnancy rate (39.2 % versus 26.5 %; $P=0.004$) than ICSI. Despite their initial poor reproductive prognosis, patients with two or more previously failed attempts benefited the most from IMSI in terms of pregnancy (29.8 % versus 12.9 %; $P=0.017$) and miscarriage rates (17.4 % versus 37.5 %).

In a meta-analysis Souza et al. initially retrieved a total of 37 studies from the literature [25]. Only five published studies, which analyzed the relationship between ICSI and IMSI outcomes, were considered for inclusion [2, 4, 6, 13, 26]. The articles were analyzed independently. The studies had to be comparative or randomized and homogenous. Three studies were retained (Bartoov et al. [4]; Berkovitz et al. [6]; Antinori et al. [13]).

The main outcome measures were fertilization, implantation, pregnancy and miscarriage rates. Two of the three studies analyzed the percentage of top-quality embryos [4, 26] and the outcome. Results demonstrated no significant difference in fertilization rate between ICSI and IMSI groups. However, a significantly improved implantation (odds ratio (OR) 2.72; 95 % confidence interval (CI) 1.50–4.95) and pregnancy rate (OR 3.12; 95 % CI 1.55–6.26) was observed in IMSI cycles. Moreover, the results showed a significantly decreased miscarriage rate (OR 0.42; 95 % CI 0.23–0.78) in IMSI as compared with ICSI cycles. In this analysis IMSI cycles they demonstrated a statistically significant improvement in implantation and pregnancy rates and a statistically significant reduction in miscarriage rates.

Interestingly, in a more recent paper the same authors [15] analyzed IMSI procedure prospectively in cases of advanced maternal age in a randomized study. They demonstrated that, in couples with advanced maternal age (≥ 37 years old), IMSI performance results in higher blastocyst formation, implantation, and clinical pregnancy rates as compared with conventional ICSI.

High spermatozoon magnification and IMSI emphasized the fact that the sperm nucleus seems to be the most important thing. However since the origin of sperm vacuoles remains unknown, some studies suggested that sperm vacuoles are a normal feature of the sperm head [9, 27], while others suggested that it is related to male subfertility, with higher incidence of chromosomal abnormalities [28, 29]; and sperm chromatin packaging/DNA abnormalities [2–4, 8, 30–35].

The impact of large nuclear vacuoles in the embryo development was widely discussed particularly by Tanaka et al. [9] who suggest that vacuoles occur naturally in a physiological process during sperm maturation. However the same author concludes that spermatozoa with large vacuoles must not be used for injection.

Montjean et al. [36] evaluated 35 sperm samples that were incubated with the follicular fluid and with hyaluronic acid and analyzed for sperm DNA condensation and morphology through

MSOME, in order to determine if there was a correlation between the presence of vacuoles and acrosome reaction. In accordance with the findings from Kacem et al. [37], the authors showed that the presence of sperm vacuoles negatively influences sperm capacity to undergo acrosome reaction and are a reflection of sperm physiology rather than an expression of abnormalities in the nucleus.

Cassuto et al. [8] investigated whether DNA damage of 26 infertile men with OAT and IVF failures were linked to sperm-head abnormalities identified at high magnification. The analysis of 10,400 spermatozoa showed that the sperm chromatin-decondensation rate of abnormal, spermatozoa (presenting abnormal head, one or several vacuoles, and an abnormal base) was twice as high as the controls (19.5 % versus 10.1 %; $P<0.0001$).

Hammoud et al. [38] recently analyzed different types of spermatozoa in eight patients with a high degree of sperm DNA fragmentation in terms of incidence; if the spermatozoon was vacuole-free it showed a significantly lower incidence of DNA fragmentation (4.1 ± 1.1 %) than the other types.

Finally in the most recent paper, and one of the most significant, Cassuto et al. [16] demonstrated that birth defects and particularly major malformations were significantly lower with IMSI (6/450, 1.33 %) versus ICSI (22/578, 3.80 %; adjusted odds ratio 0.35, 95 % confidence interval 0.14–0.87, $P=0.014$), mainly affecting boys (Adjusted odds ratio 2.84, 95 % confidence interval 1.24–6.53, $P=0.009$). The authors concluded that IMSI significantly decreased risk of major birth defects after multivariate adjustment and highlighted the beneficial effect of sperm selection at high magnification before ICSI.

Personal Data

Presented at Venice at the 15th World Congress on Human Reproduction

Prospective studies of 350 spermatozoa from infertile men were used for ICSI in women less than 36 with normal ovarian status. The spermatozoon was first selected routinely (400×), then observed at high magnification (6,100×) and scored according to our scoring system. To clarify the methodology we decided to compare scores 6+5 (Group A) versus scores 1+0 (Group B). Overall we followed 202 extreme ranges spermatozoa (Group A+B) from 350. Each oocyte was individually cultured in order to follow the outcome of each embryo until the blastocyst stage. Results: In group A, 94 injected spermatozoa permit to obtain 78 embryos, and 34 blastocysts including 14 "top blastocysts". In group B, 108 injected spermatozoa permitted to obtain 62 embryos and 24 blastocysts including 4 "top blastocysts." Comparing the two groups we found a significant difference in terms of fertilization rate ($p=0.007$) and "top" blastocysts ($p=0.01$). Regarding "top" blastocysts obtained in the two groups according to pregnancies there is a significant difference ($p=0.03$). Finally, 12 ongoing pregnancies occur in group A and only 1 in group B ($p=0.0003$). These data validate our classification and scoring system, permitting to discard the worst spermatozoa from ICSI and giving a guideline for the choice of the spermatozoa likely to be injected.

Discussion and Indications

In light of the numerous and conflicting studies described above, one might conclude that the IMSI indications remain unclear.

However, whether we refer to randomized or no randomized studies, or to selected or unselected populations, one thing remains clear: the lack IMSI's impact on fertilization rates (except in the last studies of Cassuto et al. [10, 16]). This is not surprising because the majority of studies did not rate either the spermatozoon prior to microinjection or the DNA defects. From all recent and documented studies, it is clear that the majority of authors have used the IMSI procedure mainly in case of ICSI failures.

Those most reluctant to use IMSI think that a more subtle selection of sperm does not suffice to significantly increase the chance of success compared to ICSI. These authors have generally worked on unselected populations using IMSI in first intention. In these conditions only huge numbers could reflect a difference in favor of the IMSI groups.

The last work of Cassuto et al. [16] further demonstrates a significant reduction in major birth defects after IMSI in all women under 39.

This higher risk of major malformation with ICSI, mainly affects the urogenital system and more often boys.

This argument seems crucial to us, and should be enough to convince critics of the IMSI technique as it is important to understand that, unlike the initial goal, the key is not to select the best spermatozoon, which nobody could define, but rather to discard the worst.

Moreover, it is also possible that the sperm selection under high magnification itself can account for the improvement of blastocyst quality, implantation, and pregnancy rates, regardless of sperm chromatin packaging, DNA status or oocyte capacity to repair.

We must also take into account that the « best looking » spermatozoon prior to ICSI does not necessarily reflect its DNA quality.

Consequently studies suggest that the injection of DNA-damaged spermatozoa is related to blockage of embryonic development during or after the embryos' implantation, which reflects a late paternal effect [26, 39, 40].

Sperm DNA integrity and chromosomal constitution cannot be assessed in the sperm cell used for ICSI. We have already demonstrated that sperm chromatin-decondensation rate of abnormal spermatozoa (Score 0 presenting abnormal head, one or several vacuoles and an abnormal base) was twice as high as the controls [8]. It is known that, prior to histone replacement by protamine, the nucleosomes are destabilized by hyperacetylation and DNA methylation levels rise [41, 42]. These potential epigenetic mechanisms could be implied in chromatin condensation failures.

Whereas an oocyte may partially repair sperm DNA damage, it is postulated that more extensive defects and less DNA repair will result in the introduction of mutations and these have been associated with poor fertilization or embryo development rates and recurrent miscarriages.

In this respect the recent work of Setti et al. [15] among elderly women is instructive because it authenticates the idea that lesser repair capabilities of "older" oocytes justify the use of IMSI for the sole purpose of not adding a further disadvantage.

Tanaka's endeavor to explain the presence and significance of vacuoles in the sperm nucleus: Vacuolar formation occurs naturally during the process of sperm nuclei condensation, and should not be regarded as degeneration but as physiological change. However, after ICSI/IMSI their study was not able to detect a difference because of the limited number of examinations.

After the first publication of Bartoov et al., and "a fortiori" after our ICSI failures, we tried to classify the various sperm defects on a scale from 0 to 6 [10]. It gradually became apparent that the shape head and base and structure of the sperm nucleus represented the main selection criteria. We were convinced it would be very difficult to isolate a perfectly normal sperm, because, as we explained beforehand, we had no objective certainty.

Considering only the presence or absence of vacuoles is insufficient and partly explains the discrepancies between different studies results. Only the combination of abnormalities of the sperm head and base may constitute an argument to exclude sperm usually carrying nucleic structures abnormalities.

Thus, we would recommend IMSI, firstly, for OAT with a high level of spermatozoon score 0 (more than 40 %) and/or for women over 35, and secondly for patients of all ages who have experienced unexplained ICSI failures, and early repeated abortions. This point is crucial and highlights the fact that ICSI is unable to detect the 0-rated spermatozoon in the pellet before microinjection.

Conclusion

A sperm selection method represents today diagnostic and therapeutic arguments applicable to selected populations of infertile men where most sperm characteristics cannot be tested. On the other hand, using scoring scale at high magnification prior to ICSI procedure helps eliminate the worst spermatozoon.

It is impossible to use spermatozoon for microinjection that has been tested.

The sole tool we have today is morphology. High magnification improves choice with a real impact on early embryo development.

Conflicting results were probably due to sperm inclusion criteria and women's age. More randomized trials are needed to confirm the encouraging results already obtained by several authors.

But high magnification permits to avoid immature spermatozoa with expanded chromatin, and highlights the impact of spermatozoon selection by deselecting the worse before ICSI and decreasing the risk of major malformations.

Acknowledgement J.R. Kovac is an NIH K12 scholar supported by a Male Reproductive Health Research (MRHR) Career Development Physician-Scientist Award (HD073917-01) from the Eunice Kennedy Shriver National Institute of Child Health and Human Development (NICHD) Program awarded to Dolores J. Lamb (DJL). DJL is supported by NIH grants P01HD36289 from the Eunice Kennedy Shriver NICHD and 1R01DK078121 from the National Institute of Kidney and Digestive Diseases.

References

1. Palermo G, Joris H, Devroey P, Van Steirteghem AC. Pregnancies after intracytoplasmic injection of single spermatozoon into an oocyte. Lancet. 1992;340(8810):17–8.
2. Bartoov B, Berkovitz A, Eltes F. Selection of spermatozoa with normal nuclei to improve the pregnancy rate with intracytoplasmic sperm injection. N Engl J Med. 2001;345(14):1067–8.
3. Bartoov B, Berkovitz A, Eltes F, Kogosowski A, Menezo Y, Barak Y. Real-time fine morphology of motile human sperm cells is associated with IVF-ICSI outcome. J Androl. 2002;23(1):1–8.
4. Bartoov B, Berkovitz A, Eltes F, et al. Pregnancy rates are higher with intracytoplasmic morphologically selected sperm injection than with conventional intracytoplasmic injection. Fertility and Sterility. 2003;80:1413–9.
5. Vanderzwalmen P, Hiemer A, Rubner P, Bach M, Neyer A, Stecher A, Uher P, Zintz M, Lejeune B, Vanderzwalmen S, Cassuto G, Zech NH. Blastocyst development after sperm selection at high magnification is associated with size and number of nuclear vacuoles. Reprod Biomed Online. 2008;17:617–27.
6. Berkovitz A, Eltes F, Ellenbogen E, et al. Does the presence of nuclear vacuoles in human sperm selected for ICSI affect pregnancy outcome? Human Reproduction. 2006;21:1787–90.
7. Greco E, Scarselli F, Fabozzi G, Colasante A, Zavaglia D, Alviggi E, Litwicka K, Varricchio MT, Minasi MG, Tesarik J. Sperm vacuoles negatively affect outcomes in intracytoplasmic morphologically selected sperm injection in terms of pregnancy, implantation, and live-birth rates. Fertil Steril. 2013;100(2):379–85.
8. Cassuto NG, Hazout A, Hammoud I, Balet R, Bouret D, Barak Y, Jellad S, Plouchart JM, Selva J, Yazbeck C. Correlation between DNA defect and sperm-head morphology. Reprod Biomed Online. 2012;24:211–8.
9. Tanaka A, Nagayoshi M, Tanaka I, Kusunoki H. Human sperm head vacuoles are physiological structures formed during the sperm development and maturation process. Fertil Steril. 2012;98(2):315–20.
10. Cassuto NG, Bouret D, Plouchart JM, Jellad S, Vanderzwalmen P, Balet R, Larue L, Barak Y. A new real-time morphology classification for human spermatozoa: a link for fertilization and improved embryo quality. Fertil Steril. 2009;92:1616–25.
11. Cassuto N, Le Foll N, Chantot-Bastaraud S, Balet R, Bouret D, Rouen A, Bhouri R, Hyon C, Siffroi JP. Sperm fluorescence in situ hybridization study in nine men carrying a Robertsonian or a reciprocal translocation: relationship between segregation modes and high-magnification sperm morphology examination. Fertil Steril. 2011;96(4):826–32.
12. De Vos A, Van De Velde H, Joris H, Verheyen G, Devroey P, Van Steirteghem A. Influence of individual sperm morphology on fertilization, embryo morphology, and pregnancy outcome of intracytoplasmic sperm injection. Fertil Steril. 2003;79:42–8.
13. Antinori M, Licata E, Dani G, Cerusico F, Versaci C, d'Angelo D, Antinori S. Intracytoplasmic morphologically selected sperm injection: a prospective randomized trial. Reprod Biomed online. 2008;16:835–41.
14. Wilding M, Coppola G, di Matteo L, Palagiano A, Fusco E, Dale B. Intracytoplasmic injection of morphologically selected spermatozoa (IMSI) improves outcome after assisted reproduction by deselecting physiologically poor quality spermatozoa. J Assist Reprod Genet. 2011;28(3):253–62.
15. Setti AS, Figueira RC, Braga DP, Aoki T, Iaconelli Jr A, Borges Jr E. Intracytoplasmic morphologically selected sperm injection is beneficial in cases of advanced maternal age: a prospective randomized study. Eur J Obstet Gynecol Reprod Biol. 2013;171(2):286–90.
16. Cassuto NG, Hazout A, Bouret D, Balet R, Larue L, Benifla JL, Viot G. Low birth defects by deselecting abnormal spermatozoa before ICSI. Reprod BioMed Online. 2014;28(1):47–53.
17. Simon L, Proutski I, Stevenson M, Jennings D, McManus J, Lutton D, Lewis SE. Sperm DNA damage has a negative association with live-birth rates after IVF. Reprod Biomed Online. 2013;26:68–78.
18. Aitken RJ, Nixon B. Sperm capacitation: a distant landscape glimpsed but unexplored. Mol Hum Reprod. 2013;19(12):785–93.
19. Avendano C, Oehninger S. DNA fragmentation in morphologically normal spermatozoa: how much should we be concerned in the ICSI era? J Androl. 2011;32:356–63.

20. Teixeira DM, Barbosa MA, Ferriani RA, Navarro PA, Raine-Fenning N, Nastri CO, Martins WP. Regular (ICSI) versus ultra-high magnification (IMSI) sperm selection for assisted reproduction. Cochrane Database Syst Rev. 2013; 7: CD010167
21. Klement AH, Koren-Morag N, Itsykson P, Berkovitz A. Intracytoplasmic morphologically selected sperm injection versus intracytoplasmic sperm injection: a step toward a clinical algorithm. Fertil Steril. 2013; 99(5):1290–3.
22. Marci R, Murisier F, Lo Monte G, Soave I, Chanson A, Urner F, Germond M. Clinical outcome after IMSI procedure in an unselected infertile population: a pilot study. Reprod Health. 2013;10:16.
23. De Vos A, Van de Velde H, Bocken G, Eylenbosch G, Franceus N, Meersdom S, Tistaert S, Vankelecom A, Tournaye H, Verheyen G. Does intracytoplasmic morphologically selected sperm injection improve embryo development? A randomized sibling-oocyte study. Hum Reprod. 2013;28:617–26.
24. Balaban B, Yakin K, Alatas C, Oktem O, Isiklar A, Urman B. Clinical outcome of intracytoplasmic injection of spermatozoa morphologically selected under high magnification: a prospective randomized study. Reprod Biomed Online. 2011;22:472–6.
25. Souza Setti A, Ferreira RC, de Almeida P, Ferreira Braga D, de Cassia Savio Figueira R, Iaconelli Jr A, Borges Jr E. Intracytoplasmic sperm injection outcome versus intracytoplasmic morphologically selected sperm injection outcome: a meta-analysis. Reprod Biomed Online. 2010;21:450–5.
26. Hazout A, Dumont-Hassan M, Junca AM, et al. High-magnification ICSI overcomes paternal effect resistant to conventional ICSI. Reprod Biomed Online. 2006;12:19–25.
27. Pedersen H. Ultrastructure of the ejaculated human sperm. Z Zellforsch Mikrosk Anat. 1969;94:542–54.
28. Garolla A, Fortini D, Menegazzo M, De Toni L, Nicoletti V, Moretti A, Selice R, Engl B, Foresta C. High-power microscopy for selecting spermatozoa for ICSI by physiological status. Reprod Biomed Online. 2008;17:610–6.
29. Perdrix A, Travers A, Chelli MH, Escalier D, Do Rego JL, Milazzo JP, Mousset-Simeon N, Mace B, Rives N. Assessment of acrosome and nuclear abnormalities in human spermatozoa with large vacuoles. Hum Reprod. 2011;26:47–58.
30. Berkovitz A, Eltes F, Lederman H, et al. How to improve IVF-ICSI outcome by sperm selection. Reprod Biomed Online. 2006;12:634–8.
31. Boitrelle F, Ferfouri F, Petit JM, Segretain D, Tourain C, Bergere M, Bailly M, Vialard F, Albert M, Selva J. Large human sperm vacuoles observed in motile spermatozoa under high magnification: nuclear thumbprints linked to failure of chromatin condensation. Hum Reprod. 2011;26:1650–8.

32. Franco Jr JG, Baruffi RL, Mauri AL, Petersen CG, Oliveira JB, Vagnini L. Significance of large nuclear vacuoles in human spermatozoa: implications for ICSI. Reprod Biomed Online. 2008;17:42–5.
33. Franco Jr JG, Mauri AL, Petersen CG, Massaro FC, Silva LF, Felipe V, Cavagna M, Pontes A, Baruffi RL, Oliveira JB, Vagnini LD. Large nuclear vacuoles are indicative of abnormal chromatin packaging in human spermatozoa. Int J Androl. 2012;35:46–51.
34. Oliveira JB, Massaro FC, Baruffi RL, Mauri AL, Petersen CG, Silva LF, Vagnini LD, Franco Jr JG. Correlation between semen analysis by motile sperm organelle morphology examination and sperm DNA damage. Fertil Steril. 2010;94:1937–40.
35. Watanabe S, Tanaka A, Fujii S, Mizunuma H, Fukui A, Fukuhara R, Nakamura R, Yamada K, Tanaka I, Awata S, Nagayoshi M. An investigation of the potential effect of vacuoles in human sperm on DNA damage using a chromosome assay and the TUNEL assay. Hum Reprod. 2011;26:978–86.
36. Montjean D, Belloc S, Benkhalifa M, Dalleac A, Menezo Y. Sperm vacuoles are linked to capacitation and acrosomal status. Hum Reprod. 2012;27: 2927–32.
37. Kacem O, Sifer C, Barraud-Lange V, Ducot B, De Ziegler D, Poirot C, Wolf J. Sperm nuclear vacuoles, as assessed by motile sperm organellar morphological examination, are mostly of acrosomal origin. Reprod Biomed Online. 2011;20:132–7.
38. Hammoud I, Boitrelle F, Ferfouri F, Vialard F, Bergere M, Wainer B, Bailly M, Albert M, Selva J. Selection of normal spermatozoa with a vacuole-free head (·6300) improves selection of spermatozoa with intact DNA in patients with High sperm DNA fragmentation rates. Andrologia. 2013;45:163–70.
39. Tesarik J, Greco E, Mendoza C. Late, but not early, paternal effect on human embryo development is related to sperm DNA fragmentation. Human Reproduction. 2004;19:611–5.
40. Borini A, Tarozzi N, Bizzaro D, Bonu MA, Fava L, Flamigni C, Coticchio G. Sperm DNA fragmentation: paternal effect on early post-implantation embryo development in ART. Hum Reprod. 2006;21: 2876–81.
41. Miller D, Brinkworth M, Iles D. Paternal DNA packaging in spermatozoa: more than the sum of its parts? DNA, histones, protamines and epigenetics. Reproduction. 2010;139:287–301.
42. Palermo GD, Neri QV, Takeuchi T, Squires J, Moy F, Rosenwaks Z. Genetic and epigenetic characteristics of ICSI children. Reprod Biomed Online. 2008;17: 820–33.
43. Setti AS, Ferreira Braga DP, Iaconelli A, Aoki T, Borges E. Twelve years of MSOME and IMSI: a review. Reproductive BioMedicine Online. 2013;27: 338–52.

Genomic and Proteomic Approaches in the Diagnosis of Male Infertility

17

Jason R. Kovac, Ryan P. Smith, and Dolores J. Lamb

Abbreviations

AZF	Azoospermia factor
CGH	Comparative genomic hybridization
CNV	Copy number variation
HBPs	Heparin-binding proteins
NOA	Nonobstructive azoospermia
OA	Obstructive azoospermia
SNP	Single nucleotide polymorphisms

Introduction

Despite rapid growth in the understanding of the genetic basis for male infertility, much remains poorly defined. Current estimates indicate that genetic abnormalities contribute to 15–30 % of male infertility [1, 2]. Many men have their conditions uncharacterized and are subsequently diagnosed as idiopathic infertility. It has been postulated that these men actually have unrecognized genetic aberrations [1, 2]. Unfortunately, even with the current genetic tools at a clinician's disposal (i.e., karyotype, Y-chromosome microdeletion assay, cystic fibrosis testing), there are many genetic causes that remain unrecognized.

Men with oligospermia and non-obstructive azoospermia (NOA) have a known predisposition to genetic abnormalities and comprise 40–50 % of all infertile men [3]. Current guidelines recommend genetic testing when either sperm density is <5 million/mL, NOA is present, or there are clinical signs of an abnormality [4]. The limitations of contemporary testing are reflected in the growth of recognized genomic and proteomic contributors towards male infertility [2]. Indeed, while much work needs to be done, it appears that future utilization of genetic evaluations will be determined with more direct delineation. As such, the current chapter aims to provide a background regarding the genetic tests that are currently available to clinicians investigating male infertility. Furthermore, advanced methodologies are discussed with recent advances in genomics and proteomics highlighted.

J.R. Kovac, MD, PhD, FRCSC
D.J. Lamb, PhD (✉)
Scott Department of Urology, Department of Molecular and Cellular Biology, The Center for Reproductive Medicine, Baylor College of Medicine, 1 Baylor Plaza, Alkek Building, Alkek Building, N730, Houston, TX 77030, USA
e-mail: Jason.r.kovac@gmail.com; dlamb@bcm.edu

R.P. Smith, MD
The Department of Urology, University of Virginia, PO Box 800422, Charlottesville, VA 22908, USA
e-mail: rps2k@virginia.edu

Genomics: Chromosomal Abnormalities

Karyotype

The advent of modern genetic techniques has led to a rapid proliferation of tests and technologies that have the potential to alter the treatment of male infertility. However, in spite of large numbers of individuals affected by male infertility, genetic analysis has been slow to identify causes. The ability to identify genetic causes of male infertility is beneficial several reasons. First, by understanding the genetic basis of disease, one can hope to develop novel treatments for the future. Second, determination of signal transduction pathways underlying male infertility may yield better comprehension of mechanisms of disease. Importantly, investigators today believe that the majority of male infertility has a genetic basis [5]. Lastly, when using in vitro fertilization, natural selection is bypassed, thus opening up the possibility of transmitting unknown diseases to offspring. If clinicians can identify and control for these changes, risks for transmission would be decreased.

With respect to genetic testing, the karyotype was one of the earliest techniques developed for assessing human chromosomes. Using light microscopy, the number and appearance of chromosomes as well as variations in DNA composition of >4 megabases (Mb) in size became possible [6]. The technique documented the basics of human disease with the identification of numerical defects such as Down's syndrome (extra chromosome 21) and Turner's syndrome (XO) identified in the early 1950s [7, 8]. With regards to male subfertility, karyotypic chromosomal abnormalities was shown to occur at 5 times greater rates compared to the normal population [9]. In men with NOA, the prevalence numerical and structural chromosomal abnormalities is ~10–15 % [10] whereas in men with severe oligospermia (defined as <5 million sperm/mL), this rate correspondingly decreases and approaches ~5 % [11, 12]. Over the years, as the technology and accuracy has expanded, these numbers have increased. Most recently, Yatsenko and colleagues recorded that >11 % of men with NOA had abnormalities identified on karyotype [10]. Interestingly, men with normal sperm concentrations demonstrated <1 % prevalence of karyotype-associated abnormalities [11, 12] while the frequency of karyotypic abnormalities amongst infertile men is ~12.6 % [13].

Karyotype is currently recommended in men with NOA or severe oligospermia (<5 million/mL) [4]. In azoospermic men, sex chromosome abnormalities predominate, whereas in oligospermic men, autosomal anomalies (i.e., Robertsonian and reciprocal translocations) are more frequent [11]. Chromosomal inversions in autosomes 1, 3, 4, 6, 9, 10, and 21 are also more common in infertile men [14].

Klinefelter's syndrome (KS) represents the most common genetic cause and karyotypic abnormality found in infertile men (47, XXY). Present in 11 % of men with azoospermia, KS occurs in 1 of 500 live births [11, 15, 16]. The majority (95 %) of affected males present in adulthood with infertility [17]. Most will have normal libido and erectile function with only 25 % demonstrating characteristic KS features of gynecomastia, tall stature, and small firm testes (8–10 cm^3) [18, 19].

KS results from a meiotic nondisjunction event in most cases; however, up to 3 % of men with KS are mosaic 46,XX/47,XXY [15, 18]. Mosaic males tend to have less severe phenotypic changes and many may be fertile. Spermatogenesis is typically profoundly affected in non-mosaic KS resulting in azoospermia in most with ~8.4 % of men may having sperm in the ejaculate [20–22]. In addition, follicle stimulating hormone (FSH) and luteinizing hormone (LH) levels are markedly increased. FSH is increased in response to abnormal spermatogenesis with an increase in LH reflecting maximal simulation of Leydig cells to produce androgen [20–23].

Karyotypic diagnosis is essential when KS is suspected since these patients are at increased risk for breast cancer, non-Hodgkin lymphoma, extragonadal germ cell tumors, and likely lung cancer [24–26]. Spermatogenic potential declines with advancing age in KS patients; however, the best approach to the adolescent with KS and adequate virilization is currently unclear [19, 27–29]. Some have suggested testicular sperm extraction with cryopreservation of sperm or testicular tissue [30] while others have argued in favor of waiting for extraction in coordination with IVF-ICSI when paternity is desired [31]. Another concern in men with KS is the high rates of sperm aneuploidy [27, 31–33]. Despite these issues, many 46, XX and 46, XY live births have been reported in the literature [34–36]. Micro-TESE, coupled with ICSI, has proven to be a successful strategy for the majority of patients with azoospermia and KS [15].

There are no universally agreed-upon clinical or laboratory findings that predict successful sperm retrieval in KS; however, testis volume, testosterone level and age <35 are generally thought to be positive indices [19, 29, 37, 38]. Unfortunately, the primary difficulty with karyotypic analysis is that baseline resolution of the technique is unable to detect small DNA aberrations and as personalized medicine comes to the forefront, newer techniques are supplementing the karyotype.

Fluorescence In Situ Hybridization

A more advanced test compared to the karyotype focuses on fluorescent probes that are able to detect and localize specific DNA sequences on chromosomes [39]. This technique, termed Fluorescence in situ Hybridization (FISH), was developed to detect sperm aneuploidy as well as to determine the presence/absence of specific DNA sequences [40]. Sperm FISH is unaffected by functional deficiencies [39] and while it assesses defects in men with normal karyotypes (described above), it is limited by the cost of commercially available probes. Specifically, chromosomes X, Y, 13, 18, and 21 are the main probes used in sperm FISH since alterations in these chromosomes results in viable offspring [6]. The test is thus unable to detect aberrations in other chromosomes beyond these limited few, because of cost constraints.

As a method of further clarifying genetic abnormalities, FISH is used clinically as an adjunct to the karyotype. Some have proposed that FISH should be used to more accurately identify men with mosaic Klinefelter's syndrome [41]. Indeed, retrospective and prospective studies have noted that elevated aneuploidy obtained via sperm FISH correlated to fetal aneuploidy and IVF failure [39, 42, 43]. At the present time, sperm FISH is used as a screening tool as well as for patient counseling and clinical decision making. In certain situations and depending upon the clinical diagnosis, preimplantation genetic diagnosis and ICSI could be used to select genetically unaffected embryos.

Genomics: Gene Mutations

Cystic Fibrosis

Congenital bilateral absence of the vas deferens (CBAVD) is found in ~1 % of infertile males and up to 6 % of those with obstructive azoospermia [1, 19]. CBAVD is due to a mutation in the *CFTR* (Cystic Fibrosis Transmembrane Conductance Regulator) gene located on chromosome 7 [44, 45] and results from gene mutations that cause cystic fibrosis (CF) or alterations in the genetic mechanisms controlling mesonephric duct differentiation [19]. CF is an autosomal recessive disease, affecting 1 in 1,600 people of Northern European background. It occurs with variable frequency in different geographic and ethnic populations. Genetic testing typically accounts for ethnicity and recognizes >850 genetic variants associated with CF [23, 46–50]. Most cases of CBAVD result from mutations in both the maternal and paternal copies of the genes that encode for the CFTR. Eighty percent of azoospermic men with CBAVD and one-third of men with unexplained obstruction will have CFTR mutations [51, 52]. The prevalence of CFTR mutations is increased in men with azoospermia related to congenital bilateral obstruction of the epididymis and those with unilateral vasal agenesis [4].

CBAVD is reliably diagnosed on physical exam with vasa absent bilaterally and seminal vesicles classically absent or atrophic.

Occasionally, the seminal vesicles can be large and cystic [19]. Testis size is also preserved and correspondingly, spermatogenesis is unaltered. The efferent ductules and caput of the epididymis are present and full with fluid from the testis. Transrectal ultrasound may reveal absence of the ampullae of the vas deferens or seminal vesicle abnormalities [53].

CFTR encodes an ion channel that maintains the viscosity of epithelial secretions via regulation of the sodium/chloride balance [19]. Analysis of the ejaculate will reveal thin, watery, low volume (<1.5 mL), and acidic (pH 6.5–7.0) fluid, as it is comprised primarily of prostatic secretions [19]. Pulmonary and pancreatic function in patients with CBAVD is unaltered [44]. Nearly all men with clinically detected CF demonstrate CBAVD [23, 54].

Significant genotypic differences are seen in CF and CBAVD. In males with CBAVD, the majority (~88 %) has a severe mutation resulting in absent CFTR function in combination with an allelic mutation that preserves some CFTR function [23, 55–57]. A three-base-pair deletion of CFTR, termed ΔF508, is the most common mutation found in both CF and CBAVD [19, 57]. When the patient is ΔF508 homozygous, clinical CF is apparent whereas CBAVD commonly results from a polymorphism within intron 8, sometimes termed the 5T allele, coupled with a ΔF508 mutation [19, 57, 58]. Several studies have demonstrated variable penetrance of the 5T allele, which results in a lowered efficiency of splicing that subsequently lowers levels of CFTR mRNA and protein required for maintenance of normal function [23, 55–57].

Failure of appropriate mesonephric duct differentiation before week 7 of gestation may underlie a second genetic etiology of CBAVD [19, 59]. If an isolated, unilateral injury occurs to one of the developing mesonephric ducts, unilateral renal and vasal agenesis may be present. In contrast, the presence of a genetic aberration that compromises mesonephric duct differentiation would affect both renal and reproductive ductal units, as in Potter's syndrome [19, 59]. Indeed, some patients may have unilateral vasal agenesis due to a non-cystic-fibrosis mediated embryologic defect, which is associated with unilateral absence of the kidney. A renal ultrasound is therefore indicated in these patients [60]. Unilateral renal atrophy/dysgenesis can also be associated with ipsilateral hydroureter and ectopic insertion into other genitourinary structures such as the seminal vesicles [61].

In patients found to have an abnormality on CFTR testing, the partner should similarly be screened. Microsurgical or percutaneous sperm retrieval in coordination with in vitro fertilization and intracytoplasmic sperm injection (IVF-ICSI) remains an option for these couples. If the partner is a carrier of a CF mutation, preimplantation genetic diagnosis can be employed to prevent the transfer of any embryos that will be predicted to have CF or CBAVD. Failure to detect a CFTR mutation in either partner does not exclude the presence of a mutation, which is not identifiable by routine analysis performed by most clinical genetics laboratories for diagnosing CF and not CBAVD, and therefore the progeny of the couple remains at some risk unless the entire gene is sequenced. Patients demonstrating CFTR mutations should therefore be referred for genetic counseling prior to IVF [62, 63].

Genomics: Y-Chromosome Microdeletions

The Y chromosome contains 60 million base pairs and is composed of a short arm (Yp) and a long arm (Yq). The *SRY* gene is located on Yp and is essential to sex-specific embryogenesis and determination of the bipotential gonad [19, 64–66]. The male-specific region of the Y-chromosome (MSY) is the chromosomal material bridging the two polar pseudoautosomal regions, located at the tips of Yp and Yq, and comprises 95 % of the entirety of the Y chromosome [64, 65]. Many of the genes in this MSY region are poorly characterized but are involved in spermatogenesis. Included in the MSY region are three important zones that influence spermatogenesis. These Azoospermia Factor (AZF) regions are recognized as AZFa, (proximal), AZFb (central), and AZFc (distal). Known spermatogenesis genes within these confines include *USP9Y* and *DBY* in AZFa and *DAZ*, *RBMY1*, and *BPY2* in AZFb and AZFc [19, 64–66].

There are eight palindromic sequences throughout the length of the Yq and, as the MSY region has no genetic partner sequence to pair or repair, it is postulated that this organization helps to maintain the genetic integrity of the Y chromosome [19, 64–67]. Sub-segments within these palindromic sequences, known as amplicons, can occasionally fuse resulting in loss of all intervening chromosomal material [19, 64, 65, 67]. When this occurs, it is termed a microdeletion, as despite the loss of a large magnitude of genetic material, it is undetectable on a karyotypic analysis [19, 67]. The subsequent genes within this sequence are lost, resulting in impaired spermatogenesis and possibly other undefined consequences.

The overall prevalence of Y chromosome microdeletions in patients with sperm counts greater than 5×10^6/mL is low (~0.7 %) [68]. A rate that increases to 4 % in oligospermic men and 11 % in azoospermic men [68]. Other studies have identified microdeletions in 6–12 % of men with impaired spermatogenesis—a value that can increase to 16 % in men with azoospermia [69]. Within the AZF regions, AZFc deletions are the most common, being seen in 13 % of men with NOA and 6 % of severely oligospermic men [19, 70, 71]. The *DAZ* (Deleted in Azoospermia) gene, which encodes a transcription factor present in men with normal fertility, resides in the AZFc region. In contrast, microdeletions within the AZFa region occur in approximately 1 % of NOA men and do not involve any of the aforementioned palindromic sequences [19].

The location of AZF deletions impacts the likelihood of spermatogenesis and is prognostic in regards to the success of micro-TESE. Men with AZFc microdeletions have quantitatively impaired spermatogenesis with either severe oligospermia or azoospermia. The quality of sperm produced is typically normal in terms of fertilization, embryo development, and live birth [19, 72]. The level of spermatogenesis is typically stable among individuals, and micro-TESE with ICSI remains a therapeutic option [4, 19, 73]. In contrast, deletions of the AZFa or AZFb regions portend a very poor prognosis for sperm retrieval [19, 74, 75]. In a study by Hopps et al. [76], a total of 78 men with AZF deletions were analyzed with respect to the ability to identify sperm following diagnostic testes biopsies or TESE. Men with an isolated AZFc deletion had sperm identified in 56 % of cases [76].

With regards to heredity, men with Y-chromosome microdeletions will pass the abnormality to their sons who consequently may also be infertile. Although limited data exists, microdeletions of the Y-chromosome are known to have minor somatic health consequences (i.e., permanent tooth size [77] and short stature [78]) or testicular abnormalities [19]. It is possible however, that transmission of AZF microdeletions may have unrecognized consequences to offspring. Couples may elect to forgo use of the partner's sperm, utilize the ejaculated or testicular sperm for IVF-ICSI or elect for preimplantation genetic screening to transfer only female embryos. Therefore, men exhibiting NOA or severe oligospermia should be offered a Y-chromosome microdeletion assay and genetic counseling prior to pursuing micro-TESE for IVF-ICSI [19]. Indeed, molecular studies of patients with Y-chromosome microdeletions have shown previously unknown Y structural variations in NOA men [79].

Infertile men can have other Y chromosome structural abnormalities including, ring Y, truncated Y, isodicentric Y and various other mosaic states which may be present on karyotype analysis [10, 11, 19, 80, 81]. Early work hypothesized that the Y-chromosome contained a region that was initially thought to contain no X-Y crossing over; however, it has recently been shown to have extensive recombination and is termed the male-specific region (MSY) [64]. This area is flanked by pseudoautosomal regions (PAR) where X-Y crossing over is normal [64]. Indeed, Y-chromosome microdeletions can also include PAR defects causing genetic disorders such as SHOX [82]. The sequencing of the MSY region has been conducted [64] and further studies have found that high mutation rates resulting in structural polymorphisms in the human Y-chromosome exist with selective constraints possible [83].

In all cases, a Y-chromosome microdeletion assay is a necessary complementary test to determine the presence of the AFZ regions and direct counseling [10, 11, 19, 80].

Genomics: Advanced Techniques

Given the limits of detection and resolution of the above-mentioned techniques (karyotype, FISH, etc.), new approaches are being developed that test the current limits of genomic resolution. One of these involves detection of Copy number variations (CNVs). CNVs are defined as small (~1 kb) pieces of DNA that vary between individuals. Affecting ~20 % of the human genome, CNVs are either additions/duplications or deletions within the genome [84] that are critical sources of genetic diversity. Given that they lie within regions that are potentially invisible to karyotype analysis, novel techniques were developed to assess the impact of CNVs on human disease.

Array comparative genomic hybridization (aCGH) is one approach that focuses on single nucleotides in the human genome. It has the capacity to identify both small and large-scale changes by examining the relative quantities of DNA between samples. Gene copy number are optimally analyzed and depicted as a function of chromosome location with fluorescence identifying copy number gain or loss [85]. In the context of the microarray platform, resolution of aCGH has improved to <1 kb [86] with the ability to scale the testing in order to perform thousands of experiments in a single run [6]. Indeed, genome-wide assays are gradually replacing karyotyping for prenatal genetic diagnoses [87].

While aCGH has been applied to numerous malignancies including those of the breast, nasopharynx, ovary, stomach and bladder, others are using the technology to probe for alterations in infertile men [88]. Array CGH has already been used in the context of male infertility to identify Y-chromosome microdeletions in infertile males [82]. An earlier study ascertained whether CNVs were involved in patients with oligospermia/azoospermia compared to controls [89]. Several genes and genomic regions were identified on autosomes and sex-chromosomes that were theorized to be involved in spermatogenesis [89]. While the authors could not identify any large CNV (>1 Mb) variants between men with infertility; 11 CNVs in severe oligospermia and 4 CNVs in men with azoospermia (i.e., *EPHA3, PLES, DDX11, ANKS1B*) were identified in more than one patient suggesting that these regions were potential candidates for infertility genes [89]. Defects in the pseudoautosomal regions (PARs) of the Y-chromosome cause genomic disorders such as SHOX that can be affiliated with infertility, mental and stature disorders and subsequently transmitted to offspring [82].

Another technique that has recently benefitted from significant technological improvement is gene-expression DNA microarray. The primary advantage of DNA microarray technology is the ability to perform simultaneous analysis of thousands of genes at the same time [90]. By generating a large amount of data, DNA-microarrays require modern computational and statistical bioanalytic and bioinformatics approaches. The power of the technique lies in the ability to provide a snapshot of all transcriptional activity in a sample.

Preliminary studies by Sha et al. [91] utilizing cDNA microarrays identified 101 candidate fertility genes. Lin et al. [92] expanded on these early findings by pooling cDNA from testicular biopsy samples grouped by pathology. More recently, Malcher et al. [93] utilized testicular biopsy samples from controls and men with NOA. Gene expression found 4,946 differentially expressed genes with SPACA4 and CAPN11 significantly downregulated in infertile patients [93]. Interestingly, SPACA4 (or SAMP14) has been found in the sperm acrosome and postulated to be involved with sperm–egg interactions [94] with CAPN11 potentially involved in cytoskeletal remodeling during spermatogenesis [93, 95].

Unfortunately, previous studies examining gene expression have been mostly conducted in cellular homogenates obtained from testicular biopsy specimens. As such, the comparisons between patients with SCO and controls are essentially classifying cellular heterogeneity. Indeed, given that spermatocytes and spermatids have high rates of RNA synthesis [96], their presence in the control population affects all genetic outputs analyzed [97]. Interestingly, Yatsenko et al. [98] previously assessed genes involved in meiosis for mutations using the long-living residual RNA found in mature sperm from semen ejaculate. If examining whole-system alterations, an alternative approach would be to examine tissue fibroblasts. This method allows determination of conserved pathways to be more thoroughly examined while not being affected by the presence, or absence of germ cells [97]. Future studies using DNA microarrays are currently being conducted with results poised to highlight signal transduction pathways unique to human male infertility.

Genomics: Epigenetics

Epigenetics, the study of genetic alterations due to indirect modifications of the DNA sequence, is gaining prominence as a mechanism to regulate male fertility. Since it is crucial for sperm to be correctly arranged and programmed, epigenetic modifications have the potential to evoke system-wide changes. For example, DNA-binding proteins as well as DNA methylation are just two of the epigenetic variations that have the potential to alter genetic code without directly affecting the DNA sequence. In this context, the regulation of transcription and gene expression can be appropriately, or inappropriately, modified.

The most well described epigenetic factors in the realm of male infertility has so far focused on protamines and packaging of the sperm genome [99–101]. Indeed, a critical component of spermatogenesis involves chromatin packaging during which ~85 % of the histones are replaced with protamines [102]. Alterations in protamine [103] may thus result in improper post-translational processing and subsequently decreased sperm counts, motility, morphology and increased DNA fragmentation [100, 101, 103]. Two types of human protamines (PRM), PRM-1 and PRM-2, have been identified [103] with alterations in the timing or ratio of expression resulting in arrested spermatogenesis and infertility [100, 101]. Indeed, men with asthenospermia have been shown to have lower levels of PRM-1 and PRM-2 messenger RNA [104] with altered protamination inversely associated functionally and fertilization ability [105]. Histones that are not replaced by protamine during chromatin packaging are termed "retained histones" and have been found to contain both activating and silencing epigenetic influences making them ready for rapid gene activation or inhibition. DNA to histone binding is also affected by the methylation of genomic DNA with several genes, including IGF2 and MEST affected in oligozoospermic men [106].

Maternal or paternal imprinting is the result of DNA methylation that subsequently regulates embryonic gene expression. Methylation is another important source of epigenetic modification. Occurring by the addition of a methyl ($-CH_3$) group to a cytosine to a CpG site within DNA, the ability to alter genetic profiles with DNA methylation may hold the key to epigenetic control of male infertility [107]. Indeed, aberrant patterns of methylation in differentially methylated regions (DMRs) of DNA have been found in men with moderate to severe oligospermia [108]. Abnormal germ-line epigenetic reprogramming was proposed as a possible mechanism affecting spermatogenesis [109]. Wide-ranging erasure of DNA methylation followed by sex-specific patterns of de-novo DNA methylation with subsequent incomplete reprogramming of male germ cells was found to alter sperm DNA methylation; thus worsening spermatogenesis outcomes [109]. More recently, DNA methylation profiling using a Methylation array identified 471 CpG sites encompassing 287 genes that were differentially methylated between men with infertility and fertile controls [110]. The fact that sperm DNA methylation profiles are consistent over time and highly reproducible [111] makes this an interesting and promising avenue of future research.

Proteomics

The study of the human proteome lies in the interface between genes and their protein products. By examining the function of proteins in the context of the expressed complement of the human genome, an indication of active cellular protein content can be ascertained. This is important in the context that while distinct genes are expressed in a cell-dependent manner, protein expression can vary under different times, physiological states and environmental conditions [2]. Alternative splicing of a gene transcript can also yield unique isoforms of a given gene [112]. Moreover, given that messenger RNA is not always translated to protein, proteomic analysis of specific products in exact disease states has the potential to provide accurate biomarkers; especially in the realm of male infertility.

Currently, semen analysis is the best tool physicians have to assess male fertility potential; however, many cases of male infertility remain undiagnosed. Proteomics has made rapid progress over the years and by understanding the types and amounts of proteins as well as their modifications (i.e., acetylaction, glycosylation), the potential for the field are enormous. While it is challenging to sort through the vast amounts of data collected in proteomic analyses to select the handful of genes, several novel biomarkers have already been proposed.

In the context of male fertility, the most difficult challenges lay in the composition of the biological fluid itself and the variability of the possible changes. Semen is made up of sperm and seminal plasma and contains products from multiple different organs including the prostate, seminal vesicles, and bulbourethral glands [113]. The fact that variations in semen occur seasonally and with age makes analysis difficult. Post-ejaculation, variable proteins are activated during coagulation and liquefaction making the generation of a proteomic profile distinct to men with NOA exceptionally challenging.

Research on protein products contained in the seminal plasma began early in the 1940s. Advancements in the field eventually came following the identification of a germ cell binding, Sertoli cell secreted protein, transferrin [114]. Proteolytic breakdown of seminal plasma proteins was examined by two-dimensional (2D) electrophoresis followed by silver staining and found to be accelerated in oligospermic men compared to azoospermic and normospermic cohorts [115]. The development and use of mass-spectrometric techniques allowed more thorough investigations of complex body fluids. Using this technology, in combination with 2D gel electrophoresis, a more detailed characterization of the proteins involved in male infertility was conducted [116]. Differences were identified between men with Sertoli Cell Only (SCO) Syndrome and vasectomized men [116]. Further studies on a single individual using this technology found 923 unique proteins in seminal plasma and provided an accurate and in-depth inventory of proteins in this biological substance [117]. While only 10 % of the reported proteins were known as originating from the male reproductive tract, they encompassed nearly all the proteins identified by two previous studies [118, 119]. Investigators then assessed the seminal proteins of fertile men, and found ~919–1,487 unique proteins in each individual with 83 common in all fertile men [120]. Of these, human cationic microbial protein (hCAP18) was present in the human epididymis and the seminal plasma while spindlin1 was also implicated given its localization to the tails of murine sperm and previously known involvement with spermatogenesis [120, 121].

Batruch [122] expanded this work by examining the constituents of seminal plasma from control men compared to those men who had vasectomies. In post-vasectomy (PV) men, the testicular and epididymal secretions were physically blocked from reaching the ejaculate and as such, the investigators were able to assess proteins originating from different areas of the reproductive tract. These authors identified 32 proteins unique to controls and 4 unique to PV patients [122]. From these, TEX101, the "testis expressed 101" gene located at chromosome 19q13.31 was noted to be one of the leading biomarker candidates. TEX101, a glycosylphosphatidylinositol (GPI)-anchored protein is essential for the production of fertile mouse spermatozoa [123]. Indeed, via interaction with ADAM3 (A disintegrin and metallopeptidase domain 3), a sperm membrane protein critical for both sperm migration into the oviduct [124] and sperm binding to the zona pellucida [125] TEX101 has the potential to be a regulator of male fertility.

Further work from the same authors compared the proteome of NOA men [126] to their previously published results [122] finding several proteins that were elevated (Control vs. NOA, $n=34$; NOA vs. PV, $n=59$) and others that were decreased (Control vs. NOA, $n=18$; NOA vs. PV, $n=16$). Given that several of these proteins were from the male reproductive tract and have previously been linked to fertility, it is tempting to speculate that many of these proteins play important roles in male infertility.

Several other proteins that are of interest as potential biomarkers of male fertility include Heparin binding proteins (HBPs) and prolactin inducible protein (PIP). HBPs are glycosaminoglycans that are potent enhances of sperm capacitation in animals [127]. Purification of seven HBPs from human seminal plasma identified them as semenogelin 1 and 2 as well as PSA and zinc finger protein. PIP, a 17-kDa glycoprotein, is also increased in azoospermic men and, as an abundant seminal plasma protein, it also has a role in capacitation and acts to improve sperm motility [128].

In summary, proteomic analysis of seminal plasma, while at its infancy, is currently expanding the scope of potential male infertility biomarkers. While much work still needs to be conducted, the premise of the research is exciting.

Acknowledgement JRK is an NIH K12 Scholar supported by a Male Reproductive Health Research Career (MHRH) Development Physician-Scientist Award (HD073917-01) from the Eunice Kennedy Shriver National Institute of Child Health and Human Development (NICHD) Program (awarded to DJL).

References

1. Ferlin A, Raicu F, Gatta V, Zuccarello D, Palka G, Foresta C. Male infertility: role of genetic background. Reprod Biomed Online. 2007;14:734–45.
2. Kovac JR, Pastuszak AW, Lamb DJ. The use of genomics, proteomics, and metabolomics in identifying biomarkers of male infertility. Fertil Steril. 2013;99:998–1007.
3. Thonneau P, Marchand S, Tallec A, Ferial ML, Ducot B, Lansac J, et al. Incidence and main causes of infertility in a resident population (1,850,000) of three French regions (1988-1989). Hum Reprod. 1991;6:811–6.
4. Practice Committee of American Society for Reproductive M. Diagnostic evaluation of the infertile male: a committee opinion. Fertil Steril. 2012;98: 294–301.
5. Matzuk MM, Lamb DJ. The biology of infertility: research advances and clinical challenges. Nat Med. 2008;14:1197–213.
6. Pastuszak AW, Lamb DJ. The genetics of male fertility–from basic science to clinical evaluation. J Androl. 2012;33:1075–84.
7. Jacobs PA, Strong JA. A case of human intersexuality having a possible XXY sex-determining mechanism. Nature. 1959;183:302–3.
8. Ford CE, Jones KW, Polani PE, De Almeida JC, Briggs JH. A sex-chromosome anomaly in a case of gonadal dysgenesis (Turner's syndrome). Lancet. 1959;1:711–3.
9. Chandley AC, Edmond P, Christie S, Gowans L, Fletcher J, Frackiewicz A, et al. Cytogenetics and infertility in man. I. Karyotype and seminal analysis: results of a five-year survey of men attending a subfertility clinic. Ann Hum Genet. 1975;39:231–54.
10. Yatsenko AN, Yatsenko SA, Weedin JW, Lawrence AE, Patel A, Peacock S, et al. Comprehensive 5-year study of cytogenetic aberrations in 668 infertile men. J Urol. 2010;183:1636–42.
11. Van Assche E, Bonduelle M, Tournaye H, Joris H, Verheyen G, Devroey P, et al. Cytogenetics of infertile men. Hum Reprod. 1996;11 Suppl 4:1–24. discussion 5-6.
12. Ravel C, Berthaut I, Bresson JL, Siffroi JP. Genetics Commission of the French Federation of C. Prevalence of chromosomal abnormalities in phenotypically normal and fertile adult males: large-scale survey of over 10,000 sperm donor karyotypes. Hum Reprod. 2006;21:1484–9.
13. Nakamura Y, Kitamura M, Nishimura K, Koga M, Kondoh N, Takeyama M, et al. Chromosomal variants among 1790 infertile men. Int J Urol. 2001;8: 49–52.
14. Lee JY, Dada R, Sabanegh E, Carpi A, Agarwal A. Role of genetics in azoospermia. Urology. 2011; 77:598–601.
15. Schiff JD, Palermo GD, Veeck LL, Goldstein M, Rosenwaks Z, Schlegel PN. Success of testicular sperm extraction [corrected] and intracytoplasmic sperm injection in men with Klinefelter syndrome. J Clin Endocrinol Metab. 2005;90:6263–7.
16. Harari O, Bourne H, Baker G, Gronow M, Johnston I. High fertilization rate with intracytoplasmic sperm injection in mosaic Klinefelter's syndrome. Fertil Steril. 1995;63:182–4.
17. Yoshida A, Miura K, Nagao K, Hara H, Ishii N, Shirai M. Sexual function and clinical features of patients with Klinefelter's syndrome with the chief complaint of male infertility. Int J Androl. 1997;20:80–5.
18. Burrows PJ, Schrepferman CG, Lipshultz LI. Comprehensive office evaluation in the new millennium. Urol Clin North Am. 2002;29:873–94.
19. Oates RaL D. Genetic aspects of infertility. In: Lipshultz L, Howards S, Niederberger C, editors.

Infertility in the male. Cambridge, UK: Cambridge University Press; 2009. p. 251–76.
20. Groth KA, Skakkebaek A, Host C, Gravholt CH, Bojesen A. Clinical review: Klinefelter syndrome—a clinical update. J Clin Endocrinol Metab. 2013;98:20–30.
21. Oates RD. Clinical and diagnostic features of patients with suspected Klinefelter syndrome. J Androl. 2003;24:49–50.
22. Wikstrom AM, Dunkel L, Wickman S, Norjavaara E, Ankarberg-Lindgren C, Raivio T. Are adolescent boys with Klinefelter syndrome androgen deficient? A longitudinal study of Finnish 47, XXY boys. Pediatr Res. 2006;59:854–9.
23. Hotaling J. Genetics of male infertility. Urol Clin North Am. 2014;41:1–17.
24. Aguirre D, Nieto K, Lazos M, Pena YR, Palma I, Kofman-Alfaro S, et al. Extragonadal germ cell tumors are often associated with Klinefelter syndrome. Hum Pathol. 2006;37:477–80.
25. Swerdlow AJ, Hermon C, Jacobs PA, Alberman E, Beral V, Daker M, et al. Mortality and cancer incidence in persons with numerical sex chromosome abnormalities: a cohort study. Ann Hum Genet. 2001;65:177–88.
26. Swerdlow AJ, Schoemaker MJ, Higgins CD, Wright AF, Jacobs PA, UKCC Group. Cancer incidence and mortality in men with Klinefelter syndrome: a cohort study. J Natl Cancer Inst. 2005;97:1204–10.
27. Arnedo N, Templado C, Sanchez-Blanque Y, Rajmil O, Nogues C. Sperm aneuploidy in fathers of Klinefelter's syndrome offspring assessed by multicolour fluorescent in situ hybridization using probes for chromosomes 6, 13, 18, 21, 22, X and Y. Hum Reprod. 2006;21:524–8.
28. Eskenazi B, Wyrobek AJ, Kidd SA, Lowe X, Moore 2nd D, Weisiger K, et al. Sperm aneuploidy in fathers of children with paternally and maternally inherited Klinefelter syndrome. Hum Reprod. 2002;17:576–83.
29. Okada H, Goda K, Yamamoto Y, Sofikitis N, Miyagawa I, Mio Y, et al. Age as a limiting factor for successful sperm retrieval in patients with nonmosaic Klinefelter's syndrome. Fertil Steril. 2005;84:1662–4.
30. Damani MN, Mittal R, Oates RD. Testicular tissue extraction in a young male with 47, XXY Klinefelter's syndrome: potential strategy for preservation of fertility. Fertil Steril. 2001;76:1054–6.
31. Aksglaede L, Wikstrom AM, Rajpert-De Meyts E, Dunkel L, Skakkebaek NE, Juul A. Natural history of seminiferous tubule degeneration in Klinefelter syndrome. Hum Reprod Update. 2006;12:39–48.
32. Bakircioglu ME, Ulug U, Erden HF, Tosun S, Bayram A, Ciray N, et al. Klinefelter syndrome: does it confer a bad prognosis in treatment of nonobstructive azoospermia? Fertil Steril. 2011;95:1696–9.
33. Foresta C, Galeazzi C, Bettella A, Marin P, Rossato M, Garolla A, et al. Analysis of meiosis in intratesticular germ cells from subjects affected by classic Klinefelter's syndrome. J Clin Endocrinol Metab. 1999;84:3807–10.
34. Bourne H, Stern K, Clarke G, Pertile M, Speirs A, Baker HW. Delivery of normal twins following the intracytoplasmic injection of spermatozoa from a patient with 47, XXY Klinefelter's syndrome. Hum Reprod. 1997;12:2447–50.
35. Hinney B, Guttenbach M, Schmid M, Engel W, Michelmann HW. Pregnancy after intracytoplasmic sperm injection with sperm from a man with a 47, XXY Klinefelter's karyotype. Fertil Steril. 1997;68:718–20.
36. Komori S, Horiuchi I, Hamada Y, Hasegawa A, Kasumi H, Kondoh N, et al. Birth of healthy neonates after intracytoplasmic injection of ejaculated or testicular spermatozoa from men with nonmosaic Klinefelter's syndrome: a report of 2 cases. J Reprod Med. 2004;49:126–30.
37. Lin YM, Huang WJ, Lin JS, Kuo PL. Progressive depletion of germ cells in a man with nonmosaic Klinefelter's syndrome: optimal time for sperm recovery. Urology. 2004;63:380–1.
38. Madgar I, Dor J, Weissenberg R, Raviv G, Menashe Y, Levron J. Prognostic value of the clinical and laboratory evaluation in patients with nonmosaic Klinefelter syndrome who are receiving assisted reproductive therapy. Fertil Steril. 2002;77:1167–9.
39. Hwang K, Weedin JW, Lamb DJ. The use of fluorescent in situ hybridization in male infertility. Ther Adv Urol. 2010;2:157–69.
40. Holmes JM, Martin RH. Aneuploidy detection in human sperm nuclei using fluorescence in situ hybridization. Hum Genet. 1993;91:20–4.
41. Abdelmoula NB. Amouri A, Portnoi MF, Saad A, Boudawara T, Mhiri MN, et al. Cytogenetics and fluorescence in situ hybridization assessment of sex-chromosome mosaicism in Klinefelter's syndrome. Ann Genet. 2004;47:163–75.
42. Nagvenkar P, Zaveri K, Hinduja I. Comparison of the sperm aneuploidy rate in severe oligozoospermic and oligozoospermic men and its relation to intracytoplasmic sperm injection outcome. Fertil Steril. 2005;84:925–31.
43. Carrell DT, Wilcox AL, Udoff LC, Thorp C, Campbell B. Chromosome 15 aneuploidy in the sperm and conceptus of a sibling with variable familial expression of round-headed sperm syndrome. Fertil Steril. 2001;76:1258–60.
44. Oates RD, Amos JA. The genetic basis of congenital bilateral absence of the vas deferens and cystic fibrosis. J Androl. 1994;15:1–8.
45. Anguiano A, Oates RD, Amos JA, Dean M, Gerrard B, Stewart C, et al. Congenital bilateral absence of the vas deferens. A primarily genital form of cystic fibrosis. JAMA. 1992;267:1794–7.
46. Dayangac D, Erdem H, Yilmaz E, Sahin A, Sohn C, Ozguc M, et al. Mutations of the CFTR gene in Turkish patients with congenital bilateral absence of the vas deferens. Hum Reprod. 2004;19:1094–100.

47. Sakamoto H, Yajima T, Suzuki K, Ogawa Y. Cystic fibrosis transmembrane conductance regulator (CFTR) gene mutation associated with a congenital bilateral absence of vas deferens. Int J Urol. 2008; 15:270–1.
48. Strausbaugh SD, Davis PB. Cystic fibrosis: a review of epidemiology and pathobiology. Clin Chest Med. 2007;28:279–88.
49. Southern KW. Cystic fibrosis and formes frustes of CFTR-related disease. Respiration. 2007;74:241–51.
50. Zielenski J. Genotype and phenotype in cystic fibrosis. Respiration. 2000;67:117–33.
51. Danziger KL, Black LD, Keiles SB, Kammesheidt A, Turek PJ. Improved detection of cystic fibrosis mutations in infertility patients with DNA sequence analysis. Hum Reprod. 2004;19:540–6.
52. Jarvi K, Zielenski J, Wilschanski M, Durie P, Buckspan M, Tullis E, et al. Cystic fibrosis transmembrane conductance regulator and obstructive azoospermia. Lancet. 1995;345:1578.
53. Carter SS, Shinohara K, Lipshultz LI. Transrectal ultrasonography in disorders of the seminal vesicles and ejaculatory ducts. Urol Clin North Am. 1989; 16:773–90.
54. Samli H, Samli MM, Yilmaz E, Imirzalioglu N. Clinical, andrological and genetic characteristics of patients with congenital bilateral absence of vas deferens (CBAVD). Arch Androl. 2006;52:471–7.
55. Claustres M. Molecular pathology of the CFTR locus in male infertility. Reprod Biomed Online. 2005;10:14–41.
56. Claustres M, Guittard C, Bozon D, Chevalier F, Verlingue C, Ferec C, et al. Spectrum of CFTR mutations in cystic fibrosis and in congenital absence of the vas deferens in France. Hum Mutat. 2000;16:143–56.
57. Uzun S, Gokce S, Wagner K. Cystic fibrosis transmembrane conductance regulator gene mutations in infertile males with congenital bilateral absence of the vas deferens. Tohoku J Exp Med. 2005;207: 279–85.
58. Lebo RV, Grody WW. Variable penetrance and expressivity of the splice altering 5 T sequence in the cystic fibrosis gene. Genet Test. 2007;11:32–44.
59. McCallum TJ, Milunsky JM, Cunningham DL, Harris DH, Maher TA, Oates RD. Fertility in men with cystic fibrosis: an update on current surgical practices and outcomes. Chest. 2000;118:1059–62.
60. Schlegel PN, Shin D, Goldstein M. Urogenital anomalies in men with congenital absence of the vas deferens. J Urol. 1996;155:1644–8.
61. Kovac JR, Golev D, Khan V, Fischer MA. Case of the month # 168: seminal vesicle cysts with ipsilateral renal dysgenesis. Canadian Association of Radiologists journal =. J Assoc Can Radiol. 2011; 62:223–5.
62. McPherson E, Carey J, Kramer A, Hall JG, Pauli RM, Schimke RN, et al. Dominantly inherited renal adysplasia. Am J Med Genet. 1987;26:863–72.
63. McCallum T, Milunsky J, Munarriz R, Carson R, Sadeghi-Nejad H, Oates R. Unilateral renal agenesis associated with congenital bilateral absence of the vas deferens: phenotypic findings and genetic considerations. Hum Reprod. 2001;16:282–8.
64. Skaletsky H, Kuroda-Kawaguchi T, Minx PJ, Cordum HS, Hillier L, Brown LG, et al. The male-specific region of the human Y chromosome is a mosaic of discrete sequence classes. Nature. 2003; 423:825–37.
65. Tilford CA, Kuroda-Kawaguchi T, Skaletsky H, Rozen S, Brown LG, Rosenberg M, et al. A physical map of the human Y chromosome. Nature. 2001; 409:943–5.
66. Jobling MA, Tyler-Smith C. The human Y chromosome: an evolutionary marker comes of age. Nat Rev Genet. 2003;4:598–612.
67. Repping S, Skaletsky H, Lange J, Silber S, Van Der Veen F, Oates RD, et al. Recombination between palindromes P5 and P1 on the human Y chromosome causes massive deletions and spermatogenic failure. Am J Hum Genet. 2002;71:906–22.
68. Foresta C, Moro E, Ferlin A. Y chromosome microdeletions and alterations of spermatogenesis. Endocr Rev. 2001;22:226–39.
69. Pryor JL, Kent-First M, Muallem A, Van Bergen AH, Nolten WE, Meisner L, et al. Microdeletions in the Y chromosome of infertile men. N Engl J Med. 1997;336:534–9.
70. Reijo R, Lee TY, Salo P, Alagappan R, Brown LG, Rosenberg M, et al. Diverse spermatogenic defects in humans caused by Y chromosome deletions encompassing a novel RNA-binding protein gene. Nat Genet. 1995;10:383–93.
71. Reijo R, Alagappan RK, Patrizio P, Page DC. Severe oligozoospermia resulting from deletions of azoospermia factor gene on Y chromosome. Lancet. 1996;347:1290–3.
72. Mulhall JP, Reijo R, Alagappan R, Brown L, Page D, Carson R, et al. Azoospermic men with deletion of the DAZ gene cluster are capable of completing spermatogenesis: fertilization, normal embryonic development and pregnancy occur when retrieved testicular spermatozoa are used for intracytoplasmic sperm injection. Hum Reprod. 1997;12:503–8.
73. Oates RD, Silber S, Brown LG, Page DC. Clinical characterization of 42 oligospermic or azoospermic men with microdeletion of the AZFc region of the Y chromosome, and of 18 children conceived via ICSI. Hum Reprod. 2002;17:2813–24.
74. Krausz C, Quintana-Murci L, McElreavey K. Prognostic value of Y deletion analysis: what is the clinical prognostic value of Y chromosome microdeletion analysis? Hum Reprod. 2000;15:1431–4.
75. Brandell RA, Mielnik A, Liotta D, Ye Z, Veeck LL, Palermo GD, et al. AZFb deletions predict the absence of spermatozoa with testicular sperm extraction: preliminary report of a prognostic genetic test. Hum Reprod. 1998;13:2812–5.
76. Hopps CV, Mielnik A, Goldstein M, Palermo GD, Rosenwaks Z, Schlegel PN. Detection of sperm in men with Y chromosome microdeletions of the

AZFa, AZFb and AZFc regions. Hum Reprod. 2003; 18:1660–5.
77. Alvesalo L, de la Chapelle A. Permanent tooth sizes in 46, XX-males. Ann Hum Genet. 1979;43:97–102.
78. El Awady MK, El Shater SF, Ragaa E, Atef K, Shaheen IM, Megiud NA. Molecular study on Y chromosome microdeletions in Egyptian males with idiopathic infertility. Asian J Androl. 2004;6:53–7.
79. Jorgez CJ, Weedin JW, Sahin A, Tannour-Louet M, Han S, Bournat JC, et al. Y-chromosome microdeletions are not associated with SHOX haploinsufficiency. Hum Reprod. 2014;29:1113–4.
80. Lange J, Skaletsky H, van Daalen SK, Embry SL, Korver CM, Brown LG, et al. Isodicentric Y chromosomes and sex disorders as byproducts of homologous recombination that maintains palindromes. Cell. 2009;138:855–69.
81. Lehmann KJ, Kovac JR, Xu J, Fischer MA. Isodicentric Yq mosaicism presenting as infertility and maturation arrest without altered SRY and AZF regions. J Assist Reprod Genet. 2012;29:939–42.
82. Jorgez CJ, Weedin JW, Sahin A, Tannour-Louet M, Han S, Bournat JC, et al. Aberrations in pseudoautosomal regions (PARs) found in infertile men with Y-chromosome microdeletions. J Clin Endocrinol Metab. 2011;96:E674–9.
83. Repping S, van Daalen SK, Brown LG, Korver CM, Lange J, Marszalek JD, et al. High mutation rates have driven extensive structural polymorphism among human Y chromosomes. Nat Genet. 2006;38:463–7.
84. Lee C, Iafrate AJ, Brothman AR. Copy number variations and clinical cytogenetic diagnosis of constitutional disorders. Nat Genet. 2007;39:S48–54.
85. Kallioniemi A, Kallioniemi OP, Sudar D, Rutovitz D, Gray JW, Waldman F, et al. Comparative genomic hybridization for molecular cytogenetic analysis of solid tumors. Science. 1992;258:818–21.
86. Lucito R, Healy J, Alexander J, Reiner A, Esposito D, Chi M, et al. Representational oligonucleotide microarray analysis: a high-resolution method to detect genome copy number variation. Genome Res. 2003;13:2291–305.
87. Evangelidou P, Alexandrou A, Moutafi M, Ioannides M, Antoniou P, Koumbaris G, et al. Implementation of high resolution whole genome array CGH in the prenatal clinical setting: advantages, challenges, and review of the literature. BioMed Res Int. 2013; 2013:346762.
88. Shaffer LG, Bejjani BA. A cytogeneticist's perspective on genomic microarrays. Hum Reprod Update. 2004;10:221–6.
89. Tuttelmann F, Simoni M, Kliesch S, Ledig S, Dworniczak B, Wieacker P, et al. Copy number variants in patients with severe oligozoospermia and Sertoli-cell-only syndrome. PLoS One. 2011; 6:e19426.
90. Slonim DK, Yanai I. Getting started in gene expression microarray analysis. PLoS Comput Biol. 2009;5:e1000543.

91. Sha J, Zhou Z, Li J, Yin L, Yang H, Hu G, et al. Identification of testis development and spermatogenesis-related genes in human and mouse testes using cDNA arrays. Mol Hum Reprod. 2002;8:511–7.
92. Lin YH, Lin YM, Teng YN, Hsieh TY, Lin YS, Kuo PL. Identification of ten novel genes involved in human spermatogenesis by microarray analysis of testicular tissue. Fertil Steril. 2006;86:1650–8.
93. Malcher A, Rozwadowska N, Stokowy T, Kolanowski T, Jedrzejczak P, Zietkowiak W, et al. Potential biomarkers of nonobstructive azoospermia identified in microarray gene expression analysis. Fertil Steril. 2013;100:1686-94.e1–7.
94. Shetty J, Wolkowicz MJ, Digilio LC, Klotz KL, Jayes FL, Diekman AB, et al. SAMP14, a novel, acrosomal membrane-associated, glycosylphosphatidylinositol-anchored member of the Ly-6/urokinase-type plasminogen activator receptor superfamily with a role in sperm-egg interaction. J Biol Chem. 2003;278:30506–15.
95. Ben-Aharon I, Brown PR, Shalgi R, Eddy EM. Calpain 11 is unique to mouse spermatogenic cells. Mol Reprod Dev. 2006;73:767–73.
96. Geremia R, Boitani C, Conti M, Monesi V. RNA synthesis in spermatocytes and spermatids and preservation of meiotic RNA during spermiogenesis in the mouse. Cell Differ. 1977;5:343–55.
97. Kovac JR, Lamb DJ. Male infertility biomarkers and genomic aberrations in azoospermia. Fertil Steril. 2014;101(5):e31.
98. Yatsenko AN, Roy A, Chen R, Ma L, Murthy LJ, Yan W, et al. Non-invasive genetic diagnosis of male infertility using spermatozoal RNA: KLHL10 mutations in oligozoospermic patients impair homodimerization. Hum Mol Genet. 2006;15:3411–9.
99. Carrell DT, Aston KI. The search for SNPs, CNVs, and epigenetic variants associated with the complex disease of male infertility. Syst Biol Reprod Med. 2011;57:17–26.
100. Carrell DT, Emery BR, Hammoud S. Altered protamine expression and diminished spermatogenesis: what is the link? Hum Reprod Update. 2007;13:313–27.
101. Carrell DT, Liu L. Altered protamine 2 expression is uncommon in donors of known fertility, but common among men with poor fertilizing capacity, and may reflect other abnormalities of spermiogenesis. J Androl. 2001;22:604–10.
102. Aoki VW, Carrell DT. Human protamines and the developing spermatid: their structure, function, expression and relationship with male infertility. Asian J Androl. 2003;5:315–24.
103. Iguchi N, Yang S, Lamb DJ, Hecht NB. An SNP in protamine 1: a possible genetic cause of male infertility? J Med Genet. 2006;43:382–4.
104. Kempisty B, Depa-Martynow M, Lianeri M, Jedrzejczak P, Darul-Wasowicz A, Jagodzinski PP. Evaluation of protamines 1 and 2 transcript contents in spermatozoa from asthenozoospermic men. Folia Histochem Cytobiol. 2007;45 Suppl 1:S109–13.

105. Aoki VW, Liu L, Jones KP, Hatasaka HH, Gibson M, Peterson CM, et al. Sperm protamine 1/protamine 2 ratios are related to in vitro fertilization pregnancy rates and predictive of fertilization ability. Fertil Steril. 2006;86:1408–15.
106. Poplinski A, Tuttelmann F, Kanber D, Horsthemke B, Gromoll J. Idiopathic male infertility is strongly associated with aberrant methylation of MEST and IGF2/H19 ICR1. Int J Androl. 2010;33:642–9.
107. O'Flynn O'Brien KL, Varghese AC, Agarwal A. The genetic causes of male factor infertility: a review. Fertil Steril. 2010;93:1–12.
108. Kobayashi H, Sato A, Otsu E, Hiura H, Tomatsu C, Utsunomiya T, et al. Aberrant DNA methylation of imprinted loci in sperm from oligospermic patients. Hum Mol Genet. 2007;16:2542–51.
109. Houshdaran S, Cortessis VK, Siegmund K, Yang A, Laird PW, Sokol RZ. Widespread epigenetic abnormalities suggest a broad DNA methylation erasure defect in abnormal human sperm. PLoS One. 2007;2:e1289.
110. Friemel C, Ammerpohl O, Gutwein J, Schmutzler AG, Caliebe A, Kautza M, et al. Array-based DNA methylation profiling in male infertility reveals allele-specific DNA methylation in PIWIL1 and PIWIL2. Fertil Steril. 2014;101(4):1097–1103.e1.
111. Cortessis VK, Siegmund K, Houshdaran S, Laird PW, Sokol RZ. Repeated assessment by high-throughput assay demonstrates that sperm DNA methylation levels are highly reproducible. Fertil Steril. 2011;96:1325–30.
112. Kovac JR, Preiksaitis HG, Sims SM. Functional and molecular analysis of L-type calcium channels in human esophagus and lower esophageal sphincter smooth muscle. Am J Physiol Gastrointest Liver Physiol. 2005;289:G998–1006.
113. Duncan MW, Thompson HS. Proteomics of semen and its constituents. Proteomics Clin Appl. 2007;1:861–75.
114. Holmes SD, Bucci LR, Lipshultz LI, Smith RG. Transferrin binds specifically to pachytene spermatocytes. Endocrinology. 1983;113:1916–8.
115. Ayyagari RR, Fazleabas AT, Dawood MY. Seminal plasma proteins of fertile and infertile men analyzed by two-dimensional electrophoresis. Am J Obstet Gynecol. 1987;157:1528–33.
116. Starita-Geribaldi M, Poggioli S, Zucchini M, Garin J, Chevallier D, Fenichel P, et al. Mapping of seminal plasma proteins by two-dimensional gel electrophoresis in men with normal and impaired spermatogenesis. Mol Hum Reprod. 2001;7:715–22.
117. Pilch B, Mann M. Large-scale and high-confidence proteomic analysis of human seminal plasma. Genome Biol. 2006;7:R40.
118. Utleg AG, Yi EC, Xie T, Shannon P, White JT, Goodlett DR, et al. Proteomic analysis of human prostasomes. Prostate. 2003;56:150–61.
119. Fung KY, Glode LM, Green S, Duncan MW. A comprehensive characterization of the peptide and protein constituents of human seminal fluid. Prostate. 2004;61:171–81.
120. Milardi D, Grande G, Vincenzoni F, Messana I, Pontecorvi A, De Marinis L, et al. Proteomic approach in the identification of fertility pattern in seminal plasma of fertile men. Fertil Steril. 2012;97:67–73.e1.
121. Zhang KM, Wang YF, Huo R, Bi Y, Lin M, Sha JH, et al. Characterization of Spindlin1 isoform2 in mouse testis. Asian J Androl. 2008;10:741–8.
122. Batruch I, Lecker I, Kagedan D, Smith CR, Mullen BJ, Grober E, et al. Proteomic analysis of seminal plasma from normal volunteers and post-vasectomy patients identifies over 2000 proteins and candidate biomarkers of the urogenital system. J Proteome Res. 2011;10:941–53.
123. Fujihara Y, Tokuhiro K, Muro Y, Kondoh G, Araki Y, Ikawa M, et al. Expression of TEX101, regulated by ACE, is essential for the production of fertile mouse spermatozoa. Proc Natl Acad Sci U S A. 2013;110:8111–6.
124. Li W, Guo XJ, Teng F, Hou XJ, Lv Z, Zhou SY, et al. Tex101 is essential for male fertility by affecting sperm migration into the oviduct in mice. J Mol Cell Biol. 2013;5:345–7.
125. Fujihara Y, Okabe M, Ikawa M. GPI-anchored protein complex, LY6K/TEX101, is required for sperm migration into the oviduct and male fertility in mice. Biol Reprod. 2014;90:60.
126. Batruch I, Smith CR, Mullen BJ, Grober E, Lo KC, Diamandis EP, et al. Analysis of seminal plasma from patients with non-obstructive azoospermia and identification of candidate biomarkers of male infertility. J Proteome Res. 2012;11:1503–11.
127. Parrish JJ, Susko-Parrish J, Winer MA, First NL. Capacitation of bovine sperm by heparin. Biol Reprod. 1988;38:1171–80.
128. Davalieva K, Kiprijanovska S, Noveski P, Plaseski T, Kocevska B, Broussard C, et al. Proteomic analysis of seminal plasma in men with different spermatogenic impairment. Andrologia. 2012;44:256–64.

Index

A

aCGH. *See* Array comparative genomic hybridization (aCGH)
Acrosomal enzymes, 114–115
Adaptive Electronic Condenser (AEC)™, 107
Amplicons, 171
Aneuploid spermatozoa, 152
Animal sperm, chemotaxis of, 54
Apoptosis, 138
    abortive, 69
    on ART clinical outcomes, 72
    changes in sperm, 71
    in human spermatozoa, 69–70
    impact of, 72
Array comparative genomic hybridization (aCGH), 172
Assisted reproductive techniques (ART), 5, 41, 112, 149
    effects on clinical, 75–76
    outcome
        electrophoretic method and, 48
        sperm apoptosis on, 72
        zeta method and, 46
Azoospermia, 8, 10, 16
Azoospermia Factor (AZF)
    deletions, 171
    regions, 170

B

Biomarkers, 30, 32, 174, 175
Birefringence technique, 29
Birth defects, 162, 163
Blastocyst culture, 115–116
Bromodomain testis-specific protein (BRDT), 114

C

Caspase-activated deoxyribonuclease (CAD), 71
Caspase (CP) activation, 71–72
CBAVD. *See* Congenital bilateral absence of the vas deferens (CBAVD)
CD52, 42, 43
Centrifugation, swim-up and isopycnic, 51
Cephalic vacuoles, 112
CFTR gene. *See* Cystic Fibrosis Transmembrane Conductance Regulator (CFTR) gene

Chemotaxis, 56
    of animal sperm, 54
    integration of, 54–55
Chromatin
    packaging, 113, 115, 117
    structural morphology, 128–130
Chromatin condensation, 140
    vs. sperm head vacuoles, 130–134
Chromosome abnormalities
    karyotype, 168–169
    male infertility and, 152
    MSOME and, 152–154
Clinical varicocele, treatment of, 4–5
CNVs. *See* Copy number variations (CNVs)
Congenital bilateral absence of the vas deferens (CBAVD), 169
Contemporary testing, limitations of, 167
Copy number variations (CNVs), 172
Cryopreservation, sperm, 124–125
Cumulus cells, 54
Cystic fibrosis (CF), 169–170
Cystic Fibrosis Transmembrane Conductance Regulator (CFTR) gene, 169
Cytoplasmic changes, in sperm, 71–72
CytoScreen™, 106, 107
CytoScreen Flex™, 107, 108
Cytotoxic sperm assessment, 150

D

Deleted in Azoospermia (DAZ) gene, 171
Density gradient centrifugation (DGC)
    techniques, 13
    zeta *vs.* MACS-DGC, 45–46
Differential Interference Contrast (DIC), 102
    components, 95
        analyzer, 96–97
        compensator for bias retardation, 97
        condenser prism, 95–96
        linear polarizer, 95
        objective prism, 96
    optics, 158
Differentially methylated regions (DMRs), 173
Digital imaging system, camera and, 99–100
DNA damage, 45, 160

DNA fragmentation, sperm, 24–25, 72, 113, 115, 116
    biological considerations, 140–141
    clinical considerations, 141–143
    diagnosis and treatment of, 143
    etiology of, 137–138
    evaluation of, 138
    and fertility, 138–139
DNA integrity, 113
DNA methylation, 114, 163, 173
DNA microarray, 31–32
    technology, 172

E
Early paternal effect, 137
Electrophoresis
    advantage and disadvantage of, 48
    and ART outcome, 48
    sperm quality, 47–48
    sperm selection based on, 46, 47
Embryo cleavage, 137
Embryo development
    MSOME and, 86–87
    vacuole-like structure and, 115–116
Enzymes, acrosomal, 114–115
Epididymal hamster spermatozoa, 8
Epigenetics, 173
Externalization of phosphatidylserine (EPS), 44, 45, 71

F
Fertilization rates, 10
Fluorescence in situ hybridization (FISH), 152, 169
Follicular fluid, 54
Freezing–thawing process, 124

G
Gamete formation, in males, 151
Gamete micromanipulation techniques, 7
Gene mutations, 169–170
Genomics, 31–32
    advanced techniques, 172–173
    epigenetics, 173
    gene mutations, 169–170
    karyotype, 168–169
    proteomics, 173–175
    Y-chromosome microdeletions, 170–171
Germ cells, 69, 138
Glycocalyx, 42
Glycosylphosphatidylinositol (GPI)-anchored protein, 42, 174

H
HA. *See* Hyaluronic acid (HA)
HBA. *See* Hyaluronic acid binding assay (HBA)
Hemizona assay (HZA), 60–62
Hemi-zona-index (HZI), 62
Heparin binding proteins (HBPs), 175

High magnification
    of spermatozoon, 157
    sperm cells selection in, 87
    sperm-head abnormalities at, 162
    sperm selection under, 163
    as tool, 160
Hoffman modulation contrast (HMC), in ICSI, 92–95
Human cationic microbial protein (hCAP18), 174
Human spermatozoa, 106, 151
    apoptosis in, 69–70
    components of, contributing, 149
Hyaluronic acid (HA), 14, 63
    binding test, 26
    vs. zeta method, 45
Hyaluronic acid binding assay (HBA), 60, 62–64
HZA. *See* Hemizona assay (HZA)
HZI. *See* Hemi-zona-index (HZI)

I
ICSI. *See* Intracytoplasmic sperm injection (ICSI)
IMSI. *See* Intracytoplasmic morphologically selected sperm injection (IMSI)
Infertile men, semen from, 71
Infertility, 1
    male, 8, 14
        and chromosome abnormalities, 152
        diagnosis of, 3–4
        epigenetic factors in, 173
        genetic causes of, 168
Intracytoplasmic morphologically selected sperm injection (IMSI), 13, 14, 91, 116, 127
    advanced system, 105–108
    advantage of, 139
    differential interference contrast in, 95–98
    discussion and indications, 162–163
    literature and results, 160–162
    microscope body considerations, 98–99
    modern microscope intended for, 106
    prospective studies, 162
    spermatozoon selection, 158–159
    sperm DNA structure, impact of, 159–160
    sperm morphology, impact of, 159
    sperm preparation and technical considerations, 157–158
Intracytoplasmic sperm injection (ICSI), 5, 8–9, 41, 43, 48, 91, 111, 116
    clinical outcome, 9–12
    conventional, 137, 139
    efficacy and safety of, 153
    Hoffman modulation contrast (HMC) in, 92–95
    safety and conclusions, 16–17
    spermatozoa chosen for, 159, 160
    with unselected spermatozoa, 14–15
    utilization of, 60
Intrauterine insemination (IUI), 5, 9, 60
In vitro formation, of vacuole-like structure, 115
In vitro models, 74
In vivo formation, of vacuole-like structures, 112
Isopycnic centrifugation, 51
IUI. *See* Intrauterine insemination (IUI)

Index

K
Karyotype, chromosomal abnormalities, 168–169
Klinefelter's syndrome (KS), 168–169

L
Laser photoablation, of zona, 7
Late paternal effect, 137, 139, 141

M
Magnetic activated cell sorting (MACS)
    DGC *vs.* DGC-zeta, 45–46
    integration of, 76
    for selection of non-apoptotic spermatozoa, 73
    as sperm selection method, 74
        effects on clinical ART, 75–76
Magnetic cell selection, of non-apoptotic sperm, 75
Male fertility, biomarkers of, 32, 175
Male infertility, 8, 14
    and chromosome abnormalities, 152
    diagnosis of, 3–4
    epigenetic factors in, 173
    genetic causes of, 168
Manual for Examining Semen Analysis, 5th Edition, 2–3
Maternal imprinting, 173
Methylation, DNA, 114, 163, 173
Microarrays, DNA, 31–32
Microdeletions, Y-chromosome, 170–171
Microflow®, practical approach to, 46–47
Microfluidic chemoattractant gradient generator, 54
Microfluidics devices
    integration of chemotaxis into, 54–55
    for sperm selection, 52–54
Microfluidic sperm sorter, 52, 53
Microinjectors, 101
Micromanipulators, 101
MicroRNA (miRNA), 32
Mitochondrial changes, in sperm, 71
Mitochondrial membrane potential (MMP), 25–26, 71
Molecular techniques, omics as, 30
Motile sperm organelle morphology examination (MSOME), 13, 24, 26–27, 81–83, 91, 112, 115
    and chromosome abnormalities, 152–154
    concept of, 139
    and conventional semen analysis, 123–124
    criteria for selected sperm cells, 83–84
    damaged DNA detected by, 139–140
    and diagnosis of sperm DNA fragmentation, 143
    and embryo development, 86–87
    magnification for, 98
    to microinjection, 95–98
    microscopy equipment for, 83
    for routine laboratory semen analysis, 87–88
    and sperm cryopreservation, 124–125
    and sperm manipulation, 124
    and sperm nuclear vacuoles, 85–86
    and sperm preparation, 83, 124
    and treatment of sperm DNA fragmentation, 143
Mutations, gene, 169–170

N
Natural barriers, of spermatozoa selection, 111
Nikon Advanced Modulation Contrast (NAMC) system, 93, 94
Nikon DIC system, 96
Nikon/Narishige NT88 V3 Micromanipulator System, 101
Nomarski system, 157, 158
Non-apoptotic spermatozoa
    MACS for selection of, 73
    magnetic cell selection of, 75
    rationale for selection of, 72–73
Nuclear, abnormalities of, 85
Nuclear changes, in sperm, 72
Nuclear chromatin, abnormalities of, 85
Nuclear dysfunction, vacuole-like structure and, 113–114

O
OCTAX® Microscience GmbH, 106
Oligozoospermia, 152
Omics, as molecular techniques, 30
Oocyte viability, temperature, 100–101
Oxidative stress, 138

P
Papanicolaou (PAP) staining, 29
Partial zona dissection (PZD), 7
Paternal effect, 137, 139, 141
Paternal imprinting, 173
Phosphatidylserine (PS), externalization of, 71
Photolithography, 54
Physiologic ICSI (PICSI), 14
Plasma membrane changes, in sperm, 71
Pneumatic microinjector, 101
Polydimethylsiloxane (PDMS), 52, 53
Post-vasectomy (PV) men, 174
Pregnancy rates, 10
Preimplantation genetic diagnosis (PGD), 9
Progenitor, germ cells, 69
Programmed cell death. *See* Apoptosis
Protamines (PRM), 173
Proteomics, 30, 173–175
    analysis
        of seminal plasma, 30
        of spermatozoa, 31
Pseudoautosomal regions (PARs), defects in, 172
PZD. *See* Partial zona dissection (PZD)

Q
Quantitative ultramorphological sperm analysis, 112

R
Reactive oxygen species (ROS), determination of, 24, 27–29
Research Instruments Ltd Integra 3™, 101, 102

S

SCD test. *See* Sperm chromatin dispersion (SCD) test
SCSA. *See* Sperm chromatin structure assay (SCSA)
Semen
    from infertile men, 71
    preparation of, 52, 55
Semen analysis, 1
    conventional, 123–124
    history of modern, 1–2
    MSOME for routine laboratory, 87–88
Semen parameters, 1, 2
    of fertile men, distribution, 4
    limitations, 3
Seminal plasma, proteomics analysis of, 30
Sertoli Cell Only (SCO) Syndrome, 174
Sias, membrane negative charge, 42
Sperm apoptosis, on ART clinical outcomes, 72
Spermatogenesis, 151
Spermatozoa
    aneuploid, 152
    apoptosis in, 69–71
    assessment, cytotoxic, 150
    epididymal hamster, 8
    genetic and epigenetic assessment of, 15
    under high-magnification, 88
    human apoptosis in, 69–70
    ICSI with unselected, 14–15
    motility, 54
    non-apoptotic
        MACS for selection of, 73
        rationale for selection of, 72–73
    normal, 83–84
    proteomics analysis of, 31
    swimming, 54
Spermatozoal parameters, 10
Spermatozoon
    high magnification of, 157
    quest for ideal, 12–14
Sperm chromatin condensation, 140
    vs. sperm head vacuoles, 130–134
Sperm chromatin decondensation, 74, 162
Sperm chromatin dispersion (SCD) test, 13, 25, 141
Sperm chromatin, remodeling, 138
Sperm chromatin structure assay (SCSA), 13, 25
Sperm chromosomal analysis, 151–152
Sperm chromosomal constitution, 150–151
Sperm cryopreservation, 124–125
Sperm DNA fragmentation, 72
    biological considerations, 140–141
    clinical considerations, 141–143
    diagnosis and treatment of, 143
    etiology of, 137–138
    evaluation of, 138
    and fertility, 138–139
Sperm DNA integrity, 13, 138, 141, 143
Sperm head, 157, 161
    abnormalities, 162
    vacuoles *vs.* sperm chromatin condensation status, 130–134

Sperm intranuclear vacuoles, 140
Sperm manipulation, 124
Sperm-microcapture channels, 115
Sperm morphology, 91, 111
    evaluation of, 123
    grading, 60
    visualization of, 142
Sperm motility, 54
Sperm nuclear vacuoles, MSOME and, 85–86
Spermocytogramme, 111
Sperm parameter, 4
Sperm plasma membrane, 42–43
Sperm quality, 47–48, 91
SpermSep®, practical approach to, 46–47
Sperm sorter, microfluidic, 52, 53
Sperm viability, temperature, 100–101
Sperm–zona pellucida binding assays, 60
Suboptimal spermatozoa, 9, 16
Subzonal sperm injection (SUZI), 7, 8
Swimming, sperm, 54
Swim-up centrifugation, 51

T

TAC. *See* Total antioxidant capacity (TAC)
Testicular biopsy, 8
Testicular blood barrier, 69
Testis-specific histone 2B (TH2B), 114
Testis, structure of, 71
Thermosafe mechanism, 101
Tokai Hit's Thermo Plate, 100
Total antioxidant capacity (TAC), 24, 27–29
TUNEL (terminal deoxynucleotidyl transferase-mediated dUTP nick-end labeling) assay, 25, 72, 87, 138

U

Ubiquitinated sperm, 44
Ultramorphological sperm analysis, quantitative, 112

V

Vacuole-like structure
    and embryo development, 115–116
    and nuclear dysfunction, 113–114
    and postnatal data, 116–117
    pregnancies, and miscarriages, 116
    receptacle of acrosomal enzymes, 114–115
    in vitro formation of, 115
    in vivo formation of, 112
Vacuoles, 123, 124
    cephalic, 112
    structural aspects of, 128–130
Varicocele
    AUA guidelines for treating, 4
    clinical, treatment of, 4–5

Index

W
Washing technique, 12
World Health Organization (WHO)
  Manual for Examining Semen Analysis, 5th Edition, 2–3
  reference values on
    assisted reproductive technologies (ART), 5
    clinical practice, 3–4
    treatment of clinical varicocele, 4–5
  semen parameters, limitations, 3

Y
Y-chromosome microdeletions, 170–171

Z
Zeta method
  advantage and disadvantage of, 46
  and ART outcome, 46
  vs. HA-binding, 45
  practical approach to, 43–44
  sperm quality following, 44–45
  sperm selection based on, 43
Zeta potential, 42
  formation of, 42
  sperm selection, 74
Zona-binding assays, 60
Zona drilling (ZD), 7

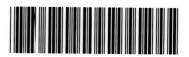